Claus Petersen, Benno M. Ure (Eds.)

Thoracic Surgery in Children and Adolescents

Claus Petersen, Benno M. Ure (Eds.)

Thoracic Surgery in Children and Adolescents

DE GRUYTER

Editors
Prof. Dr. med. Claus Petersen
Hanover Medical School
Center for Pediatric Surgery
Carl-Neuberg-Str. 1
30625 Hanover
e-mail: petersen.claus@mh-hannover.de

Prof. Dr. med. Benno M. Ure
Hanover Medical School
Center for Pediatric Surgery
Carl-Neuberg-Str. 1
30625 Hanover
e-mail: ure.benno@mh-hannover.de

ISBN: 978-3-11-042529-1
e-ISBN (PDF): 978-3-11-041982-5
e-ISBN (EPUB): 978-3-11-042002-9

Library of Congress Cataloging-in-Publication Data
A CIP catalog record for this book has been applied for at the Library of Congress.

Bibliographic information published by the Deutsche Nationalbibliothek
The Deutsche Nationalbibliothek lists this publication in the Deutsche Nationalbibliografie; detailed bibliographic data are available in the Internet at http://dnb.dnb.de.

Typesetting: Compuscript Ltd., Shannon, Ireland
Printing and Binding: CPI books GmbH, Leck
Cover image: Daria Dmitrieva/iStock/Thinkstock
∞ Printed on acid-free paper
Printed in Germany

www.degruyter.com

Prolog

Thoracic surgery in children and adolescents is no longer the same as 20 years ago. Antenatal detection of structural abnormalities has preponed diagnostic and therapeutic procedures and surgical as well as interventional techniques have undergone considerable development. Furthermore, substantial progress has been made in practitioners' general understanding of congenital thoracic malformations, in minimally invasive approaches to the thoracic cavity and surgery of the chest wall.

Today, neonatologists, pediatric pulmonologists and pediatric as well as thoracic surgeons are involved in the treatment of patients with thoracic problems, while imaging and anaesthesiological techniques remain particularly challenging in small and premature infants. However, correction of chest wall deformities is no longer recommended before puberty and transition of those patients has become a reality. As a consequence, the diagnosis and treatment of thoracic disorders are crossing borders and interdisciplinary cooperation has become mandatory.

Taking this evolution into account, the time for an innovative textbook of thoracic surgery for the first two decades of life has arisen. The idea behind this book is new: address to on experts and newcomers profit from an interactive concept.

We are very thankful that numerous well-known specialists have contributed to this book, be it through introducing topics, presenting their individual views or discussing some of the more controversial aspects related to this field. Recommended papers for further reading are included, and supplementary material can be found on the publisher's website. In addition to presenting the work, ideas and research of experts, this textbook opens the door for an interactive exchange between author and reader.

Claus Petersen
Benno M. Ure

Contents

Authors and contributors

Anesthesia and Analgesia for Thoracic Surgery
Christian Seefelder
Department of Anesthesiology, Perioperative and Pain Medicine, Boston Children's Hospital, Boston, MA, USA
Christian.Seefelder@childrens.harvard.edu

Robert Sümpelmann
Clinic of Anaesthesiology, Hanover Medical School, Hanover, Germany
suempelmann.robert@mh-hannover.de

Approaches to the Thoracic Cavity
Marcus Krüger, Taufiek Konrad Rajab
Department of Cardiothoracic, Transplantation and Vascular Surgery, Hanover Medical School, Hannover, Germany; Department of Surgery, Brigham and Women's Hospital and Harvard Medical School, Boston, USA
Marcus.Krueger@Martha-Maria.de, trajab@rics.bwh.harvard.edu

Jens Dingemann, Benno M. Ure
Department of Pediatric Surgery, Hanover Medical School, Hanover, Germany
ure.benno@mh-hannover.de, Dingemann.Jens@mh-hannover.de

Nicolaus Schwerk
Department of Pediatric Pneumology, Allergology and Neonatology, Hanover Medical School, Hannover, Germany
schwerk.nicolaus@mh-hannover.de

Rolf Oerter
Department of Thoracic Surgery, University Rostock, Germany
rolf.oerter@med.uni-rostock.de

Hartmut Grasemann
Division of Respiratory Medicien, Department of Paediatrics, The Hospital for Sick Children, Toronto, Canada
hartmut.grasemann@sickkids.ca

Pierre Goussard
Department of Pediatrics and ChildHealth, Stellenbosch University, Tygerberg Children's Hospital, Cape Town, South Africa
pgouss@sun.ac.za

Steve Cunningham
Dept. of Respiratory & Sleep Medicine, Royal Hospital for Sick Children, Edinburgh, UK
steve.cunningham@nhs.net

Jacques de Blic
Service Pneumologie et Allergologie Pédiatriques, Hôpital Universitaire Necker Enfants Malades, Paris, France
j.deblic@aphp.fr

Bronchopulmonary Diseases
Ernst Eber
Division of Paediatric Pulmonology and Allergology, Department of Paediatrics and Adolescent Medicine, Medical University of Graz, Austria
ernst.eber@medunigraz.at

Steven Rothenberg
Department of Pediatric Surgery and Pediatrics, Rocky Mountain Hospital for Children in Denver, USA
steverberg@aol.com

Mark Davenport
Department of Pediatric Surgery, King's College Hospital, London, UK
markdav2@ntlworld.com

Konrad Hoetzenecker, Walter Klepetko
Department of Thoracic Surgery, Medical University Vienna, Austria
walter.klepetko@meduniwien.ac.at, konrad.hoetzenecker@meduniwien.ac.at

Martin Lacher, Oliver J. Muensterer
Department of Pediatric Surgery, University of Leipzig, Germany; Department of Pediatric Surgery, University Medicine of the Johannes Gutenberg University Mainz, Germany
martin.lacher@uniklinik-leipzig.de, oliver.muensterer@unimedizin-mainz.de

Lung Transplantation

Clemens Aigner, Walter Klepetko
Department of Thoracic Surgery, Medical University Essen, Germany; Department of Thoracic Surgery, Medical University Vienna, Austria
clemens.aigner@rlk.uk-essen.de, walter.klepetko@meduniwien.ac.at

Axel Haverich
Department of Cardiac, Thoracic, Transplantation and Vascular Surgery, Hanover Medical School, Hanover, Germany
Haverich.Axel@mh-hannover.de

Tumors

Jochen Hubertus, Dietrich von Schweinitz
Department of Pediatric Surgery, Dr. von Haunersches Kinderspital, Munich, Germany
Jochen.Hubertus@med.uni-muenchen.de, Dietrich.Schweinitz@med.uni-muenchen.de

Diaphragm

Dick Tibboel, René Wijnen, Hanneke IJsselstijn
Intensive Care and Department of Pediatric Surgery, Erasmus MC – Sophia Children's Hospital, Rotterdam, The Netherlands
d.tibboel@erasmusmc.nl, r.wijnen@erasmusmc.nl

Anne Schneider, Francesca Borruto, Francois Becmeur
Department of Pediatric Surgery, University Hospital Strasbourg, Strasbourg, France
Francois.Becmeur@chru-strasbourg.fr

Thoracic Wall

Hans Pilegaard
Department of Cardiothoracic and Vascular Surgery, Aarhus University Hospital, Denmark
pilegaard@dadlnet.dk

Caroline Fortmann, Claus Petersen
Department of Pediatric Surgery, Hanover Medical School, Hanover, Germany
fortmann.caroline@mh-hannover.de, petersen.claus@mh-hannover.de

Haiko K Jahn, Sebastian van As
Trauma Unit Red Cross Children's Hospital, Cape Town, South Africa
Sebastian.vanas@uct.ac.za

Frederic Lavrand
Department of Pediatric Surgery, Pellegrin-Enfant Hospital, Bordeaux, France
frederic.lavrand@chu-bordeaux.fr

Hyung Joo Park
Department of Thoracic and Cardiovascular Surgery, Seoul St. Mary's Hospital, Seoul, South Korea
hyjpark@catholic.ac.kr

Donald Nuss
Childrens' Hospital of The King's Daughters, Eastern Virginia Medical School, Norfolk, Virginia, USA
dnuss@umd.edu

Claus Petersen
Department of Pediatric Surgery, Hanover Medical School, Hanover, Germany
petersen.claus@mh-hannover.de

Horatio Abramson
Hospital del Tórax Antonio A. Cetrángolo, Universidad de Buenos Aires, Argentina
habramson@intramed.net.ar

Francis Robicsek
Department of Thoracic and Cardiovascular Surgery, University of North Carolina, Charlotte, USA
Francis.Robicsek@carolinashealthcare.org

Marcelo Martínez Ferro
Division Department of Surgery, Fundación Hospitalaria Children's Hospital, Ciudad Autónoma de Buenos Aires, Argentina
m.martinezferro@gmail.com

Robert E. Kelly
Childrens' Hospital of The King's Daughters, Eastern Virginia Medical School, Norfolk, Virginia, USA
Robert.Kelly@chkd.org

Jean-Marie Wihlm
Department of Thoracic Surgery, University Hospital Cochin, Paris, France
jmwihlm@gmail.com

Dawn E. Jaroszewski
Cardiothoracic Surgery, Mayo Clinic, Arizona, USA
Jaroszewski.Dawn@mayo.edu

Miscellaneous Infections

Juan Tovar
Emeritus Professor, Department of Pediatric Surgery, Hospital Universitario La Paz, Madrid, Spain
juan.tovar@salud.madrid.org

Akin Kuzucu
Department of Thoracic Surgery, Turgut Ozal Medical Center, Inonu University School of Medicine, Malatya, Turkey
akin.kuzucu@inonu.edu.tr

Thomas Junghans
Section Clinical Tropical Medicine Department Infectious Diseases, University Hospital Heidelberg, Germany
thomas.junghanss@urz.uni-heidelberg.de

Marija Stojkovic
Section Clinical Tropical Medicine Department Infectious Diseases, University Hospital Heidelberg, Germany
marija.stojkovic@med.uni-heidelberg.de

Anja Bialkowski, Christian Poets
Department of Neonatology, Tuebingen University Hospital, Tuebingen, Germany
anja.bialkowski@gmx.de,
christian-f.poets@med.uni-tuebingen.de

Bethany J. Slater, Steven S. Rothenberg
Rocky Mountain Pediatric Surgery, Denver, Colorado, USA
bjslater1@gmail.com, steverberg@aol.com

Hanmin Lee, Lan Vu
Fetal treatment center, San Francisco, USA
hanmin.Lee@ucsf.edu, lan.vu@ucsf.edu

Jose Ribas Milanez de Campos
Department of thoracic and Pediatric Surgery, University of Sao Paulo,
Brazil, jribas@usp.br

Marcus Krüger
Department of Cardiothoracic, Transplantation and Vascular Surgery, Hanover Medical School, Hanover, Germany
Krueger.Marcus@mh-hannover.de

Christian Seefelder, Robert Sümpelmann

1 Anesthesia and analgesia for thoracic surgery

1.1 Introduction

The unpleasant times of years gone by when surgeons and anesthesiologists found themselves in conflict over competing perceptions of their respective importance and relevance are hopefully consigned to the past. Today, interdisciplinary collaboration and close cooperation are critical to ensuring that all patients are provided with the best practice and levels of care. This is particularly true when treating low-weight prematures or performing minimally invasive procedures in the thoracic cavity. In the following chapter, **Christian Seefelder** focuses not only on appropriate procedures and techniques, but also on perioperative pain management.

1.2 Anesthesia for pediatric thoracic surgery

The advances in pediatric surgery have resulted in the desire by the pediatric surgeon, by families and by medical consultants for earlier, more definitive, often video-assisted, "minimally invasive" surgery in younger and sicker patients than a decade ago. Anesthesia care for small, young and sick patients may have become safer more through better understanding, improved monitoring and more courage than through improvements in drugs, advances in technology or innovation in management. Pediatric anesthesiologists need intimate knowledge and understanding of the (congenital) surgical lesion and its pathophysiology, of the associated medical disorders and of the surgical procedure. In turn, pediatric surgeons need knowledge and understanding of the anesthetic techniques, concerns and limitations such as neurotoxicity of anesthesia in neonates, infants and young children, the difficulty of lung isolation in small patients or the physiologic challenges of minimally invasive surgery in pediatric patients.

1.2.1 Neurotoxicity of anesthesia in neonates, infants and young children

Animal and human data suggest that anesthesia in young animals as well as in human neonates, infants and young children may have unfavorable effects on the developing brain. The initial animal studies provoked disbelief, as a human neonate could not just be equated with a rat pup. Subsequently, clinical studies disturbingly confirmed the concerns rather than dispelling them [1, 2]. Further data are eagerly awaited by the pediatric anesthesia community, while surgeons not uncommonly have remained unaware of the whole discussion.

1.2.1.1 Animal data

Solid data from animal models suggest that exposure of neonatal animals to agents used in human anesthesia results in accelerated or premature neuroapoptosis and neurodevelopmental disadvantages. Common criticism of these studies includes the difficulty extrapolating from animal data to humans, difficulty comparing doses required for animals and humans, difficulty comparing animal outcomes to human outcomes, difficulty excluding the effect of disease and surgery requiring anesthesia on neurodevelopment and impossibility of providing necessary surgery without anesthesia. At the same time, suspicion has been brought forward that it is less the anesthetic agent than the physiologic milieu created that may be responsible for the changes (i.e. hypotension, desaturation). A clear recommendation regarding a safe or advantageous general anesthetic technique or agent is missing, but dexmedetomidine may be less detrimental than other anesthetic agents in regards to neurotoxicity.

1.2.1.2 Human data

Human data from retrospective and database studies indicate a neurodevelopmental disadvantage in children who have undergone (multiple) anesthetics as neonates, infants or young children compared to matched controls, siblings or twins without anesthesia. First results of a prospective randomized controlled study comparing one hour of sevoflurane anesthesia with awake/regional anesthesia for hernia repair in infants did not show a difference in neurodevelopmental outcomes at the 2-year follow-up [3]. Further information is sought through studies of neurodevelopment after intrauterine exposure to anesthesia, studies of sedation of neonates in the intensive care unit and studies of retinal apoptosis as “windows into the brain”.

1.2.2 Basic anesthetic techniques in pediatric anesthesia

While thoracic surgery is performed under general anesthesia, there is often a misunderstanding by patients, families, medical specialists and surgeons about the degree of sedation for other studies and procedures. Not uncommonly, it has been agreed upon that a procedure can be done “under local” or “light sedation”, but at the same time the patient has been promised to be “asleep” and the surgeon or radiologist expects the patient to be “not moving”.

Few children are interested in being awake and aware and in lying still for procedures or studies. Small infants can sometimes be fed and bundled up and sleep through non-stimulating studies such as MRI. Distraction and entertainment with videos can be offered and parents can be present for reassurance for older children to undergo unsedated imaging studies or procedures such as lumbar puncture, bone marrow aspirate or central line placement under topical or local anesthesia.

Although light and moderate sedation with low doses of sedatives or systemic analgesics administered enterally or parenterally may relieve anxiety, by definition patients will respond to commands and stimulation and some children may move and cry, sometimes are disinhibited and may become more restless and less cooperative with the risk of escalating dosing of drugs.

For adequate surgical conditions and for imaging studies requiring immobility, deep sedation or general anesthesia are necessary; while spontaneous respirations may be maintained, concerns are progression to apnea, loss of protective airway reflexes, increasing airway obstruction and hemodynamic compromise.

1.2.3 Age at and timing of surgery

Cardiothoracic surgical intervention may occur as early as in utero, for example for aortic stenosis with evolving hypoplastic left heart syndrome, life threatening congenital pulmonary airway malformation or severe congenital diaphragmatic hernia. Some patients may require ex utero intra partum treatment or "EXIT" procedures with surgical intervention or placement on extracorporeal membrane oxygenation (ECMO) during birth and while on placental support. Anesthesia, monitoring and resuscitation of the fetus is provided by fetal anesthesia subspecialists while the mother is anesthetized and monitored by the obstetric anesthesiologist. Emergent or urgent neonatal thoracic surgery is required for large or enlarging congenital pulmonary lesions, for tracheo-esophageal fistula (TEF) and congenital diaphragmatic hernia. Many lung biopsies and tumor resections need to be performed whenever the patient presents. Given the neurodevelopmental risks of anesthesia in young patients, elective pediatric surgery should be postponed, but the age by which anesthesia in children is safe remains elusive. Irrespective of the neurodevelopmental concerns, the risk of anesthesia-related complications is highest in the youngest [4].

Surgical pathology in children is dominated by congenital abnormalities or pediatric-specific acquired disorders. Pediatric anesthesia and surgery provide care to patients from the 0.5 kg 24-week premature neonate to the 100 kg teenager. While "a child is not just a small adult", the main difference and the anesthetic implication for older children lie mostly in the psychological issues as well as in issues of equipment-size. For premature and term neonates as well as infants, drugs, equipment or technologies may not be available, formally approved or scientifically validated. The difference in physiology of the neonate and infant from the physiology of older children and adults is characterized by immaturity of the function of all organs and systems (central nervous, cardiovascular, respiratory system, renal, hepatic, endocrine, metabolic, gastrointestinal function, pharmacology, immunology, hematology), all of which need to be considered by the pediatric anesthesiologist during anesthesia in this patient population.

1.2.4 Preoperative evaluation and workup

The typical evaluation and workup will include all aspects of the history and physical exam, with focus on the thoracic pathology in question, specifically any respiratory symptoms and distress, stridor and any signs or symptoms indicating difficult airway management or risk of respiratory obstruction during anesthesia and surgery. Most studies will have been ordered by surgeons and pediatric specialists but should be reviewed by the pediatric anesthesiologist, including chest x-ray, computed tomography (CT), magnetic resonance imaging (MRI), angiograms, ventilation/perfusion scans, cardiologic studies, lung function tests, laboratory results, cultures and biopsies. Of particular importance is consultation with other pediatric specialists such as pediatric pulmonologists, cardiologists, hematologists, oncologists, endocrinologists and radiologists to optimize preoperative workup, evaluation, management and communication.

Especially in younger children with limited cooperation, many types of studies such as lung function tests may not be possible at all. Others such as CTs, MRIs, angiographies or biopsies will require the involvement of the anesthesiologist for sedation or anesthesia. To provide the patient with a safe anesthetic and a satisfactory study, requesting service, surgeon, radiologist and anesthesiologist should communicate before the study to understand each other's concerns and objectives. While case to case assessment and discussion are important, agreeing on a protocol across departments allows input from all specialties ahead of time and decreases case to case confrontation. Protocols appear reasonable for imaging studies in patients with anterior mediastinal masses or tracheomalacia. Early involvement has the advantage of familiarizing the anesthesiologist with the patient's airway anatomy and management and physiologic response to anesthesia prior to major thoracic surgery.

1.2.5 Intraoperative monitoring

Standard monitoring includes electrocardiogram (ECG), non-invasive blood pressure (NIBP), pulse oximetry, patient temperature, inspiratory oxygen concentration (F_iO_2) and end-tidal CO_2 concentration ($ETCO_2$). It may be difficult to establish all monitors prior to induction in children.

Invasive arterial monitoring allows arterial blood gas sampling and immediate recognition of hemodynamic effects of surgical retraction, mechanical arrhythmias or air embolism. It is indicated in lobectomy or pneumonectomy, in thoracic tumor resections, major neonatal thoracic surgery for congenital diaphragmatic hernia or TEF repair, in infant thoracoscopy or for the patient's general medical condition. Lung isolation in itself is not an indication for placement of an arterial catheter, and it may not be necessary for simple lung wedge resections or biopsies, thoracoscopic pleurodesis or pectus repair. Risks include ischemic complications from local skin necrosis to loss of an extremity. Placement aids for small patients are transillumination, Doppler and more recently ultrasound.

Central venous pressure monitoring may not be reliable in situations of an open chest, retraction of cardiovascular structures and capnothorax but may have a place for perioperative monitoring. A central venous catheter also serves as secure perioperative venous access and for the administration of vasoactive agents and should be considered whenever their need is anticipated.

Pulse oximeters, arterial catheter and blood pressure cuff are distributed over several extremities. In neonates, pre- (right arm) and post-ductal (lower extremity) oxygen saturation should be monitored to detect right to left shunting across the ductus arteriosus. Electroencephalographic monitors are available for anesthetic depth, seizure and ischemia monitoring. Transesophageal echocardiography is available for children, non-invasive cardiac output monitors are being evaluated, pulmonary arterial catheters are used less commonly in the pediatric population.

Cerebral blood flow can be monitored via transcranial Doppler, and near-infrared spectroscopy (NIRS) measures brain oxygenation. In particular cerebral or somatic tissue oxygenation monitoring is rapidly gaining importance and popularity, since hemodynamic parameters alone do not reflect actual end organ supply. Intraoperative decreases of regional brain oxygenation must be responded to promptly by improving hemodynamics and cerebrovascular perfusion but also by correcting surgical maneuvers such as retraction, increased intrathoracic pressure or hypercarbia from CO_2 insufflation.

1.2.6 Lung isolation and one lung ventilation in children [5, 6]

Indications for lung isolation with double lumen tubes include protection of one lung from bleeding or contamination from the other lung and bronchopleural fistula with inability to ventilate. More commonly, the indication for lung isolation is a relative indication to provide an immobile surgical field, in particular for surgery of the lung and thoracoscopic surgeries. While double lumen tubes are not available for small children, non-ventilation of one lung may be achieved with bronchial blockers and main stem intubation. Both can easily dislodge, initial deflation of the non-ventilated lung may be delayed, and easy re-expansion and re-isolation of the non-ventilated lung may not be possible. This isolation technique can be time consuming and requires patience by surgeon and anesthesiologist. For non-pulmonary thoracic surgery, surgical immobilization of the lung by retraction or packing and creating a capnothorax for thoracoscopic surgery is therefore often applied.

Main stem intubation is achieved over a flexible or rigid bronchoscope or with fluoroscopic guidance. The main stem bronchi are smaller than the trachea and a smaller or uncuffed tube is selected for successful endobronchial intubation. The proximity of the right upper lobe bronchus to the carina (Fig. 1.2.1; 1.2.2) makes this technique less successful for ventilating the right than the left lung, as loss of the right upper lobe ventilation may result in unacceptable desaturation. However, ventilating the left lung via main stem intubation with non-ventilation of the right lung is quite successful due to the length of the left main stem bronchus and left main stem intubation is practiced widely for right thoracoscopic surgery.

Tab. 1.2.1: Options for lung isolation and single lung ventilation at different ages.

Age	Weight	Endotracheal tube size	Cuff type[1]	Main stem intubation tube size	Bronchial blocker type[2]	Blocker inside / outside the tube	Bronchial blocker size (French)	Univent™ tube size (mm inner diameter)[3]	Double lumen tube size (French)[4]
neonate	3 kg	3.0 cuffed 3.5 uncuffed	LoPro Microcuff	3 uncuffed	Fogarty	outside	2–4		
<6 months	3–6 kg	3.5 uncuffed/ cuffed	LoPro Microcuff	3 uncuffed/ cuffed	Arndt	outside	5		
6–12 months	6–10 kg	3.5–4 uncuffed/ cuffed	LoPro Microcuff	3–3.5 uncuffed/ cuffed	Arndt	outside	5		
1–2 years	<15 kg	4–4.5 uncuffed/ cuffed	LoPro Microcuff	3.5 uncuffed/ cuffed	Arndt	outside	5		
2–4 years	<20 kg	4.5–5 cuffed	LoPro Microcuff	4–4.5 cuffed	Arndt	inside/outside	5		
4–6 years	<25 kg	5–5.5 cuffed	LoPro Microcuff	4.5–5 cuffed	Arndt	inside outside	5 5, 7		
6–8 years	<30 kg	5.5–6 cuffed	LoPro Microcuff	5 cuffed	Arndt	inside outside	5 7	3.5	
8–10 years	>30 kg	6 cuffed	HiLo Microcuff		Arndt	inside outside	5 7	3.5	26
10–12 years	<40 kg	6.5 cuffed	HiLo		Arndt	inside	7	4.5	26–28
12–14 years	40–50 kg	6.5 cuffed	HiLo		Arndt	inside	7	4.5	28

Tab. 1.2.1 (continued)

Age	Weight	Endotracheal tube size	Cuff type[1]	Main stem intubation tube size	Bronchial blocker type[2]	Blocker inside / outside the tube	Bronchial blocker size (French)	Univent™ tube size (mm inner diameter)[3]	Double lumen tube size (French)[4]
14–16 years	>50 kg	6.5–7 cuffed	HiLo		Arndt	inside	7	6	32
Adult female	>60 kg	6.5–7 cuffed	HiLo		Arndt	inside	7	6.5	32–35
Adult male	>70 kg	7–7.5 cuffed	HiLo		Arndt Cohen EZ-Blocker™	inside	9 9 7	7	35–37

[1] Microcuff tube, Halyard Health Care, formerly Kimberly-Clark®, HiLo = high volume low pressure cuffs, LoPro = low profile cuffs, Medtronic, Covidien, formerly Mallinckrodt™; [2] Arndt Endobronchial Blocker: 5, 7, 9F, Cohen Endobronchial Blocker: 9F: Cook® Medical; Uniblocker™: 5, 9F: Teleflex®, formerly Fuji Systems, EZ-Blocker™ Endobronchial Blocker, Teleflex®, formerly Rüsch®; [3] Univent™, Teleflex®, formerly Fuji Systems; [4] 26F DLT, Teleflex®, formerly Rüsch® (modified from Table 6, page 1428 in: Hammer GB, Fitzmaurice BG, Brodsky JB. Methods for Single-Lung Ventilation in Pediatric Patients. Anesth Analg 1999;89:1426–9) [5].

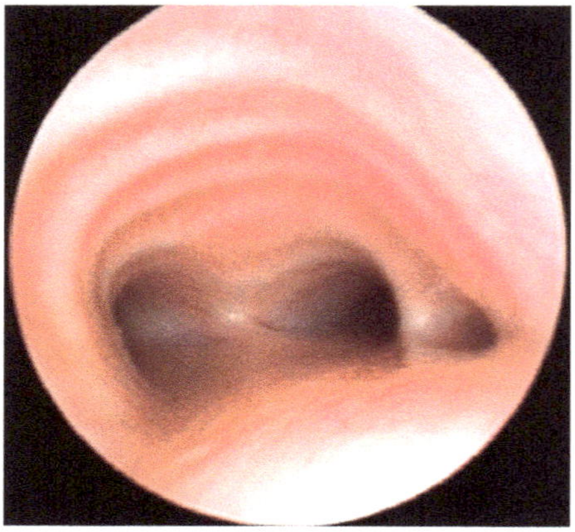

Fig. 1.2.1: Bronchoscopic view of the distal trachea and carina of an infant with the right upper lobe bronchus coming off the trachea (pig bronchus).

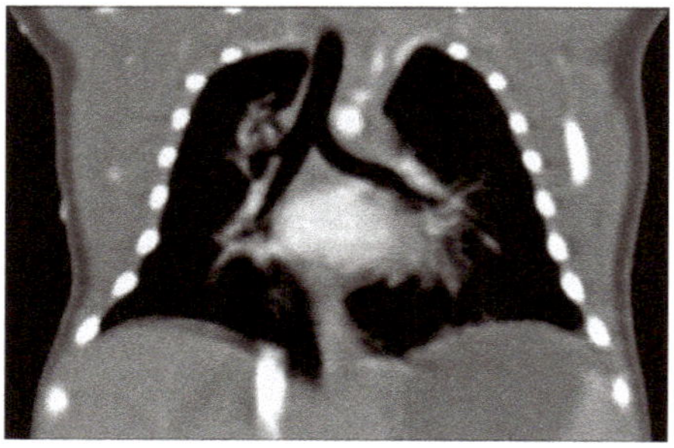

Fig. 1.2.2: Chest CT of an infant showing proximal take-off of the right upper lobe bronchus.

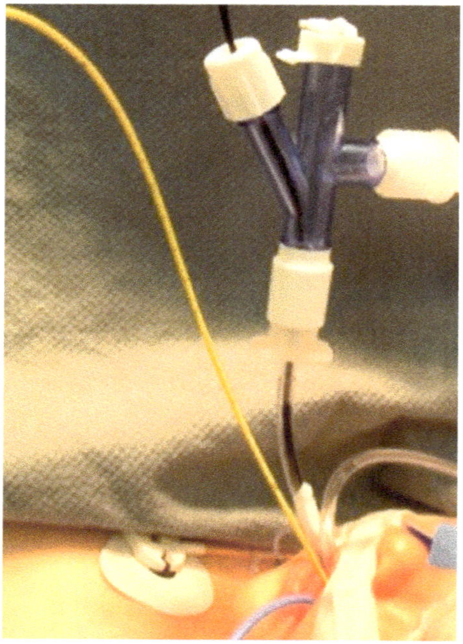

Fig. 1.2.3: Placement of an extraluminal bronchial blocker: Fiberoptic bronchoscopy through the adjustable lumen port of the triple port adaptor of an Arndt Endobronchial Blocker while the bronchial blocker is entering the airway parallel to the endotracheal tube.

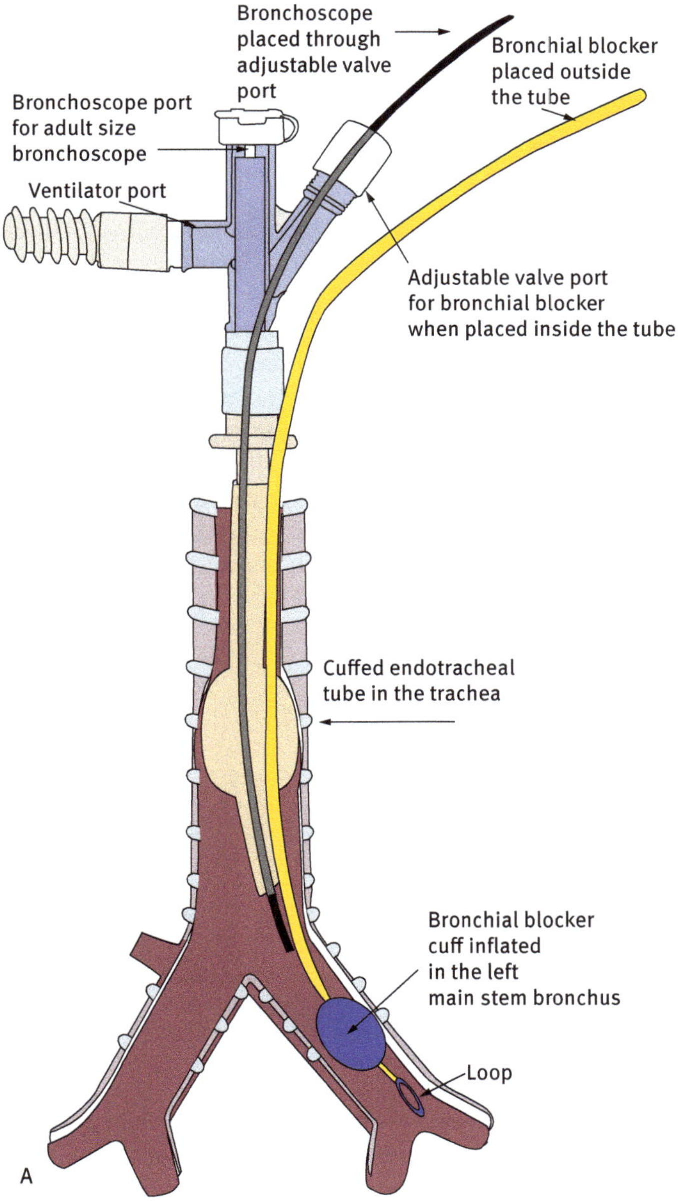

Fig. 1.2.4: Depiction of the extraluminal placement of a bronchial blocker in infants and young children.

Bronchial blockers, for example the Arndt endobronchial blocker from Cook or the Uniblocker from Fuji, available in 5, 7 and 9 French (F), or Fogarty catheters in sizes 2, 3 and 4 F can be used for lung isolation [7]. The bronchial blocker can be placed outside the endotracheal tube in infants and young children (Fig. 1.2.3; 1.2.4).

Video showing the placement of extraluminal 5F bronchial blocker into the left main stem bronchus of an infant guided with 2.2 mm fiberoptic bronchoscope. https://www.degruyter.com/view/supplement/9783110419825_placement_bronchial_blocker.mp4

Although the blocker naturally enters the right main stem more readily, it can be directed into the left main stem under fiberoptic control (supplementary video online). Due to the longer left main stem, lung isolation is more likely to be successful with a blocker in the left main stem, allowing ventilation of the right lung and non-ventilation of the left lung (Fig. 1.2.5; 1.2.6). Conversely, placement of the bronchial blocker into the right main stem is more likely to result in incomplete lung isolation due to the proximity of the right upper lobe bronchus to the carina, or in dislodgement of a very proximally placed blocker into the trachea with loss of isolation and obstruction to ventilation via the endotracheal tube. In older patients, use of the bronchial blocker through the endotracheal tube is the recommended technique. The 9 F Rüsch® EZ-Blocker™ with two balloons is an option not available in pediatric sizes at this time.

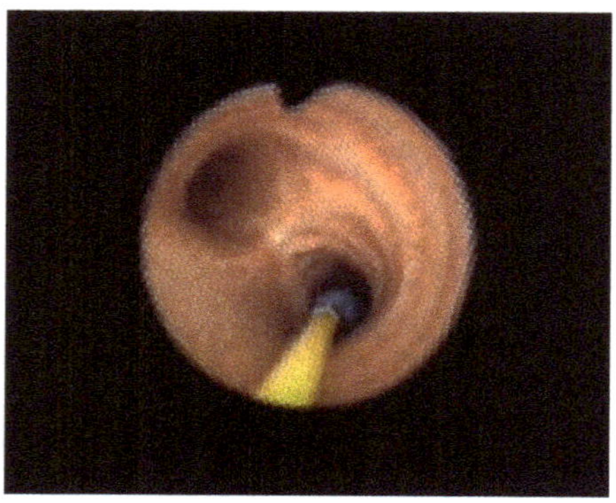

Fig. 1.2.5: Endobronchial blocker placed outside the endotracheal tube and entering the right main stem bronchus of an infant.

The Univent™ Inoue tube from Fuji has a channel for a bronchial blocker incorporated into the wall of the tube. Even though pediatric sizes are available, they appear to have an unfavorable ratio between inner and outer diameters: the “3.5 ID” uncuffed tube has a 7.5–8 mm outer diameter, the “4.5 ID” cuffed tube 8.5–9 mm. These tubes therefore are only suitable for older children and adolescents.

Double lumen tubes are commercially available from size 26 F. This smallest tube fits patients above 8 years of age, 30 kg weight and 130 cm height [8]. Marraro custom-made a double lumen tube for neonates and infants, which consists of two attached small tubes, and some practitioners have used two separate small tubes for selective lung ventilation in infants.

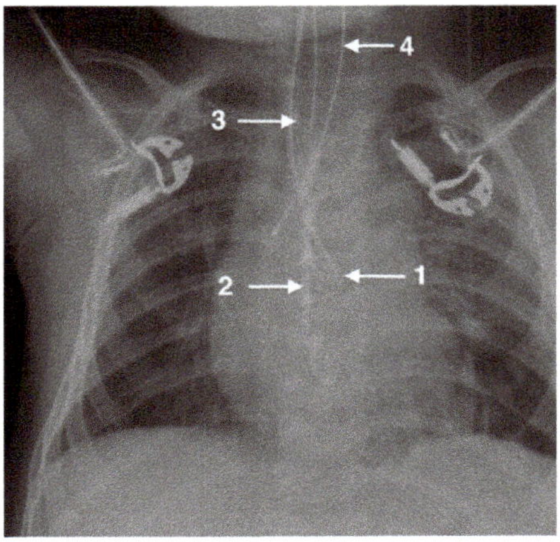

Fig. 1.2.6: Chest x-ray of an infant showing endobronchial blocker in the left main stem bronchus (1), epidural catheter and epidural contrast (2), endotracheal tube in the trachea (3), and temperature probe in the esophagus (4).

Lastly, if lung separation is necessary but technically not possible, the use of **ECMO or cardiopulmonary bypass** has been reported, for example for whole lung lavage in infants and small children.

1.2.6.1 Surgical capnothorax

Commonly, pediatric thoracic surgeons insufflate CO_2 into the pleural cavity, creating a surgical capnothorax to improve the work space for thoracoscopic procedures and to accelerate lung collapse of the non-ventilated lung. Hypercarbia results from increased CO_2 absorption and impaired ventilation due to decreased compliance and formation of atelectasis of the ventilated dependent lung. Capnothorax and hypercarbia have been shown to be associated with decreased cerebral blood flow, decreased cerebral oxygenation and severe acidosis in thoracoscopic repair of congenital diaphragmatic hernia (CDH), although increased cerebral oxygenation has also been seen, likely related to hypercarbia induced cerebral vasodilation. NIRS monitoring of cerebral oxygenation is indicated. Increased intrathoracic pressure can also result in decreased venous return with hypotension and increased venous bleeding [9, 10, 11].

Generally, in neonates and in patients with successful lung isolation, pressures of 2–3 cm H_2O should suffice, occasionally pressures of 4–5 cm H_2O may be helpful. Only on rare occasions do pressures need to be increased above 5 cm H_2O, for example to assist in reducing abdominal content during thoracoscopic CDH repair. This should be temporary and always be discussed between surgeon and anesthesiologist who will monitor ventilation, oxygenation and hemodynamics. These higher pressures may be tolerated hemodynamically while they are immediately noticeable through worsening compliance and hypercarbia.

Occasionally, the surgeon will flush CO_2 through the pleural cavity to scavenge electrocautery smoke without actually establishing pressure. This is tolerated well with less hypercarbia, but may result in more temperature or moisture loss. CO_2 insufflators with the capability to warm and humidify the insufflated CO_2 are available.

1.2.6.2 Ventilation during one lung ventilation

Decompression of the non-ventilated lung in main stem intubation and with bronchial blockers may be slow. Use of 100% oxygen or oxygen/nitrous oxide prior to isolation rather than oxygen/air accelerates lung collapse through the faster absorption of oxygen and nitrous oxide than nitrogen from the non-ventilated lung.

Pressure control ventilation is preferred over volume control ventilation to optimize tidal volumes while limiting ventilation pressures. Peak inspiratory pressures (PIPs) are chosen to achieve a desirable tidal volume of 5–8 ml/kg. Especially with the use of bronchial blockers, PIPs should be limited due to the risk of exceeding balloon seal and trapping ventilation in the non-ventilated lung. Positive end expiratory pressure (PEEP) of 3 to 5 cm H_2O helps to reduce the risk of atelectasis in the dependent/ventilated lung due to positioning, surgical compression and capnothorax.

Intraoperative hypercarbia is managed with limited increase in tidal volume by increasing peak inspiratory pressure or inspiratory time, and by increasing respiratory rate. Minimizing dead space and using low-compliance circuits may prove beneficial. Intraoperative flexible fiberoptic bronchoscopy, for example during tracheopexy, increases resistance to ventilation and may need to be limited if hypercarbia is difficult to manage. If CO_2 elimination by ventilation is difficult, avoiding patient hyperthermia helps limiting endogenous CO_2 production from increased patient metabolism. As CO_2 insufflation into the pleural cavity by the surgeon is the major contributor of hypercarbia during thoracoscopy, limiting insufflation pressures or avoiding insufflation is the best option to reduce hypercarbia.

In the absence of other contraindications to hypercarbia such as pulmonary hypertension or need for low pulmonary vascular resistance (Fontan circulation), some degree of temporary permissive hypercarbia may be reasonable and tolerated, but the degree of acceptable hypercarbia remains undefined. p_aCO_2 below 50 mm Hg is likely unproblematic and up to 60 mm Hg probably acceptable. It is important to correlate endtidal CO_2 with p_aCO_2 to be able to track changes.

1.2.6.3 Physiology of one lung ventilation [12]

When lung isolation is initiated and one lung ventilation commences, the non-ventilated lung initially remains perfused and the oxygen in the lung gradually is absorbed. Due to their higher oxygen requirement and lower oxygen reserve in the lung, this process is markedly shorter in infants and small children than in older patients, similar to the apnea time in infants. With the complete removal of the alveolar oxygen, shunting becomes obvious and oxygen desaturation can be noted. Hypoxic pulmonary vasoconstriction HPV is activated, resulting in a decreased perfusion of the non-ventilated lung and a reduction in the shunt fraction. Oxygenation and oxygen saturation improve again. Degree and duration of desaturation are variable, but transient desaturation into the 80s is not uncommon even while ventilating with 100% oxygen. Ample literature discusses influences on HPV with opportunities for intervention in adults. This is less well documented in children. In general, vasodilators including inhalational agents may impair HPV and intravenous anesthesia has been considered favorable for maintaining HPV and decreasing shunting. High PEEP or mean airway pressures may divert blood flow from the ventilated to the non-ventilated lung.

Intraoperative desaturation in pediatric thoracic anesthesia is managed similar to adults. Inspiratory oxygen concentration is increased and normoventilation is attempted. Lateral positioning, padding, surgical retraction and pressure may result in intraoperative atelectasis of the ventilated dependent lung and contribute to pulmonary desaturation. Gentle recruitment breaths can be attempted remembering the possible loss of lung isolation when bronchial blockers or main stem intubation are used and the ventilation pressures exceed the cuff pressure. PEEP is added to the dependent lung or increased. Secretions or blood may block the airway. However, suctioning any pediatric endotracheal tube and in particular suctioning during one lung ventilation may result in rapid desaturation, which may be slow to recover. Double lumen tubes and some bronchial blockers allow upper-lung CPAP (continuous positive airway pressure) and recovery of oxygenation albeit at the price of a distended lung which may not please the surgeon. Nitric oxide may improve ventilation/perfusion matching of the dependent lung. Changing the anesthetic to an intravenous technique supports HPV in adults. Finally, clamping of the pulmonary artery, especially when lobectomy or pneumonectomy are performed, (temporarily) aborting one lung ventilation, and considering ECMO or cardiopulmonary bypass would restore oxygenation.

1.2.7 Anesthetic implications for specific disorders

1.2.7.1 Congenital lung lesions in neonates and infants

These lesions can overlap and are congenital pulmonary airway malformation (CPAM, connected to the airway), including previously termed congenital cystic adenomatoid malformation (CCAM), pulmonary sequestration (PS, not connected to the airway, systemic blood supply), congenital lobar emphysema (CLE, connected to the airway with large bullae), bronchogenic and enteric duplication cysts (cysts not connected to the airway).

Expanding lesions in the neonate

Large or expanding congenital lobar emphysema or congenital pulmonary airway malformation can cause mediastinal shift and respiratory distress or produce high output cardiac failure and may require urgent surgery in the neonate. Positive pressure ventilation increases the risk of further distention, but patients are often intubated preoperatively for respiratory distress, they may be on high frequency oscillatory ventilation

(HFOV) or may required ECMO. Nitrous oxide is avoided. If the patient is unstable, anesthesia time between induction and incision should be minimized and open repair should be pursued expeditiously. Surgical "rescue" during problems under anesthesia is thoracotomy and delivery of the mass to allow the remainder of the lung to be ventilated. An arterial line and good venous access should be established and blood products should be available. Regional anesthesia may be placed postoperatively and the patient will be monitored in an intensive care unit (ICU) postoperatively.

Stable lesions

Most patients with congenital lung lesions are stable and elective thoracoscopic resection is scheduled in infancy [13]. Routine echocardiographic workup is not indicated. Postnatal imaging can help to characterize the lesion. Anesthesia induction can be performed by inhalation or intravenously. Positive pressure ventilation is of no concern in pure pulmonary sequestration and bronchogenic cysts without connection to the airway, but in patients with congenital pulmonary airway malformation or congenital lobar emphysema, positive pressure ventilation should be carried out gently, as these lesions could still expand. Solid venous and arterial access is indicated especially for lobectomy, pneumonectomy, resection of pulmonary sequestration with blood supply from the aorta, and any thoracoscopy in neonates and infants. Bleeding, air embolism and inadvertent tension capnothorax are specific risks. Lung isolation via main stem intubation or bronchial blocker is helpful. Regional anesthesia can be added for intra- and postoperative analgesia. Postoperative monitoring of respiratory sufficiency and pain control should occur in an ICU for young patients.

1.2.7.2 Esophageal atresia and tracheo-esophageal fistula repair in the neonate [14, 15]

The most common variants of congenital tracheo-esophageal anomalies and the most relevant for anesthesia management are pure esophageal atresia (EA), proximal EA with distal TEF, and H-type fistula between trachea and esophagus. Patients with EA may have polyhydramnios on prenatal ultrasound and postnatally present with coughing and signs and symptoms of aspiration when feeding. A nasogastric tube will fail to pass into the stomach and can be seen curled in the proximal esophagus on a chest x-ray.

The high association of tracheo-esophageal anomalies with other congenital anomalies such as congenital heart disease and VACTERL association (**v**ertebral, **a**no-rectal, **c**ardiac, **t**racheo-**e**sophageal, **r**enal, **l**imb abnormalities) makes a preoperative workup advisable. An echocardiogram is performed to exclude or define congenital heart disease and to identify the position of the aortic arch (left arch, right thoracic approach and vice versa). A babygram will be evaluated for gas in the stomach and intestines (presence of a TEF), pulmonary infiltrates, heart size, vertebral anomalies or the double bubble of duodenal atresia. Duodenal atresia or imperforate anus require additional procedures at the time of a TEF repair (duodenal atresia repair, gastrostomy, colostomy). Workup for renal pathology and spinal anomalies are often delayed until after TEF repair.

Tracheo-esophageal fistula (TEF)

Patients with pure EA (gas free abdomen) can be subjected to positive pressure ventilation as necessary. In the presence of a TEF, the abdomen is gas filled and pronounced gastric distention may exist, if positive pressure ventilation was performed during neonatal resuscitation. The patient should not be intubated electively preoperatively, spontaneous respirations should be maintained as long as possible. Positive pressure ventilation during anesthetic management can similarly distend the stomach, impair diaphragmatic excursion, limit ventilation and result in hypercarbia and desaturation. Management varies by institution, and anesthesiologist and surgeon should discuss their plans preoperatively.

One possible approach is to induce anesthesia maintaining spontaneous respirations. Topical anesthesia is administered to the vocal cords and to supra- and infraglottic structures with direct laryngoscopy, keeping the maximum allowed local anesthetic dose in mind. Number and location of the fistula(s) is then identified by (rigid) bronchoscopy. If the fistula is located distal in the trachea or at the level of the carina, a Fogarty catheter can be passed through the fistula into the stomach, inflated and withdrawn (Fig. 1.2.7; 1.2.8). This provides some intraoperative guidance to the location of the fistula and at the same time a modest seal if low pressure positive pressure ventilation is performed. If positive pressure ventilation has resulted in massive gastric distention, gastrostomy tube decompression may be required. TEFs higher in the trachea can be occluded by a 3.0 mm inner diameter (ID) cuffed endotracheal tube. If right thoracoscopic TEF repair is planned, the left main stem bronchus is intubated with a 3.0 mm ID uncuffed endotracheal tube.

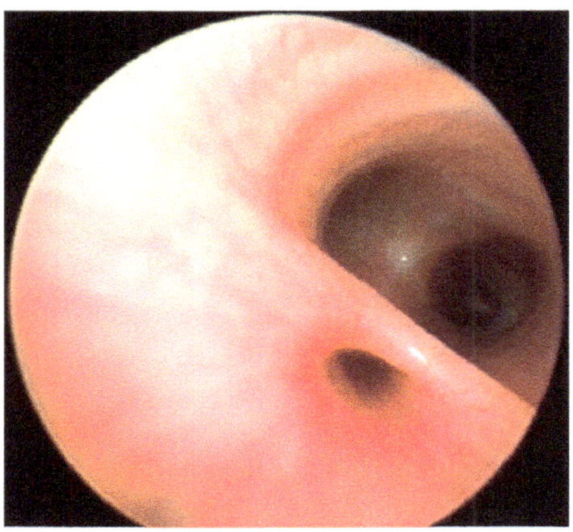

Fig. 1.2.7: Bronchoscopic view of the carina with a tracheo-esophageal fistula.

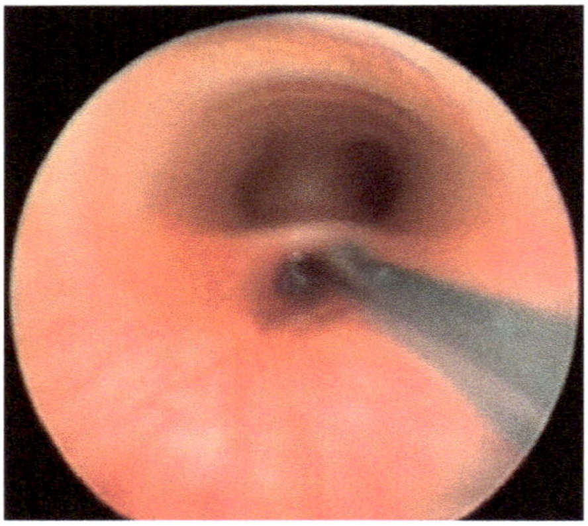

Fig. 1.2.8: Bronchoscopic view of a Fogarty catheter entering the tracheo-esophageal fistula.

At least two peripheral intravenous lines (iv) and ideally an arterial catheter are placed for anesthetic management. A 10% dextrose containing electrolyte solution is infused at a maintenance rate with drips including dopamine as indicated, while additional fluids, colloids and blood products can be administered through the second iv. The patient will be placed in a left lateral position for the right thoracotomy and in an exaggerated left lateral position for thoracoscopic repair of a TEF with a left sided aortic arch. Pre- and post-ductal pulse oximetry and brain oxygenation monitoring (NIRS) are added to standard monitors.

Intraoperative events to be expected include desaturations, hypercarbia, hypotension and arrhythmias, related to endotracheal tube migration, surgical compression of airway, lungs, heart and venous return, or airway obstruction by blood and secretions. The surgeon may request manipulation of the Fogarty catheter or of an oro- or nasogastric tube under the drapes.

To minimize the time before ligation of the fistula, regional anesthesia or central line placement may be performed postoperatively. In the absence of contraindications such as vertebral anomalies on the babygram, epidural catheters, commonly in this age as caudal catheters threaded to the appropriate thoracic level, or paravertebral catheters may be offered for postoperative analgesia. Although extubation at the end of the surgery can be considered after uneventful surgery in stable neonates, brief postoperative ventilation in the NICU after several hours of thoracic surgery with lung collapse in a just hours old neonate seems reasonable. In the presence of a new esophageal anastomosis or tracheal fistula ligation, reintubation may be anxiety provoking to the anesthesiologist, surgeon and neonatologist.

Long gap esophageal atresia

In long gap esophageal atresia, primary anastomosis of the esophageal ends is not feasible or successful. Patients need the proximal esophageal pouch drained temporarily via an oral or nasal Replogle-type suction tube, or longer term via a cervical spit fistula. A gastrostomy provides access for enteral feeding. Surgical approaches to long gap esophageal atresia repair include various techniques of esophageal stretching maneuvers, interposition of stomach, jejunum or colon or growth induction with open or thoracoscopically placed internal or external traction to the proximal and distal esophageal pouches over days and weeks with eventual esophageal anastomosis.

Typically at the time of surgical repair of long gap esophageal atresia, any tracheo-esophageal fistula has been closed and positive pressure ventilation on induction is not concerning, but mask ventilation may be technically challenging in the presence of a cervical spit fistula. Anesthetic management concerns are directed at coexisting pathology (congenital heart disease), problems with access after multiple surgeries, bleeding due to adhesions, positioning problems related to long surgical times in the lateral position. Injury to lung, esophagus and airway are possible and intraoperative fiberoptic control of the airway may be requested. Not uncommonly patients remain intubated and are ventilated postoperatively to prevent tension on the anastomosis. Regional anesthesia may be helpful in reducing systemic analgesics required for sedation.

Esophageal anastomoses are at risk for dehiscence or stricture formation and not uncommonly these patients return to the operating room for esophagoscopy and esophageal dilations.

H-type tracheo-esophageal fistula

If the esophagus is primarily intact or has been repaired, fistulae connecting trachea and esophagus may exist which are termed H-type fistulae. They present in the neonatal period or later with ongoing aspiration in patients with esophageal continuity. Preoperative barium studies and esophagoscopy and bronchoscopy under anesthesia provide the diagnosis. The fistula size is typically smaller and positive pressure ventilation is not usually a problem. A cuffed endotracheal tube may be able to occlude or exclude the H-type TEF, since it is often located higher in the trachea and esophagus. H-type fistulas may even be repaired through a neck incision in which case invasive monitoring is not always necessary. Patients are still at risk for congenital heart disease and other malformations of the VACTERL association. Given the less invasive surgery, patients can commonly be extubated postoperatively.

1.2.7.3 Aortopexy and tracheopexy

Tracheo-broncho-malacia or tracheobronchial compression may be part and result of congenital tracheo-esophageal abnormalities or exist independently. They typically present in infancy with respiratory symptoms from noisy breathing and stridor to acute life threatening events, ALTEs, with severe airway obstruction, cyanosis, respiratory and cardiac arrest. Level and extent are diagnosed during bronchoscopy with spontaneous respiration and with dynamic airway CT. Airway collapse is worse with turbulent airflow such as during agitation on anesthesia emergence. Sedation, continuous positive airway pressure and positive pressure ventilation are beneficial.

Aortopexy [16] is performed in the lateral position through a (left) lateral or anterior thoracotomy or (left) thoracoscopy, or in the supine position through an upper sternotomy: the ascending aorta is "pexed" to the sternum, the anterior fixation of the aorta is expected to pull on the anterior trachea, opening and stabilizing its lumen. Posterior *tracheopexy* [17] is performed in a (left) lateral position through a (right) lateral thoracotomy: the tracheal lumen is enlarged and stabilized by attaching the posterior trachea posteriorly to the spine.

Intraoperative monitoring for these procedures should include invasive arterial blood pressure monitoring in an upper extremity, pulse oximetry monitoring on several extremities in addition to standard monitoring. Good venous access is mandatory, blood and resuscitation drugs should be available in the operating room. NIRS monitoring is used to monitor cerebral perfusion and oxygenation. Lung isolation will be useful in thoracoscopic procedures, but intraoperative fiberoptic assessment of the tracheo-bronchial lumen is required with all techniques to document the effect of the procedure and assist in defining the necessary extent of the surgery.

Intraoperative complications include surgical retraction or compression of cardiovascular structures resulting in decreased venous return, hypotension and arrhythmias, compression of aorta or its branches with hypertension or impaired cerebral blood flow. Acute and potentially massive bleeding is possible. Lung retraction may result in desaturation and hypercarbia. While eventually the airway diameter will increase and the stability improve, intraoperatively there may be continued airway compression and collapse as well as airway injury and bleeding.

Postoperative disposition should be to an intensively monitored setting to watch for cardiorespiratory changes and compromise. In small patients, not uncommonly airway swelling may initially result in increased stridor and airway compromise. Steroids should be considered intraoperatively and racemic epinephrine nebulization may reduce airway swelling after extubation. Postoperative echocardiography should document unimpaired cardiac function. Depending on the surgical approach, postoperative analgesia can utilize regional analgesia or intravenous opioids.

1.2.7.4 Congenital diaphragmatic hernia repair in neonates [18]

Neonatal congenital diaphragmatic hernia (CDH) through the posterolateral defect of Bochdalek may be associated with ipsi- (and contra-) lateral pulmonary hypoplasia and pulmonary hypertension, right to left shunting through the ductus arteriosus with desaturation, right heart failure and potentially poor outcome. Management of this type of CDH is complex and includes early intubation, spontaneous respiration with neonatal pressure support ventilation and permissive hypercarbia, adjuvant treatment with pulmonary vasodilators and nitric oxide, vasopressors, high frequency oscillatory ventilation and even placement on ECMO. Surgery may proceed after 24 hours of cardiorespiratory stability or while on ECMO. Open CDH repair is abdominal surgery with subcostal incision; minimally invasive CDH repair is typically by thoracoscopy. Patient selection for thoracoscopic CDH repair may be controversial between anesthesiologist and surgeon, but stable cardiorespiratory support with dopamine, milrinone and nitric oxide at low levels may not be a contraindication. Surgical duration is longer than with an open repair. Leaving the patient on the neonatal ICU ventilator for transport and during surgery minimizes ventilatory instability. Invasive arterial monitoring is indicated and a central line for administration of vasoactive agents is useful. Pre- and post-ductal pulse oximetry is mandatory. All preoperative infusions are continued. Dopamine and epinephrine drips and blood products should be readily available. Patient positioning for thoracoscopic CDH repair is lateral decubitus with the arm over the head. Intraoperative access to the patient will be near impossible. Anesthesia is by intravenous opioids, benzodiazepines, ketamine, dexmedetomidine or inhalational agents, if on an anesthesia ventilator, and muscle relaxation. Lung isolation is not usually necessary as the ipsilateral lung is hypoplastic and of low compliance. A contralateral pneumothorax should be suspected if there are abrupt intraoperative difficulties with oxygenation or ventilation. Surgically, insufflation for the thoracoscopy starting at 3 to 5 cm H_2O is often utilized to create a working space inside the chest, however, occasional increase in insufflation pressure to up to 10 cm H_2O facilitates reduction of abdominal contents from the chest into the abdomen. This is frequently associated with hypercarbia and respiratory acidosis although patients may remain hemodynamically remarkably stable. If spleen or liver have herniated into the chest, there is a risk of bleeding from injury during their reduction. Attention should be directed at avoiding anything that might aggravate pulmonary hypertension including light anesthesia, hypothermia and metabolic acidosis. Neonates with true CDH will be ventilated postoperatively to monitor for cardiorespiratory stability.

Many other forms of diaphragmatic hernia come to the operating room for repair. In patients outside the neonatal age, pulmonary hypertension is less likely. These patients may have respiratory symptoms or an incidental discovery of a diaphragmatic hernia. They are more likely to have an anteromedial defect of Morgagni, eventeration of the diaphragm, intestinal herniation through a hiatal hernia, or a traumatic diaphragmatic hernia. Their repair may be laparoscopically, thoracoscopically or by open repair.

1.2.7.5 Pectus excavatum repair [19]

With a risk of long term restrictive lung disease and consecutive pulmonary hypertension, pectus excavatum repair is medically indicated as well as cosmetically and psychologically desirable. Surgery is performed in adolescence and patients may be otherwise healthy, or can have connective tissue disease like Marfan's syndrome. Electrocardiogram, echocardiogram, chest X-ray, pulmonary function tests and chest CT are typically part of the preoperative evaluation. Patients are supine for surgery and require good venous access and blood typing and screening.

Open repair (Ravitch–Welsh-Rehbein) involves a transverse incision on the anterior chest wall, excision of cartilaginous ribs at multiple levels and sternal fracture to eliminate the anterior chest wall depression. A small "Adkins" bar keeps the sternum in its new position. Pectus carinatum repair may be performed similarly with additional "shaving" of the protruding bony parts of sternum and/or ribs. Open pectus repair does not require lung isolation or invasive arterial blood pressure monitoring. Complications include mechanically induced arrhythmias, bleeding from an internal mammary vessel and pneumothorax. Postoperative pain is segmental corresponding to the ribs excised and the transverse sternotomy and is well covered by epidural analgesia. The Adkins strut is removed after a few months with a small lateral incision in a minor procedure under general anesthesia.

Minimally invasive pectus excavatum repair, the "Nuss" repair, involves thoracoscopically guided dissection between heart and sternum to bring the correcting "Lorenz" bar across under the deformity which is then corrected by flipping the bar. A Rultract® Skyhook retractor assists in elevating the sternum during the dissection. Possible intraoperative complications are injury to heart, coronaries, pericardium, mammary vessels with risk of bleeding, coronary ischemia, pericardial tamponade, cardiac arrhythmias and cardiac arrest. Lung isolation is not usually required, surgical exposure is sufficient with gentle insufflation of CO_2 at a pressure below 5 cm H_2O and ventilation with low PEEP and tidal volumes. Invasive arterial blood pressure monitoring may be considered. Epidural catheters have been used for postoperative analgesia; recently, anecdotes of postoperative neurological problems have led some practitioners to use bilateral paravertebral catheters or systemic analgesia only. The Lorenz bar is removed after several years, at which time it will be quite impacted and its removal may be surgically challenging with risk of bleeding, cardiopulmonary injury and pneumothorax. Anesthesia management should include a safe airway, adequate vascular access and postoperative pain control.

1.2.7.6 Tumor surgery

Anterior mediastinal mass

Anterior mediastinal masses (AMM) are of major concern to the anesthesiologist because of the risk of cardiorespiratory impairment or collapse, spontaneously or following sedation, induction of anesthesia or muscle relaxation [20].

Common presenting ages for anterior mediastinal masses are infancy and adolescence. Typical pediatric tumors in the anterior mediastinum are lymphomas, thymomas, teratomas and other germ cell tumors. AMMs can compress trachea and bronchi, superior vena cava (SVC), heart and pulmonary artery (Fig. 1.2.9; 1.2.10). Patients may be asymptomatic and present with unrelated pathology or with enlarged extrathoracic lymph nodes, or they may be symptomatic with weight loss, sweating, dry cough or shortness of breath, in particular when lying down, have signs of "SVC syndrome" with vascular congestion of the head and arm and conjunctival swelling. There may be pleural and pericardial effusions. Patients may be at additional risk of tumor lysis syndrome at presentation or from initiation of treatment with chemotherapy or steroids.

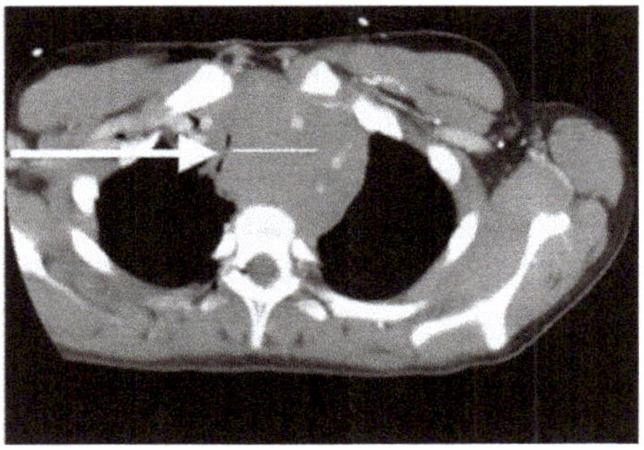

Fig. 1.2.9: Chest CT of an anterior mediastinal mass in a teenager causing displacement and near total obstruction of the trachea (arrow).

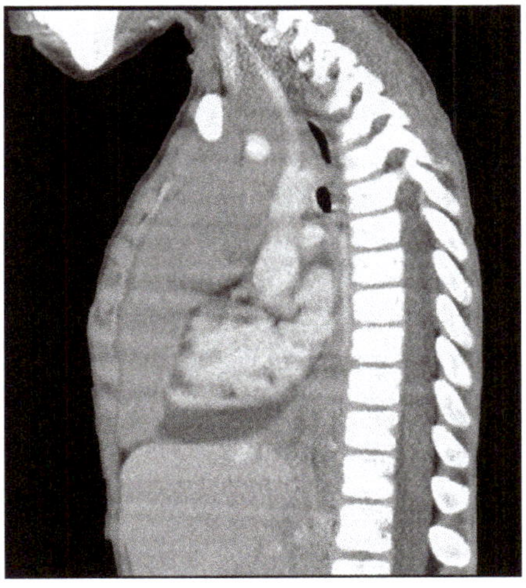

Fig. 1.2.10: Chest CT of large anterior mediastinal mass obstructing large vessels and associated with pleural and pericardial effusions.

Patients with AMM present to the anesthesiologist for diagnostic imaging studies, biopsies, line placement and potentially for resection. Anesthetic management options depend on the mass, its size, location and symptoms, the patient and patient age and the procedure.

Preoperative evaluation and workup includes a history specifically of symptoms and their deterioration in the supine position and the physical exam for airway compression and SVC syndrome. A chest X-ray gives first information of size, location of and airway compression by the mass. CTs can now be performed very quickly and may not require any type of sedation if minor motion artifacts are acceptable. A CT will further define the mass and its relationship to airway and cardiovascular structures. In cooperative patients, pulmonary function tests with peak expiratory flows in the sitting and supine position give important information about airway compression by the anterior mediastinal mass. An echocardiogram looks for pericardial effusion, compression of the SVC, heart or pulmonary artery and ventricular function. Laboratory tests should include a blood count due to possible bone marrow involvement with anemia and thrombocytopenia, as well as electrolytes, specifically potassium, uric acid, blood urea nitrogen and creatinine given possible tumor lysis.

In patients who are symptomatic and/or who have high degrees of airway compression by imaging or peak expiratory flows, SVC syndrome, pulmonary arterial compression or cardiac tamponade physiology, general anesthesia and loss of spontaneous ventilation are generally avoided [21]. The safest approach to these patients needs to be discussed between all members of the team. Occasionally treatment ex juvantibus may be required if the patient is in distress. If the patient is stable but an anesthetic is considered life threatening for the patient, a procedure such as bone marrow biopsy, lymph node biopsy, needle biopsy or pleural tap under local anesthesia without or with minimal sedation may be possible in older and cooperative patients and may yield enough information for the oncologist. Deep sedation or general anesthesia for patients with large mediastinal masses should be titrated carefully to maintain spontaneous ventilation. Anesthetic options for spontaneously breathing patients include inhalational anesthesia, propofol infusion or ketamine, low dose remifentanil or dexmedetomidine infusions. Equipment for flexible fiberoptic intubation, rigid bronchoscopy, ECMO or cardiopulmonary bypass should be available when managing large mediastinal masses in the operating room. The potential benefit of returning to spontaneous respirations and changing patient position from supine to lateral or prone should be remembered if cardiorespiratory difficulties are encountered.

Thoracic neuroblastoma

Thoracic neuroblastomas and other thoracic neural crest cell tumors in children such as ganglioneuroma and ganglioneuroblastoma typically present as posterior mediastinal masses originating from the cervicothoracic sympathetic chain. With growth, they can compress the airway and large vessels, pushing them forward or encasing them. They need to be evaluated for their effect on airway and large vessels as do anterior mediastinal masses and careful induction with slow transition to positive pressure ventilation is recommended. Large masses will more likely be resected via thoracotomy. Lung isolation is more important for thoracoscopic resection of small masses. Apical masses may involve plexus and nerves and muscle relaxation is avoided to allow intraoperative nerve stimulation. Neuroblastomas extending into the spinal canal may be a contraindication to neuraxial blocks. Resection of large posterior mediastinal masses can jeopardize spinal cord blood supply and motor evoked potential monitoring is indicated. Catecholamines (most commonly dopamine) and catecholamine metabolites (normetanephrines) are often elevated at diagnosis. Patients are not always symptomatic from excess catecholamines and preoperative chemotherapy may reduce catecholamine secretion. Patients with high catecholamine levels or symptomatic patients should undergo preoperative alpha-adrenergic receptor blockade (phenoxybenzamine, doxazosin, prazosin), adding beta-adrenergic antagonists or combined alpha/beta-adrenergic antagonists (labetalol) with tachycardia. Intraoperatively, even after blockade or in previously asymptomatic and unblocked patients, manipulation of the tumor can result in hemodynamic instability, and short-acting intravenous vasodilators (sodium nitroprusside) and beta-adrenergic antagonists (esmolol) should be readily available. Intraoperative monitoring with an arterial catheter, availability of blood and postoperative monitoring in an ICU should be considered.

Pulmonary malignancies

Primary pulmonary malignancies are rare in children. Surgical approach to resect pleuropulmonary blastoma depends on location and extent of the tumor and may be via thoracoscopic or open lobectomy or (extrapleural) pneumonectomy. Pneumonectomy is rare in children and anesthetic considerations are directed at lung isolation, appropriate lines for monitoring and management, possibility of bleeding, judicious fluid management, risk of pulmonary hypertension and right heart failure with need for appropriate pharmacologic support, need for adequate pain control including regional anesthesia to assist in postoperative chest physiotherapy to clear secretions, and postoperative critical care monitoring.

More commonly, pulmonary metastases require diagnostic or therapeutic resection. Individual well-defined lesions are resected thoracoscopically. Resection of osteosarcoma metastases often is performed as an open procedure to allow palpation by the surgeon and removal of as many suspicious lesions as possible. Bilateral metastases require successive lateral thoracotomies with positioning change or sternotomy. Lung isolation with double lumen tube, EZ-Blocker™ or sequential placement of a bronchial blocker in the two main stem bronchi is indicated. Despite the presence of a chest tube, a pneumothorax can occur on the first side during surgery on the second side. Epidural analgesia is appropriate for postoperative pain control. As in all patients with oncologic disorders, preoperative patient evaluation needs to specifically address the chemotherapeutic agents that were used and their common side effects, in particular cardiac, renal, hepatic function, bone marrow suppression and neuropathy.

Thymectomy

Thymectomy is performed for thymoma. Imaging studies are reviewed for its location, size and extension. Large thymomas need to be managed as anterior mediastinal masses but will require primary resection. Thymectomy is also offered in juvenile myasthenia gravis unresponsive to medical management with pyridostigmine, steroids and intravenous immunoglobulin [22]. Bulbar and ocular muscle weakness present with double vision and swallowing problems, generalized muscle weakness may result in problems with walking and breathing, which are reflected in decreased pulmonary function tests. Plasmapheresis is used to optimize patients perioperatively. Pyridostigmine is continued at least to the day before surgery, management on the day of surgery varies, some neurologists hold it or give it orally, some intravenously. Intraoperative severe bradycardia can occur related to pyridostigmine medication, use of opioids, neuraxial blockade, vagal stimulation from intubation or mechanical cardiac irritation. Muscle relaxants are avoided in myasthenia gravis although not contraindicated. Good venous access and invasive arterial monitoring are indicated. The choice of anesthetic drugs for thymectomy in patients with myasthenia gravis seems to matter less than careful monitoring and postoperative respiratory and pain management. Thymectomy can be performed via sternotomy, thoracotomy, thoracoscopy or mediastinoscopy. Lung isolation is not necessary for thymectomy via sternotomy. By definition these patients will have muscle weakness postoperatively, but extubation at the end of the surgery may be considered. Careful thoracic epidural analgesia can be helpful, when additional weakness of thoracic muscles is weighed against the benefit of good pain control. Postoperative ICU placement appears prudent after thymectomy for myasthenia gravis for respiratory and pain monitoring and management as well as for observation for myasthenic or cholinergic crises. Clinical improvement of myasthenic symptoms may not become apparent until weeks after the surgery.

1.3 Perioperative pain management

Effective perioperative pain management is in the surgeon's interest as much as in the patient's. Particularly for thoracic surgery, it reduces perioperative respiratory complications from atelectasis or retained secretions and may allow for earlier extubation and shorter ICU or hospital stay, resulting in overall better surgical outcome. The surgeon has an essential role in perioperative analgesia by supporting, if not participating in the process of it.

The principles of effective perioperative pain management include

- preventive analgesia: preventing the pain response by early administration of loco-regional and systemic analgesics
- multimodal analgesia: using multiple modalities of pain management including non-pharmacological as well as multiple pharmacological mechanisms
- using loco-regional anesthesia including catheter techniques whenever possible
- scheduled rather than only "as-needed" (prn) medication early after the surgery with a plan for rescue medication for break-through pain
- ready access to pain management through pediatric pain services and patient/nurse-controlled pumps for systemic or loco-regional analgesia
- monitoring of pain control and side effects of analgesic regimens to minimize both inadequate pain control and complications from analgesia.

1.3.1 Systemic analgesia

Many drugs are available for postoperative analgesia. Anesthesiologists and surgeons need to familiarize themselves with locally available drugs and the manufacturers' recommendations for dose, dosing interval or limitation of use, as well as with the side effect profile. While generally drugs from the same drug class, such as μ-agonist opioids or nonsteroidal anti-inflammatory drugs (NSAIDs), are to a degree comparable, there may be differences in side effects, formulation, indication and occasionally efficacy so that switching from one drug to another in the same group may still be reasonable. As much as possible, different drug classes should be combined, more potent drugs (opioids) should dominate the early and "weaker" analgesics (paracetamol/acetaminophen) should be reserved for late postoperative pain control. Consideration should be given to administering analgesics on a schedule immediately following surgery and changing to an "as needed" regimen only after the initial pain has been well controlled.

1.3.1.1 Available drugs

Acetaminophen/paracetamol is a common basic non-opioid, non-NSAID analgesic and antipyretic, available for enteral (oral, rectal) and parenteral (iv) dosing; with availability of the parenteral formulation, the rectal administration has lost its place in the hospital postoperative setting; it can be used over extended periods of time but the maximum daily dose, which can be as low as 30 mg/kg/d for premies and neonates, needs to be adhered to. It has no cardiorespiratory side effects but can be hepatotoxic.

NSAIDs (non-steroidal anti-inflammatory drugs: ibuprofen, diclofenac, ketorolac and others) are potent analgesic, antipyretic and anti-inflammatory drugs which work particularly well for perioperative inflammatory pain; some NSAIDs are available for parenteral application and have proven particularly helpful as adjunct analgesics in thoracic surgery to supplement regional anesthesia or to treat shoulder pain from positioning or from thoracoscopy as well as chest tube discomfort; renal toxicity, platelet inhibition and gastrointestinal problems are the main side effects; some pain protocols limit scheduled intravenous NSAIDs to a 48-hour period; although NSAIDs are used in premies to promote closure of a persistent ductus arteriosus, use as analgesic in premies and neonates is limited by immaturity of renal function.

Metamizol is a potent non-NSAID-non-opioid analgesic. It is not available in all countries but has seen a resurgence even in children despite its potentially severe side effects (including agranulocytosis).

Acetylsalicylic Acid/Aspirin is used in children for management of Kawasaki disease, its analgesic use in children generally is avoided due to the risk of Reye's syndrome.

Opioids such as the short-acting remifentanil, alfentanil, sufentanil and fentanyl are used intraoperatively, although some of them such as fentanyl patches may be indicated in chronic pain management. For postoperative analgesia, the longer acting opioids such as intravenous morphine, hydromorphone or piritramid are preferred. They can initially be ordered on a schedule, especially in the ICU setting, and also as a continuous infusion, or for suitable patients as patient-controlled analgesia (PCA). Most children over 6 years of age are able to use PCA pumps appropriately, in younger children, nurse-controlled analgesia pumps (NCA) are popular because they allow safe and frequent dosing of opioids directly at the patient's bedside without the need to go, draw up and deliver the opioid dose. After the initial postoperative period with parenteral opioids, oral opioids such as oxycodone and oral morphine or hydromorphone are used. Codeine acts as an analgesic only after metabolism to morphine and this metabolism may be lacking or accelerated in some patients, making codeine for these patients either ineffective or increasing its risk for respiratory depression; its use in children is not recommended anymore; agonist/antagonist opioids like buprenorphine or tramadol are used in older children; pethidine/meperidine is less popular in pediatric anesthesia due to its side effect profile.

NMDA receptor antagonists include the opioid methadone, the anesthetic ketamine and the electrolyte magnesium. Their analgesic effect is used intraoperatively, but also postoperatively, usually in combination with other analgesics; many studies have confirmed their efficacy at reducing postoperative opioid requirement.

Alpha-2-adrenergic agonists (clonidine and the more potent and more alpha-2-selective dexmedetomidine) are analgesics with anxiolytic and sedative quality. They may have cardiovascular side effects like hypotension and bradycardia. Neuraxial clonidine in neonates has been associated with respiratory depression, but respiratory side effects are otherwise not expected with alpha-2-adrenergic agonists. Both can be given intraoperatively in patients who require an opioid free anesthetic, to reduce intraoperative opioid requirement and to prevent emergence delirium in children from anesthesia. Their beneficial respiratory profile make them suitable drugs to assist in postoperative analgesia of patients with obstructive sleep apnea. Dexmedetomidine is frequently used as a sedative in intubated and extubated children in the ICU. Clonidine is also a component of chronic pain management and weaning schedules.

Sedatives such as benzodiazepines, although not analgesics, may be indicated in patients with high levels of anxiety or agitation, but in particular they can be part of the postoperative analgesic schedule in children who may suffer from muscle spasms following orthopedic or thoracic surgery with involvement of bones and muscles. Opioids or antihistamines such as diphenhydramine may be added for their sedative properties. For patients with spasticity, baclofen may be helpful. In the perioperative setting it is particularly important to continue its administration in patients already receiving the drug.

Others: Gabapentin is a component of the multimodal cocktail offered preoperatively to patients undergoing orthopedic surgery and can be useful in thoracic surgery as well. Dexamethasone is used as an adjunct to systemic or regional analgesia.

1.3.2 Local-regional anesthesia

Loco-regional analgesia can prevent the painful stimulus from reaching the central nervous system, reducing the negative effects of pain such as development of chronic pain states, specifically after thoracic surgery. Agents used include

- chlorprocaine as a short-acting local anesthetic is used particularly in neonates and infants for continuous infusions due to its reliable metabolic elimination
- intermediate (lidocaine, mepivacaine, prilocaine) and long-acting (bupivacaine, levo-bupivacaine, ropivacaine, tetracaine) local anesthetics are the classic local anesthetics for perioperative use
- very long-acting local anesthetics such as liposomal bupivacaine (Exparel®) or neosaxitoxin, a paralytic shellfish toxin producing local analgesia, are new and in use or under investigation in adults only
- mixtures of shorter acting, fast onset with long-acting slow onset drugs
- additives such as bicarbonate, epinephrine, clonidine, dexamethasone and opioids modify onset, duration and effect.

Especially in neonates, maximum allowed doses of local anesthetics such as bupivacaine and lidocaine may either be limited or reached quickly, so that drug doses need to be calculated to avoid overdoses and complications from local anesthetic injections.

1.3.2.1 Surgically placed loco-regional anesthesia

- **skin infiltration** with local anesthetic before incision is one of the major surgical contributions to preventive and perioperative analgesia, as are local anesthetic infiltration of trocar and instrument tracks for thoracoscopic procedures. Additionally, direct infiltration around visible nerves, or skin infiltration during closure of the surgical wound should be practiced routinely, if no formal regional anesthetic is performed or if additional volume of local anesthetic can safely be administered.
- **surgical nerve blocks** such as intercostal nerve blocks under direct vision are easy and safe, they add minutes to the procedure while adding hours to the patient's pain control. The needle is inserted as far posteriorly as possible, advanced under the rib until just external to the parietal pleura. After careful aspiration, a few milliliter of local anesthetic are injected while observing from the inside as the local anesthetic creates a wheal under the pleura. The high risk for local anesthetic toxicity is reduced by careful aspiration and injection of a small volume at different

levels. The block is performed at multiple levels covering at least one or two levels above the highest and below the lowest incisional site as well as the chest tube site.
- **surgically placed catheters** are for example subpleural or intrapleural catheters, and local anesthetic instillation through the chest tube has been used to assist with postoperative pain control, but they have a risk of high local anesthetic absorption and toxicity. Wound catheters placed into the wound during closure of an incision have proven effective for thoracotomy incisions [23].

1.3.2.2 Regional anesthesia

Anesthesia providers or regional anesthesia teams may offer epidural and paravertebral blocks and catheters for thoracic surgery. Especially in children, all continuous catheter techniques require availability of a pain management service to follow the patients and respond to analgesic insufficiency, excessive blocks or complications on short notice.

Paravertebral blockade has been used in adults for many years as a landmark technique with risks including pneumothorax. With the introduction of ultrasound in regional anesthesia, paravertebral blocks have become safer and are used increasingly in pediatric pain management as well. Under ultrasound guidance, the paravertebral space is entered at one or several levels and local anesthetic is deposited and/or a catheter introduced for continuous local anesthetic infusion. Multiple dermatomes can be covered by a single injection or catheter. Advantages of paravertebral blockade include safe placement under ultrasound guidance, one-sidedness of the block for one-sided surgery, lower incidence of hemodynamic effects due to lower risk of sympathetic blockade and avoidance of side effects of epidural blockade. There is a small failure rate of paravertebral blocks as well as a complication risk from epidural and intrathecal spread. Paravertebral blocks are popular for thoracoscopies or one-sided thoracic procedures. Midline or bilateral procedures require bilateral blocks or catheters. High procedures involving T1 and higher dermatomes may require additional blocks such as supraclavicular, interscalene or cervical plexus blocks.

Epidural or peridural catheters remain the most established regional analgesia technique after thoracic surgery. In children they need to be placed under anesthesia, either by primary thoracic placement or they can be threaded from lumbar or caudal insertion sites to mid-thoracic levels. Placement should be verified by imaging with fluoroscopy, epidurogram (Fig. 1.2.6) or ultrasound. Infusion rate of the local anesthetic determines the spread, and opioids or clonidine are often added to increase the effectiveness. Spinal cord injury or dural puncture are risks, but rare with careful technique. Thoracic epidural local anesthetic can result in sympathetic blockade in older children with hypotension and some bradycardia. High spread of local anesthetic can cause Horner's syndrome and harlequin phenomenon postoperatively. Pruritus, respiratory depression and urinary retention from epidural opioids, epidural hematoma or infection, blockade of the wrong side or block failure are other drawbacks. Epidural catheters are popular for bilateral or midline thoracic surgery including sternotomy as well as for thoracotomy and procedures requiring postoperative chest tubes. Epidural catheters have good efficacy for open or minimally invasive pectus repairs and for chest wall resections.

1.4 Further reading

[1] Backeljauw B, Holland SK, Altaye M, Loepke AW. Cognition and brain structure following early childhood surgery with anesthesia. Pediatrics 2015;136:e1–12.
[2] Lin EP, Soriano SG, Loepke AW. Anesthetic neurotoxicity. Anesthesiology Clin 2014;32:133–155.
[3] Davidson AJ, Disma N, de Graaff JC, et al. Neurodevelopmental outcome at 2 years of age after general anaesthesia and awake-regional anaesthesia in infancy (GAS): an international muticentre, randomised controlled trial. Lancet 2016;387:239–250.
[4] Flick RP, Sprung J, Harrison TE, et al. Perioperative Cardiac Arrests in Children between 1988 and 2005 at a Tertiary Referral Center. A Study of 92,881 Patients. Anesthesiology 2007;106:226–37.
[5] Hammer GB, Fitzmaurice BG, Brodsky JB. Methods for single-lung ventilation in pediatric patients. Anesth Analg 1999;89:1426–9.
[6] Hammer GB. Single-lung ventilation in infants and children. Pediatr Anesth 2004;14:98–102.
[7] Stephenson LL, Seefelder C. Routine Extraluminal Use of the 5F Arndt Endobronchial Blocker for One-Lung Ventilation in Children up to 24 Months of Age. J Cardiothorac Vasc Anesth 2011;25:683–686.
[8] Seefelder C. Use of the 26-French-double-lumen-tube for lung isolation in children. J Cardiothorac Vasc Anesth 2014;28:e19–21.
[9] Bishay M, Giacomello L, Retrosi G, et al. Decreased cerebral oxygen saturation during thoracoscopic repair of congenital diaphragmatic hernia and esophageal atresia in infants. J Pediatr Surg 2011;46:47–50.
[10] Bishay M, Giacomello L, Retrosi G, et al. Hypercapnia and acidosis during open and thoracoscopic repair of congenital diaphragmatic hernia and esophageal atresia. Ann Surg 2013;258:895–900.
[11] Witt L, Osthaus WA, Schröder T, et al. Single-lung ventilation with carbon dioxide hemipneumothorax: hemodynamic and respiratory effects in piglets. Pediatr Anesth 2012;22:793–798.
[12] Choudhry DK. Single-Lung Ventilation in Pediatric Anesthesia. Anesthesiology Clin N Am 2005;23:693–708.
[13] Choudhry M, Drake D. Antenatally diagnosed lung malformations: a plea for long-term outcome studies. Pediatr Surg Int 2015;31:439–444.
[14] Knottenbelt G, Skinner A, Seefelder C. Tracheo-oesophageal fistula (TOF) and oesophageal atresia (OA). Best Pract Res Clin Anaesthesiol 2010;24:387–401.
[15] Broemling N, Campbell F. Anesthetic management of congenital tracheoesophageal fistula. Paediatr Anaesth 2011;21:1092–9.
[16] Jennings RW, Hamilton TE, Smithers CJ, Ngerncham M, Feins N, Foker JE. Surgical approaches to aortopexy for severe tracheomalacia. J Pediatr Surgery 2014;49:66–71.
[17] Bairdain S, Smithers CJ, Hamilton TE, et al. Direct tracheobronchopexy to correct airway collapse due to severe tracheobronchomalacia: short-term outcomes in a series of 20 patients. J Pediatr Surg 2015;50:972–977.
[18] McHoney M. Congenital diaphragmatic hernia, management in the newborn. Pediatr Surg Int 2015;31:1005–1013.

[19] Mavi J, Moore DL. Anesthesia and analgesia for pectus excavatum surgery. Anesthesiology Clin 2014;32:175–184.

[20] Blank RS, de Souza DG. Anesthetic management of patients with an anterior mediastinal mass. Can J Anaesth 2011;58:853–859.

[21] Shamberger RC, Holzman RS, Griscom NT, Tarbell NJ, Weinstein HJ, Wohl ME. Prospective evaluation by computed tomography and pulmonary function of children with mediastinal masses tests. Surgery 1995;118:468–71.

[22] Stephenson L, Tkachenko I, Shamberger R, Seefelder C. Anesthesia for patients undergoing transsternal thymectomy for juvenile myasthenia gravis. Saudi J Anaesth 2011;5:25–30.

[23] Krylborn J, Anell-Olofsson ME, Bitkover C, et al. Plasma levels of levobupivacaine during continuous infusion via a wound catheter after major surgery in newborn infants. Eur J Anaesthesiol 2015;32:851–856

2 Approaches to the thoracic cavity

2.1 Introduction

Further development of technical devices facilitates surgical and interventional approaches in ever smaller intrathoracic structures. **Jens Dingemann** and **Benno Ure** provide an overview of the current status of video-assisted thoracoscopic surgery (VATS) and focus critically on the disadvantages and limitations of this technique. Despite the innovative and unstoppable shift away from conventional surgery that has been observed in recent years, open approaches to the thorax and mediastinum retain their importance, as described by **Marcus Krüger** and **Taufiek Rajab**. Their philosophy also involves consideration of surgical trauma reduction and is rounded off by valuable comments from **Rolf Oerter**

Bronchoscopy in small children represents a significant challenge, and interventional approaches are complex, as demonstrated by **Nicolaus Schwerk** and the commentators **Jacques de Blic, Steve Cunningham and Hartmut Grasemann**. Herein, it is important to stress that the treatment of those patients should ideally be restricted to specialized centers that are home to highly experienced interdisciplinary teams.

Marcus Krüger, Taufiek K. Rajab

2.2 Thoracotomy

In order to achieve optimal exposure and minimal damage to ribs, cartilages, muscles, intercostal nerves and the vasculature, several techniques and modifications of thoracotomies have been developed. The intercostal approach is the common feature of all thoracotomies. In principle, three basically different variants of thoracotomies can be distinguished – anterior thoracotomy, posterolateral thoracotomy and lateral approaches probably best described as lateral muscle sparing thoracotomy.

2.2.1 Anterior thoracotomy

Anterior thoracotomies are mainly used to control emergency situations. This refers to both cardiac emergencies and severe lung bleeding, such as after penetrating trauma. Anterior thoracotomy facilitates access to both ventricles of the heart and to the descending aorta. Life-threatening lung bleeding may be controlled by hilar clamping via this approach. Moreover, anterior thoracotomy is widely used in lung transplantation. However, these indications are not within the scope of this book. Hereafter, posterolateral thoracotomy and the lateral approaches will be discussed in more detail.

2.2.2 Posterolateral thoracotomy

Posterolateral thoracotomy provides superb exposure of the organs within the ipsilateral hemithorax. Though posterolateral thoracotomy is associated with more extensive tissue damage and supposed to contribute to negative postoperative sequelae [1], there is still uncertainty about the optimal location of the thoracotomy [1]. Standard posterolateral thoracotomy requires division of the latissimus dorsi muscle (LD), whereas the serratus anterior muscle (SA) can be mobilized without division. Although functional drawbacks of LD division are negligible, the loss of a major muscle for potential chest wall reconstruction in the future should be taken into consideration. In order to preserve the integrity of the LD a latissimus sparing thoracotomy has been described. The muscle is mobilized by blunt dissection and then retracted allowing for a nearly similar exposure of the respective hemithorax. During dissection of the LD care is taken not to divide penetrating vessels. An additional dissection of the inferior border of the SA, after retracting the LA posteriorly, allows for a total muscle sparing thoracotomy within the third to 7th intercostal space [2]. Despite a slightly longer operation time the muscle sparing approach potentially provides several advantages, such as better lung function in the early postoperative period with reduced need for opioids and less musculoskeletal sequelae.

A variety of musculoskeletal sequelae are attributed to thoracotomies, in particular to posterolateral thoracotomy, in younger children: weak elevation of the ipsilateral shoulder, winged scapula secondary to injury of the long thoracic nerve, thoracic asymmetry secondary to atrophy of the SA, fusion of ribs and to some extent thoracic scoliosis. An association between thoracotomy at a young age and scoliosis is discussed, especially in older publications. However, scoliosis may be associated with the underlying diseases, rather than to the thoracic incision itself. Concomitant spinal deformity in patients with esophageal atresia or an extensive fibrotic process due to esophageal leaks and the necessity of several thoracotomies in patients with tracheoesophageal fistulas could serve as examples. In contrast, chest wall resection is associated with a significant risk for scoliosis development. This is especially true for rib resection involving the fifth or more cranial ribs. A comparable risk exists in case of rib fusion following thoracotomy. However, a thoracotomy with uneventful postoperative healing does not seem to be associated with a higher risk of scoliosis [3].

2.2.3 Lateral muscle sparing thoracotomy (anterolateral/anteroaxillary thoracotomy)

Recent research reveals evidence that higher pain scores after posterolateral thoracotomy compared to muscle sparing lateral approaches are triggered by more severe nerve damage [4]. Therefore, these neurophysiologic investigations support the authors preference for lateral/anterolateral approaches. A variety of different muscle sparing lateral approaches has been described, such as vertical thoracotomy. In fact, main differences are related to the angle and to the length of the skin incision. Despite the modern paradigm "small cut – big surgeon", a too small skin incision should be avoided to prevent injury of the skin. Especially in case of excessive usage of the retractor, or even two retractors, impairment of skin healing is likely to occur. Landmarks for the skin incision in conventional lateral thoracotomy is a point somewhat above the inferior angle of the scapula and the inframammary crease (Fig. 2.2.1). The anterior border of the latissimus dorsi more or less predetermines the dorsal margin of the soft tissue preparation. Mobilization and dorsal retraction of the latissimus dorsi contributes little to extension of the approach, since the long thoracic nerve lies beneath the anterior border of the latissimus dorsi and injury to the long thoracic nerve should be avoided. To gain better exposure of the intrathoracic organs a steeper incision line is recommended. A gradually steeper incision results in anterolateral, anteroaxillary or vertical thoracotomies (Fig. 2.2.1). For vertical thoracotomies the skin incision follows the posterior axillary line slightly posterior to the anterior border of the LD.

Beside a better exposure of the intrathoracic organs, a steep incision line and according line of soft tissue preparation has another substantial advantage. In young female patients care must be taken to avoid breast and pectoral mal-development [5]. This risk can be limited with a steep line of the skin incision followed by meticulous preparation of the pectoralis major (Fig. 2.2.1), provided a thoracotomy not higher than in the fourth intercostal space. However, a higher thoracotomy is rarely necessary.

Alternatively, for younger children from birth until about 8 to 10 years the approach through the axillary skin crease (muscle sparing axillary skin crease incision (MSASCI) represents a promising option [6]. Especially in neonates and young infants this approach allows for a comprehensive operational exposure for a wide range of procedures including lower lobectomies [6]. In older children good access to the lung and the mediastinum via the third or fourth intercostal space is still possible.

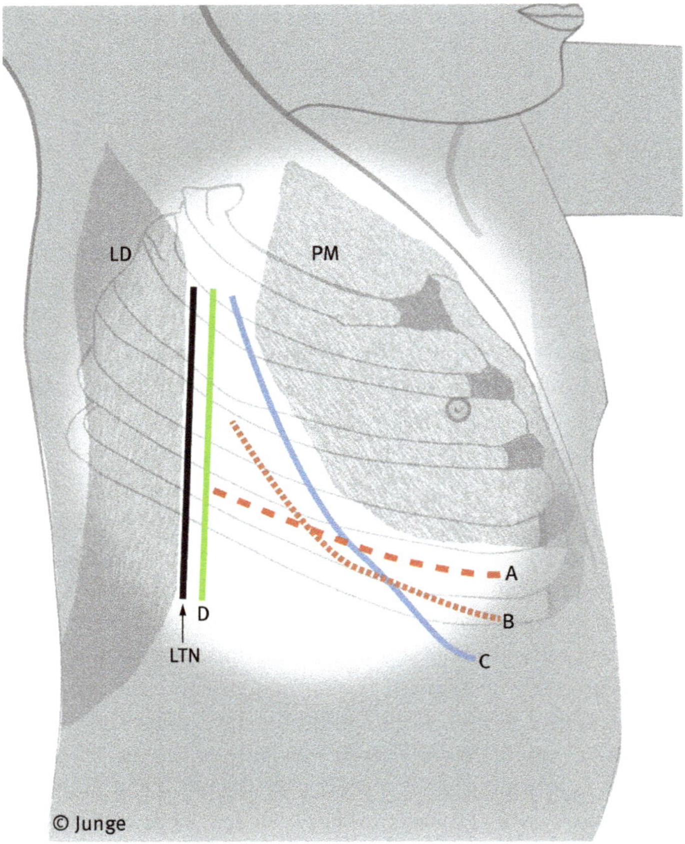

Fig. 2.2.1: Schematic diagram of skin incisions for different muscle sparing lateral approaches. A: conventional lateral thoracotomy; B: anterolateral thoracotomy; C: anteroaxillary thoracotomy; D: vertical thoracotomy. LD, latissimus dorsi muscle; PM, pectoralis major muscle; LTN, long thoracic nerve.

2.2.4 Closure of the thoracotomy with regard to postoperative pain

The appropriate technique of thoracotomy is the first step also in terms of avoiding post-thoracotomy pain syndrome (PTPS). However, closure of the thoracotomy seems of paramount importance regarding acute postoperative pain as well as long-term sequelae. The treatment of the PTPS is challenging even in the hands of specialized pain experts and with multimodal treatment schedules. Due to the difficulties in objectifying pain, data concerning the incidence of PTPS and the benefit of prophylactic and therapeutic measures strongly vary. In fact, thoracotomy is one of the surgical procedures with the highest rates of chronic postoperative pain. The incidence is as high as 30% or even 50% in adult patients. In children, acute postoperative pain plays a more prominent role while chronic pain is less common. The precise pathogenesis of PTPS is still under debate. It can be assumed with a high degree of certainty that

both neuropathic and myofascial pain components play a decisive role. Actually, different factors contribute to an elevated risk of PTPS:
- type and extent of surgery
- intraoperative and postoperative analgesia
- age of the children and underlying diseases
- nerve damage due to the metallic thoracic retractor
- damage of the intercostal nerve beneath the thoracotomy due to pericostal sutures

Some of the above mentioned features can be influenced by the treating physicians. The extent of the surgical trauma can only be influenced with respect to the surgical approach as described in the preceding chapter. Analgesia is of great significance and is discussed in the respective chapter of this book. Damage of the intercostal nerve due to pressure of the retractor was thought to be one of the main triggers for postoperative pain in particular for chronic pain syndrome. Unfortunately, the implementation of minimally invasive approaches, where the retractor is omitted, did not lead to the predicted dramatic reduction in long-term pain. According to case series, harvesting of the intercostal bundles and taking them out of the operative field before inserting the retractor reduces chronic postoperative pain.

Different technical alternatives for the re-approximation of the ribs aiming at reduced long-term pain have been described (Fig. 2.2.2). In the edge closure technique the suture is placed between the caudal edge of the distal rib and the related neurovascular bundle. For safe preservation of the neurovascular structures usage of a large blunt needle is recommended. Before suturing the inferior edge of the rib and the back of the rib are carefully freed from intercostal tissue. Especially in infants and smaller children the distal suture may be placed subperiosteally (Fig. 2.2.2). Intracostal suture technique represents a third method to prevent strangulation of the neurovascular bundle beneath the distal rib (Fig. 2.2.2). The sutures are placed through small holes drilled through the bony part of the lower rib or of both ribs. The double edge technique allows for potential protection of both neurovascular bundles involved in a thoracotomy (Fig. 2.2.2). The sutures are placed through the thin area between neurovascular structures and the lower rib and similarly between neurovascular structures and the upper rib. Harvesting an intercostal muscle flap before inserting the retractor is another way to reduce the mechanic alteration of the upper and the lower intercostal neurovascular bundles.

For all the above mentioned techniques a significant advantage regarding reduced acute and/or chronic postoperative pain could be demonstrated in case series or even small randomized trials. However, the benefit under controlled conditions could not be proven for larger series or in routine surgical practice. Therefore, it is difficult to give a definitive generally valid recommendation. Since post-thoracotomy pain syndrome is one of the major concerns in thoracic surgery, any effort should be made to reduce the risk of chronic pain through optimal closure of the thoracotomy. We feel that appropriate analgesia within the early postoperative period is of great significance. Moreover, we apply local anesthetics into the intercostal space prior to the incision. The concept behind this is a potential reduction or even elimination of the pain memory.

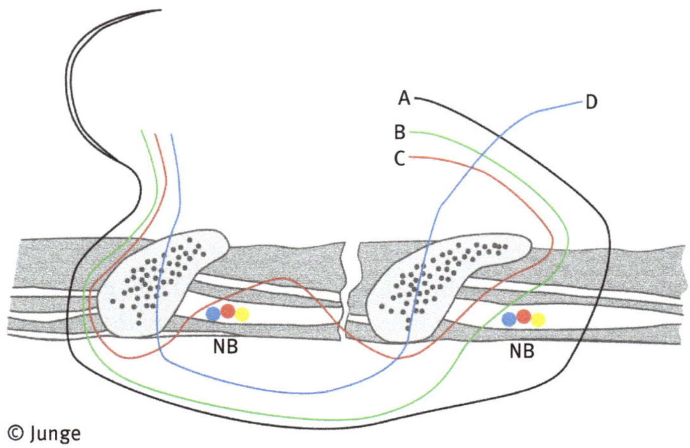

Fig. 2.2.2: Re-approximation of the ribs after thoracotomy – technical variants aiming at reduced impairment of the neurovascular bundle (NB): A – pericostal; B – edge technique; C – double edge technique; D – transcostal (drilling holes through the rib).

Ralf Oerter

Comment

The authors reveal their broad and detailed expertise in the techniques of the various approaches to the respective compartments of the thoracic cavity by open surgery.

With regard to the different size ratio in the musculo-skeletal structures of the child at different ages, the choice of the best approach is crucial. This applies for postoperative musculo-skeletal function as well as for postoperative pain connected to the type of the surgical access and closure techniques. So it does in adults and even more so in children.

As to the problem of nerve damage related postoperative pain in posterolateral and lateral thoracotomy it might be helpfull to separate the latissimus dorsi muscle below the line of skin incision as much as possible. This not alone allows for a tensionfree spontaneous retraction of the latissimus dorsi muscle without any need to keep the muscle out of the way by a retractor, jeopardizing the nervus thorakodorsalis. It also preserves a greater portion of innervated muscle without remarkable loss of function after reinsertion. Likewise best exposure can be achieved by separating the serratus anterior muscle close to its insertion at the ventral thoracic wall, leaving a small portion of the muscle for subsequent reinsertion. The complete muscle can then be "rolled" easily on the thoracic wall cephalad to the intercostal line designed for access to the thoracic cavitiy, be it the sixth, the fifth or the fourth intercostal space. No tractor is needed with its intrinsic risk of damage to the nervus thoracicus longus.

A second "pain issue" is the technique of opening and closing the intercostal space. Practising in adult thoracic surgery I observed a dramatic decrease in postoperative pain syndrome since I abandoned mid-line intercostal muscle incision with subsequent pericostal reconstruction on either side of the ICS with 4 to 5 thick single sutures. Often, in repeat surgery the respective ICS was blocked by substantial synossification of the ribs, hardly allowing for repat access to the thoracic cavity through the ICS of previous surgery.

In the new technique the intercostal layer is opened by subcostal disection preserving both neurovascular bundle and muscle but not isolating those structures from one another. Reconstruction is then rendered by a thick monofil sling thread using a running suture technique catching the upper rib pericostally and the disected muscle of the ICS below with about 8 to 10 turns. As a result of this, easy and anatomical reconstruction of the ICS is provided with little traction and friction force to periostal and muscular structures. Moreover, in cases of repeat surgery an ICS reconstructed this way often shows normal width with the intercostal muscle layer still intact without any synostosis between the ribs, allowing for repeat access through the same ICS. Also, for the time we have been appliying this technique we can observe a drastic decrease in postoperative pain, both in intensity and duration.

These considerations are drawn from practice in thoracic surgery in adults. Yet they may contribute to aspects of how and where to go into a child's thoracic cavity as profoundly discussed in Krüger's and Rajab's chapter.

Marcus Krüger, Taufiek K. Rajab

2.3 Sternotomy

In thoracic surgery, the sternotomy approach is primarily reserved for pathologies in the anterior mediastinum and for bilateral lung resections. Moreover, sternotomy allows for good exposure of the distal trachea and the main stem bronchi. For this reason, sternotomy is used less often than thoracotomy. Chronic pain after sternotomy is less common in children than in adults, but still represents a relevant complication. About 10% to 15% of pediatric patients suffer from significant long-lasting pain following sternotomy. A neuropathic pain component presumably contributes to this. Against this background, it is worth considering some technical aspects of sternotomy.

2.3.1 Median sternotomy

A skin incision is performed starting just below the sternal notch down to the tip of the xiphoid process. However, the extent of the incision can be reduced depending on the experience of the surgeon, elasticity of the skin and the nature of the planned procedure. Especially in infants and young children the approach should not be expanded too far below the xiphoid process to avoid diaphragmatic hernias. The xiphoid process can be resected or cut with a heavy pair of scissors. Leaving the xiphoid process in situ and extending the sternotomy to one side may potentially reduce the incidence of incisional hernias. During dissection in the jugular fossa, injury of the transverse venous arch can lead to significant bleeding. Therefore, these veins should be identified and clipped beforehand. After division of the interclavicular ligament the posterior surface of the sternum is freed by blunt dissection.

To avoid healing disorders of the sternum particular care should be taken to divide the sternum exactly in the midline. The midline can be easily identified by palpating the sternal borders with two fingers and marking the periosteum with electrocautery. Electrocautery is used for the division of the periosteum. The direction of sawing can be left to the surgeon's preference, since according to the literature there is no evidence to favor either direction [7]. However, before sawing from cephalad to caudad, division of the interclavicular ligament is essential. Pulling the sternal saw upwards (from dorsal to ventral) helps to avoid injury to vessels located at the backside of the sternum, such as the brachiocephalic artery and innominate vein. Deflating the lungs by disconnecting the ventilator prior to sawing is standard of care particularly in cardiac surgery. This procedure is believed to avoid accidental pleurotomy and hence to facilitate postoperative recovery. However, according to the current literature this measure cannot be supported [7]. Interestingly, the rate of inadvertent pleurotomy seems to vary significantly from surgeon to surgeon [7]. Sternopericardial ligaments should be divided before further opening of the retractor in order to reduce tension and to avoid unintended opening of the pericardium and the pleura. Periosteal bleeding is controlled by pinpoint cautery. Excessive electrocautery may interfere with sternal healing. If bone wax is applied to treat profuse bleeding from the bone marrow, it should be used sparingly since bone wax is known to interfere with the healing process. Alternatively, vancomycin paste can be used.

Cervico-sternotomies allow a safe exposure of tumors involving the thoracic inlet, such as ganglio-neuromas localized within the upper third of the posterior mediastinum (Tab. 2.3.1).

Tab. 2.3.1: Types of sternotomy and related non-cardiac exposure.

Approach	**Shape**	**Incision of the sternum (downwards)**	**Exposure (non-cardiac)**
median sternotomy	"I"	entire sternum	anterior mediastinal tumors, bilateral lung metastases, distal trachea and main stem bronchi
partial upper	"L"	third/fourth intercostal space	thymectomy, upper thoracic esophagus
partial upper	"I"	fifth intercostal space	almost exclusively heart and aorta/intrathoracic goiter
manubriotomy	"L"	second intercostal space	cervicothoracic vertebrae/ intrathoracic goiter/stenosis of supra-aortic vessels
manubriotomy	inversed "T"	second intercostal space	third cervical to fifth thoracic vertebrae/thymectomy
cervico-sternotomy	"I"	entire sternum	tumors of the superior posterior mediastinum (eg. ganglio-neuromas), scoliosis

2.3.2 Partial median sternotomy (hemisternotomy, upper sternotomy)

The skin incision extends from the sternal notch down to about 2 cm below the angle of Louis. For the division of the sternum we prefer a sternal saw. The sternum is divided from the top down to usually the third intercostal space (Fig. 2.3.1, Tab. 2.3.1). Depending on the specific clinical situation, the sternotomy may extend to the second or sometimes even to the fourth intercostal space. The L-shaped sternal division is completed to the left or more often to the right side again depending on the concrete underlying pathology. It is also possible to omit the lateral sternal incision resulting in a so called I-shaped partial median sternotomy. Even if the sternum is divided down to the fourth or fifth intercostal space, this approach allows access almost exclusively to the heart and the aorta.

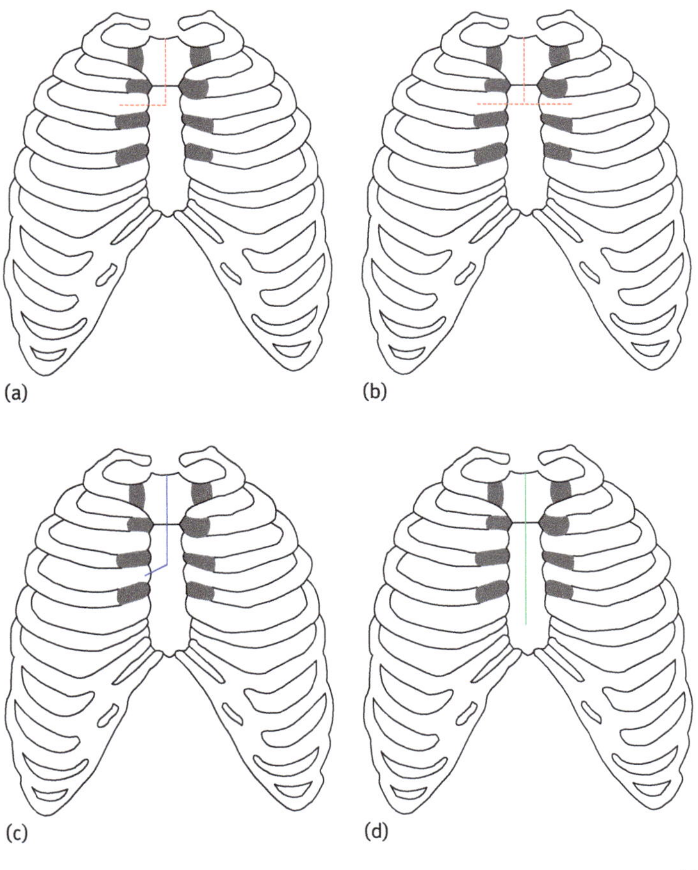

Fig. 2.3.1: Schematic diagram of different variants of partial sternotomy: (a) – L-shaped manubriotomy, (b) – inversed T-shaped manubriotomy, (c) – partial upper L-shaped sternotomy, (d) – partial upper I-shaped sternotomy.

The manubriotomy is a special version of the partial upper sternotomy. Usually, a lateral extension of the sternotomy is carried out in the second intercostal space. In older children, this allows for a 3 to 4 cm exposure width with an L-shaped incision (Fig. 2.3.1, Tab. 2.3.1) and for about 6 cm with bilateral inversed T-shaped incision (Fig. 2.3.1, Tab. 2.3.1). Examples for organs or pathologies approachable through the different sternotomy variants are summarized in Tab. 2.3.1.

2.3.3 Closure of the sternotomy

In younger patients, sternal dehiscence is rare but nevertheless a troublesome condition. Several factors, such as bone quality, comorbidites, patient age or type and duration of the surgical procedure contribute to this complication. As mentioned above meticulous midline division of the sternum and conservative hemostasis with coagulation and bone wax help to avoid healing problems. Moreover, closure of the sternotomy is the other important technical issue. Accurate approximation of the sternal halves supports proper healing.

Traditionally, non-absorbable sutures are used as standard for median sternotomy closures. In older infants steel wires are used, since tight re-approximation of the sternal halves is desired to promote uncomplicated bone healing. As a rough rule of thumb one wire or suture per 10 kg patient weight is recommended. Known disadvantages of stainless steel wires are persistent pain or discomfort, risk of breaking and erosion of dermis with subsequent infection. Alternative non-absorbable sutures, such as silk or polyester are associated with a higher risk of wound infection, whereas polypropylene leads to significant formation of granulation tissue.

Particularly in children, sternotomy closure using absorbable sutures, such as polydioxanone sutures, provides excellent results. Most studies, including several hundred pediatric patients from newborn to 17 years of age [8], confirmed good sternal stability. Advantages of these sutures compared to stainless steel wires are less chronic pain and discomfort as well as absence of an inflammatory reaction. The use of a continuous suture, figure of eight sutures or simple interrupted sutures is subject to the surgeon's preference. Due to a suspected better distribution of the sharing forces figure-of-eight sutures are recommended by some authors [8]. Even if less common in thoracic surgery, the use of sutures facilitates the approach in case of emergency re-do sternotomy.

Carefull repair of the linea alba is recommended to avoid incisional hernias. Moreover, paraxiphoid extension of the sternotomy is believed to contribute to a lower incidence of incisional hernias.

2.3.4 Extended approaches

In case of tumors involving the cervicothoracic junction or huge mediastinal tumors more extensive surgical approaches may be required such as "trap-door" and "clamshell" incisions [9] or the transmanubrial approach (TMA) [10]. Since these approaches do not fall within the scope of this textbook, the readers' attention is drawn to the respective specialized literature. According to the authors experience the transmanubrial approach allows for excellent exposure the neurovascular structures of the cervicothoracic junction with minimial osteomuscular trauma.

Jens Dingemann, Benno Ure

2.4 Video-assisted thoracoscopic surgery (VATS): Development of the operative technique

2.4.1 Introduction

Utilization of thoracoscopy has been described as early as 1910. Jacobeus [11] used a cystoscope inserted through a rigid cannula to access the pleural cavity. In a patient with pulmonary tuberculosis, pleuropulmonary adhesiolysis was performed and complete lung collapse was achieved, representing the treatment of choice in these times. Only few years later (1921), the first patient series of more than 100 patients was published by the same author [11].

Over subsequent decades, the acceptance of thoracoscopy was limited and mainly diagnostic procedures were performed. The first thoracoscopic operations in children were described in the late 1970's. Due to the limited availability of equipment suitable for minimally-invasive procedures in children, the number of procedures was still very low and mainly biopsies of intrathoracic masses were performed.

Along with the advent of laparoscopy in adults and children from the early 1990's on, VATS developed as an emerging technique and was soon employed for more advanced diagnostic and therapeutic thoracic procedures. Today, improved optical devices, small instruments and sealing devices suitable for operating in confined spaces allow most sophisticated operations even in infants and newborns.

Why VATS?

The potential of improved cosmetic results, when compared to the corresponding open operation is a common advantage VATS shares with other minimally invasive approaches. The potential avoidance of rib fusion, scoliosis and chestwall deformity make the argument for VATS even more compelling. In a recent follow-up study investigating 62 infants, we have shown that the Manchester scar assessment scores and patient's satisfaction were in favour of VATS as compared to thoracotomy. Furthermore, chest asymmetry in the horizontal plane was significantly less frequent after VATS, the incidence of scoliosis was lower after VATS and the intercostal spaces of the operated hemithoraces were narrower after thoracotomy [12].

Additionally, the technical advantages of the thoracoscopic operation including excellent visualization due to the optic magnification and collapse of the lung from the pressure of insufflation are obvious. Since the operation is performed through small incisions, ranging from 3 to 5 mm, also less postoperative pain can be anticipated. Considering these potential advantages, it is not surprising that VATS procedures represent an evolving technique in the pediatric surgical community and its acceptance for various indications is widespread today.

2.4.2 Ventilatory and pathophysiological considerations for VATS

Depending on the type of procedure performed, ventilation strategies need to be tailored to the particular patient and close teamwork between surgeon and anesthetist is essential to create space for adequate visualization, exposure, and dissection while oxygenation is maintained.

Double-lung ventilation for VATS

We routinely use low-pressure (4 mmHg) and low-flow (1 L/min) CO_2-insufflation during the procedure to keep the lung compressed. To prevent CO_2-overinsufflation in small infants and children, the use of insufflators delivering CO_2 in small controlled puffs is advocated, as these allow a better adjustment of the intrathoracic pressure in neonates and infants. If adequate visualization is not achieved, the pressure and flow may be gradually increased to obtain adequate lung collapse. Pressures of up to 8 mm Hg can be tolerated without significant respiratory or hemodynamic consequences in most cases. Small tidal volumes, low peak pressures, and a high respiratory rate facilitate the compression of the lung through CO_2 insufflation alone. This technique is usually sufficient for smaller procedures such as lung biopsy or Nuss procedure or exploratory VATS.

Single-lung ventilation for VATS

For more delicate procedures such as lobectomy where any degree of inflation can make it difficult to identify pulmonary vessels and bronchi, it is helpful to employ single-lung ventilation. We are using age-adapted devices which are inserted by fiberoptic intubation. In children <6 years of age, a conventional single lumen endotracheal tube (SLET) is inserted into the main-stem bronchus of the dependent lung. In children aged 6 to 12 years, a Univent® tube is used and the attached bronchus blocker is blocked in the main-stem bronchus of the dependent lung. Children aged 12 years or older are intubated with either a Univent® tube, a double-lumen endotracheal tube, or an Arndt endobronchial blocker.

In a clinical setting, SLV and VATS are well tolerated even by neonates. However, we have recently demonstrated that single-lung ventilation combined with a capnothorax of 5 mmHg in piglets caused a significantly higher decrease of cardiac index in comparison with singe-lung ventilation alone. This decrease was due to deterioration of the cardiac preload. The intrathoracic carbon dioxide insufflation led also to a significantly higher arterial carbon dioxide partial pressure caused by carbon dioxide absorption [13]. In accordance, McHoney et al. found an increased endtidal carbon dioxide concentration in children undergoing thoracoscopy which was higher than during laparoscopy [14]. Changes were more pronounced in smaller children undergoing single-lung ventilation. These changes may aggravate the belowmentioned intraoperative hypercapnia and acidosis in newborns undergoing VATS CDH-repair [15, 16]. Thus, it has to be emphasized that SLV in combination with VATS needs an experienced anesthetic team and a close intraoperative communication between anesthetist and pediatric surgeon.

2.4.3 Equipment

Trocars

The instrumentation for VATS is basically not different from laparoscopy. We prefer 3- to 5-mm multiuse instrumentation. To introduce the instruments and the telescope, valved ports are recommendable as compared to simple non-valved trocars to maintain the positive intrathoracic CO_2 pressure which keeps the lung compressed. We use 3- to 5-mm multiuse ports and – if needed – a 12-mm single-use valved port to introduce the 11-mm endostapler. Trocar displacement remains a problem, especially in small infants. Various trocar fixation techniques have been introduced. We fix reusable unscrewed trocars to the thoracic wall using a 2 cm sleeve of a Red Robinson catheter (27 F catheter for 5-mm trocars and 24 F catheter for 3.5-mm trocars). A 2/0 suture is passed through the catheter, the skin and through the underlying fascia to inhibit dislocation (Fig. 2.4.1 and Fig. 2.4.2). The grip of the sleeve prevents trocar dislocation and allows the trocar to slide within the sleeve [17].

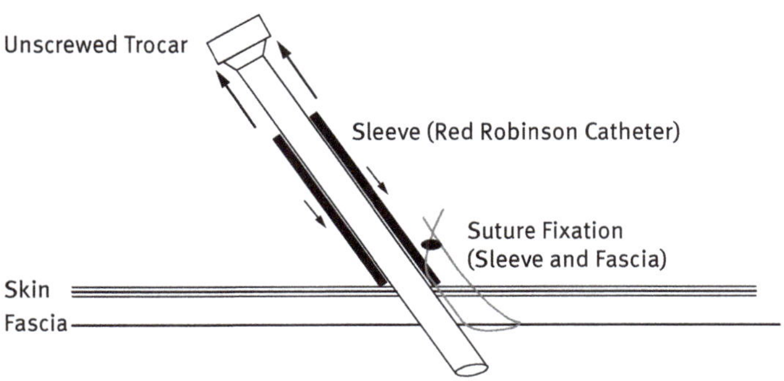

Fig. 2.4.1: Trocar fixation by a suture through the catheter sleeve, skin and fascia. The grip of the sleeve prevents trocar dislocation, and allows the trocar to slide within the sleeve. The trocar can easily be readjusted by pushing the sleeve toward the skin while gently pulling the trocar.

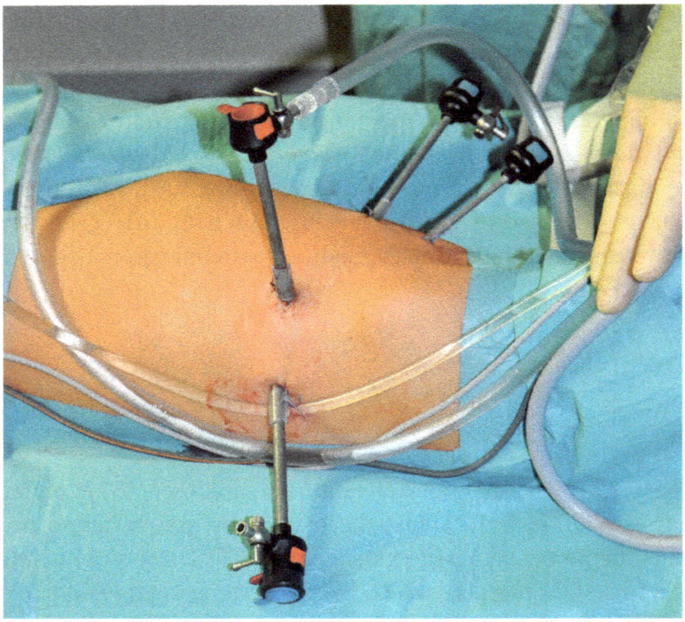

Fig. 2.4.2: Intraoperative image of trocar positioning in left lower lobectomy in a 5-year-old boy. 5-mm multiuse valved port (red valve) for introduction of the telescope below the tip of the scapula (fifth intercostal space) and three 3.5-mm multiuse valved ports (blue valves) for instrumentation. Note fascial fixation of sleeved port as described in Fig. 2.4.1.

Telescope

Our basic equipment includes 5-mm and 3.5-mm telescopes with 30° lenses. VATS procedures are best performed with a 30° lens, as the view in the confined intrathoracic spaces can be adjusted easily by the assistant surgeon. Short (16–18-cm) telescopes can be helpful to allow finer movements especially in newborns.

Instruments

Multiuse instrumentation should include 3- to 5-mm curved dissecting scissors and hooked scissors, monopolar dissecting hook, curved dissectors, atraumatic curved and straight clamps, exploratory probe, suction/irrigation tube and needle holder. In the small spaces of small children, the advantage of fan retractors is limited. Bowed and angled instruments can be helpful to advance the active range of motion within the thoracic cavity.

The basic instrumentation is completed by a variety of disposable instruments including hemostatic clips (we prefer non-absorbable "Hemolock®" clips), pretied ligatures ("Endoloop®") and endoscopic stapler. The endoscopic version of the GIA® represents an excellent tool to divide tissue and create an air- and watertight seal by laying down several rows of staples. We also use it routinely for atypical lung resection. It mostly comes as an 11-mm instrument (outer diameter) requiring a 12-mm single-use trocar, but 5-mm linear endostaplers have been developed most recently.

Various energy sources are available for dissection in pediatric VATS. We routinely use monopolar cautery and “Ligasure®” for dissection and vessel sealing. There are a multitude of other energy sources available on the market for the same purpose such as “Harmonic®” or “Ultrasonic®” shears, which may be helpful.

To secure hemostasis and sealing lung and pleural surfaces, different sealing and gluing materials are available. Fibrin sealant patches may be helpful. Certain products are available in pre-rolled forms which are suitable for a 5-mm trocar and can be inserted easily into the thoracic cavity of small children.

Insufflator, camera and screens

Not all products developed for minimally invasive surgery are suitable for pediatric VATS. The CO_2-insufflator needs to allow fine adjustment of pressure and flow between 2 and 12 mm Hg and 1–5 l/min, respectively. This is usually achieved through insufflation of CO_2 in small controlled puffs by special pediatric insufflators. The response time for the automatic pressure regulation needs to be short to prevent hemodynamic instability of the patient due to CO_2 overinsufflation. In small children, we usually establish the capnothorax with a pressure of up to 4 mmHg and a maximum flow of not more than 1 l/min. Both pressure and flow can be gradually turned up at a later stage of the operation.

High Definition cameras combined with a sufficient light source for a 5-mm telescope and wide screens (16:9) are standard equipment. It is generally advantageous to have two screens, one on either side of the table. The screens need to be movable and should be positioned somewhere between the shoulders and the hips of the patient, depending on the site of the lesion. The goal of laparoscopic surgery is true for pediatric VATS as well: the surgeon needs to work in line with the camera, the pathology and the monitor at the same time. The standard room setup for pediatric VATS is outlined in Fig. 2.4.3.

2.4.4 Positioning of the patient and trocar introduction

For most indications, a standard lateral decubitus position is preferred. We routinely place the patient on a vacuum mattress to secure the patient. The ipsilateral arm can be placed overhead in infants and newborns or hung in a sling in older children (Fig. 2.4.4). Depending on the site of the pathology, the standard positioning may be changed accordingly. A supine position with the affected side elevated 30° has proven to provide the best access to the anterior mediastinum, as the collapsed lung is retracted posteriorly by gravity. It may be used for anterior VATS procedures as thymectomy, aortopexy and anterior mediastinal masses. Access to the posterior mediastinum is

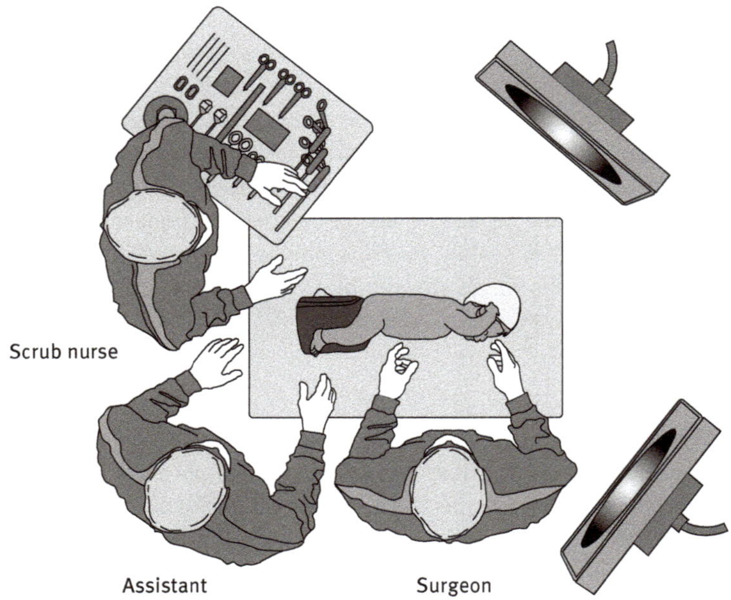

Fig. 2.4.3: Standard room setup for pediatric VATS.

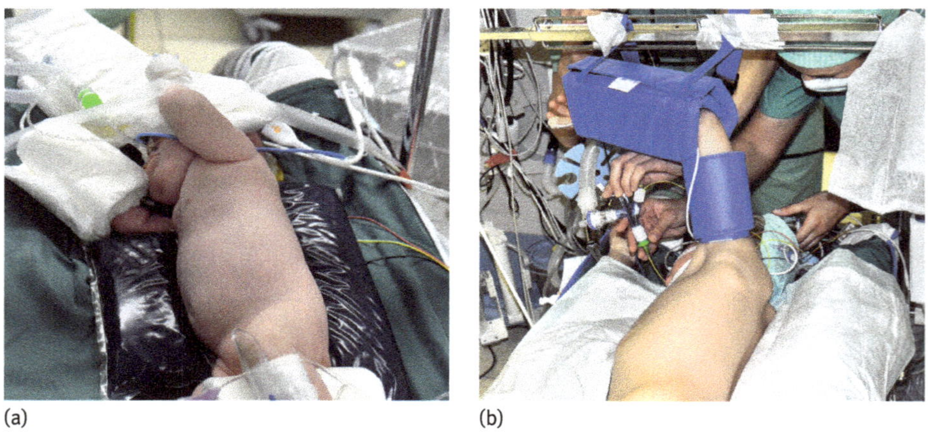

Fig. 2.4.4: Patients placed in standard lateral decubitus position for VATS with the arm overhead (a) and hung in a sling (b).

best provided in modified prone position with the affected side elevated up to 30°. This position is chosen for esophageal procedures, posterior bronchogenic cysts or foregut duplication cysts.

For introduction of the ports, an open approach is preferred. The skin is incised according to the diameter of the port and fascia and pleura are opened bluntly using a mosquito clamp. The first port is introduced blindly. In SLV, the risk of organ injury is low, as the lung is collapsed. In DLV, it is recommended to introduce the first port during a short respiratory arrest, established by the anesthesiologic team. The introduction of all further ports is safely performed under direct visualization.

No general recommendation can be given on the positioning of the ports, because the optimal arrangement varies considerably depending on the procedure performed. As compared to laparoscopy, it is even more important to plan the port placement thoughtfully. The chest wall is rigid and therefore the mobility of the instruments is certainly limited unlike in the abdomen. However, the general principles of minimally-invasive surgery are true for VATS as well. The port for the telescope is usually placed in the midaxillary line slightly above or below the pathology, dependent on the localization. The working ports are then placed somewhat closer to the pathology and with sufficient distance laterally to the camera port, so that interfering of instruments and camera is avoided. A triangular arrangement allows interchange of camera and instruments between the ports which can facilitate working in the area of interest from different directions.

Ports of 3 and 5 mm can be placed in any intercostal space in almost every position of the thoracic wall, even in neonates. In children older than 2 years, the 11-mm port required for the use of an endostapler should always be placed in the lowest costal interspace possible, as these are the widest.

For retrieval of resected tissue, a mini-thoracotomy is fashioned at one of the port sites. Even a resected lobe of a neonate may be retrieved through a 2–3-cm incision (Fig. 2.4.5). Another suitable port site can be used for insertion of a chest tube (Fig. 2.4.5).

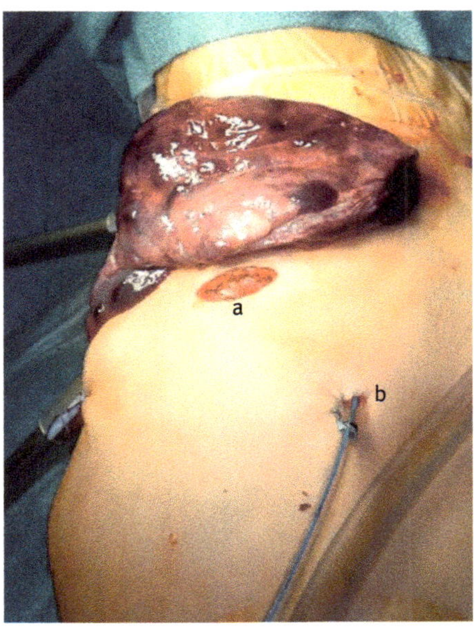

Fig. 2.4.5: Minithoracotomy for organ retrieval (a) and chest tube (b) at previous port sites.

2.4.5 Indications, pros and cons for pediatric VATS

Pediatric VATS has been applied for a considerable number of indications. It has become the gold standard for lung biopsy/pulmonary wedge resection, decortication of pleural empyema and thoracic sympathectomy for hyperhidrosis. However, also sophisticated VATS procedures, such as segmentectomy, lobectomy and resection of pulmonary sequestration are routinely performed today. VATS is also an excellent approach to the mediastinum. Biopsy and resection of mediastinal structures such as lymph nodes, thymic and thyroid structures, foregut duplication cysts, bronchogenic cysts and cystic hygromas have been performed. Besides, the thoracoscopic approach has been successfully used for repair of neonatal malformations as congenital diaphragmatic hernia, esophageal atresia/tracheoesophageal fistula and patent ductus arteriosus.

Overview of possible indications for pediatric VATS procedures in infants and children:
- Anterior spine fusion
- Aortopexy
- Bronchogenic Cyst excision
- Decortication
- Diaphragmatic hernia repair
- Diaphragmatic plication
- Esophageal atresia repair
- Tracheoesophageal fistula repair
- Esophageal resection
- Esophageal myotomy
- Foregut duplication cyst resection
- Lung biopsy/atypical lung resection
- Lobectomy
- Resection of pulmonary sequestration
- Mediastinal biopsy or mass excision
- Nuss procedure
- Patent ductus arteriosus ligation
- Pericardial window
- Pleurectomy
- Sympathectomy
- Thoracic duct ligation
- Tumor biopsy/resection
- Thymectomy

Author's experience/exemplary indications

For congenital pulmonary lesions, we have recently shown that the size of the pathology might imply useful information for decision-making on the use of VATS in infants. In a consecutive series of patients, the mean relative size of the pulmonary pathology at preoperative imaging was 0.34 in patients who received successful VATS, 0.57 in converted cases and 0.68 in infants who underwent primary thoracotomy. In our opinion, a lesion size of less than half of the thoracic diameter indicates a good feasibility for VATS resection [18].

The role of VATS for thoracic malignancies in children remains limited. The feasibility of VATS tumor biopsy is excellent with a success-rate of 93%. However, only 22% of thoracic tumors in our series were deemed suitable for VATS resection and only 14% could actually be resected via this approach (conversion rate 36%). The main reason for conversion from a VATS procedure to an open operation in this series was limited visibility [19].

VATS repair of esophageal atresia has been associated with a higher rate of anastomotic leak and recurrent fistula in some studies. We have recently published our series using distinct selection criteria for the VATS approach. Our concept for the indication for VATS EA repair included restriction to short-gap esophageal atresia, birthweight ≥ 2,000 g, cardiorespiratory stability, ≤ one major associated malformation and low threshold for conversion to thoracotomy (in cases of any intraoperative adverse events, lack of progress for 15 min or anastomosis under tension). Using this selective approach, we achieved excellent results and a low rate of complications [20].

Advantages of VATS over open surgery: What is evidence based?

We have recently reviewed the literature available for pediatric thoracoscopic procedures focussing on comparative studies investigating VATS versus open procedures and the classification of these publications according to the criteria of evidence based medicine [21]. Endpoints were defined as advantages and disadvantages of VATS as compared to the open procedure.

According to the recent classification of "Oxford Centre of Evidence Based Medicine" (CEBM), no studies of Level 1 or 2 were identified. Three meta-analyses (MA) and 18 retrospective comparative studies (RCS) investigating five different VATS procedures (repair of congenital diaphragmatic hernia (CDH), repair of oesophageal atresia/tracheoesophageal fistula (EA/TOF), lung resection, treatment of pneumothorax and resection of neuroblastoma) were included in the study. All studies were classified as CEBM Level 3. The advantages of VATS were less postoperative pain (CDH repair, OA/TOF repair and pneumothorax repair), shorter hospital stay (CDH repair, OA/TOF repair, lung resection and pneumothorax), shorter time of ventilation and lower pCO2 (CDH repair), shorter duration of chest drain (lung resection) and less blood loss (resection of neuroblastoma). However, disadvantages such as higher recurrence rates (CDH repair), higher pCO2 (OA/TOF repair), longer operative times (CDH and OA/TOF repair) were also identified (Tab. 2.4.1).

Tab. 2.4.1: Details of meta-analyses (CEBM Level 3a) and retrospective comparative studies (CEBM Level 3b) providing evidence for video-assisted thoracoscopic sugery (VATS) vs. open procedures in children (modified from [18]).

Procedure	CEBM Level	Advantage VATS (vs. open)	Disadvantage VATS (vs.open)
CDH repair	3a	None	– longer operative time – higher recurrence rate
	3b	– lower post OP pCO_2 – shorter ventilation – earlier return to feeds – shorter ventilation – less sedation/narcotics – less complications – less total costs	– longer operative time – higher recurrence rate
OA/TOF repair	3a	None	None
	3b	None	– longer operative time – higher intra OP pCO_2
Lung resection	3a	– shorter hospital stay – shorter duration of chest drain	None
	3b	– less regional anesthesia – shorter narcotic use – shorter hospital stay – shorter duration of chest drain – less complications	– longer operative time
Treatment of pneumothorax	3b	– shorter hospital stay – shorter narcotic use	None
Neuroblastoma resection	3b	– shorter hospital stay – less blood loss	None

What are possible downsides of VATS?

Particularly for thoracoscopic repair of congenital diaphragmatic hernia (CDH), worrying disadvantages of VATS compared to the open procedure have been reported. Higher recurrence rates were observed in a meta-analysis [22] and two recent retrospective series [23, 24]. This finding needs further investigation and more randomized controlled trials are urgently required in order to give a clear recommendation for or against VATS for CDH repair. Additionally, decreased cerebral hemoglobin oxygen saturation, increased intraoperative pCO_2 and acidosis were reported in a preliminary study investigating six patients undergoing VATS repair of CDH and esophageal atresia (EA)/tracheoesophageal fistula (TOF) [25]. In a most recently published pilot randomized controlled trial investigating 20 neonatal patients, the same authors clearly demonstrated that thoracoscopic repair of CDH is associated with prolonged and severe intraoperative hypercapnia and acidosis, compared with open surgery. These findings were not reproducible for VATS repair of EA/TOF [26]. Larger randomized controlled trials that compare open and VATS procedures are mandatory. In our center, all patients undergoing VATS procedures are thoroughly monitored for cerebral hemoglobin oxygen saturation and blood gas levels throughout the operation.

Nicolaus Schwerk

2.5 Bronchoscopy

2.5.1 Introduction

Pediatric bronchoscopy represents an established diagnostic and therapeutic technique in children and adolescents with congenital and acquired respiratory diseases. During the last few decades, improving technology has increased the versatility of diagnostic and therapeutic procedures. Especially the development of very small instruments has made the access of even very small airways possible, enabling examinations and interventions in neonates and even tiny preterm infants. In general, pediatric bronchoscopy entails two endoscopic techniques: rigid bronchoscopy and flexible bronchoscopy. Whereas the former is preferred for therapeutic interventions like foreign body removal and removal or biopsies of endobronchial tumors; the latter is preferred for diagnostic procedures. Nonetheless, flexible bronchoscopy has also been increasingly used for therapeutic procedures during the last few decades. Although severe complications are rare it has to be mentioned that bronchoscopy is an invasive procedure with potential harmful complications. Therefore, alternative less-invasive approaches must be considered, especially in critically ill children, before proceeding. Furthermore, an interdisciplinary team consisting of experienced anesthetists, pediatric pulmonologists, specialized nurses and also in some scenarios intensive care physicians, thoracic surgeons or ENT-surgeons may be required. The family and the child (when age appropriate) should be offered detailed information about the procedure; which should include discussing potential complications and obtaining written informed consent.

2.5.2 Bronchoscopes

There are several bronchoscopes available for different age groups [25]. The smallest neonatal 1.8-mm bronchoscopes have no suction channel and can only be used for the evaluation of airway abnormalities, mucus plugging, identifying functional abnormalities, the positioning of endobronchial occluders and establishing the correct position of endotracheal tubes (ETT). This can be challenging when endobronchial secretions hinder the view of the scope. The smallest bronchoscope with a working channel (1.2-mm diameter) has a distal external diameter of 2.8 mm. With such instruments, a diagnostic bronchoscopy including bronchoalveolar lavage, bronchial brushings and also endo- and transbronchial biopsies can be performed [26].

In general the smallest bronchoscope available should be used in children to avoid blockage of significant airways. Unsurprisingly this generalization does not apply when a biopsy is proposed. As the diagnostic quality of the sample depends on its size, it is wise to use the biggest biopsy forceps possible and hence utilize the biggest available instrument channel. Working channels with a diameter of 2 mm, optimal for biopsying, are available from bronchoscopes with a distal diameter of ≥4 mm. The smallest rigid bronchoscope has an outer diameter of 2.5 mm and can be used even in small neonatal patients. The biopsy forceps usable with small rigid bronchoscopes can potentially be much larger than those used with flexible bronchoscopes of the same sized working channel (e.g. 1.2 mm).

2.5.3 Sedation and anesthesia

In general bronchoscopy in children and adolescents should be performed under sedation or anesthesia. A detailed description of the different drugs used is beyond the scope of this chapter. Detailed information can be obtained from existing text books and specific guidelines [26, 27]. In some institutions, the investigating pulmonologist will not only be responsible for the sedation but also for monitoring the child during the procedure. This increases relative risks for the patient, including potentially fatal complications, and is therefore strongly not recommended. Hence optimally an experienced anesthetist together with a specialized nurse is always recommended even in spontaneous breathing children. Bronchoscopy can be performed either in spontaneous breathing patients with access to the airways via the nose, the mouth or a laryngeal mask, or in ventilated and intubated patients. A striking advantage of using access through the nose is the ability to explore the upper airways more extensively. This is especially important when the clinical presentation of a child is suggestive of supraglottic pathologies. Investigations in spontaneous breathing children are much more sensitive to detect functional abnormalities, like laryngo- or tracheomalacia. Whereas intubated children are protected from aspiration and can be ventilated in a more controlled setting. The choice of what sedation and which airway access is used will be dependent on the preference of the anesthetist, the indication for the bronchoscopy and the clinical status of the child. Rigid bronchoscopy should always be performed under general anesthesia and may also require relaxation of the patient.

2.5.4 Diagnostic procedures

Investigation of the airways

Flexible bronchoscopy allows the examination of the entire respiratory tract from the nose to the sub-segments of the bronchi, enabling the investigating pulmonologist to detect structural and/or functional pathologies [26]. Furthermore the extent of a lesion can be visualized, giving helpful information as to whether a special treatment is required, and if so, what treatment will be necessary. Bronchoscopy can also be useful during or before surgical procedures of the respiratory tract. In children with oesophageal atresia it can be helpful to exclude an additional proximal trachea-esophageal fistula (Fig. 2.5.1) before the child is intubated for the operation.

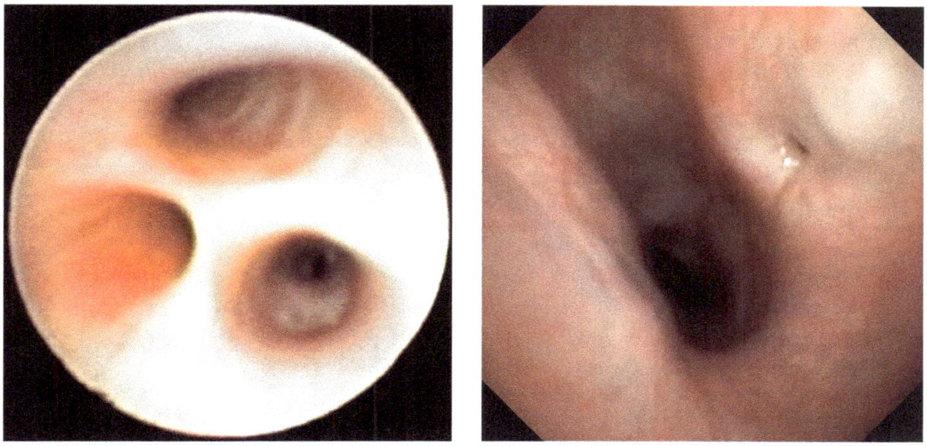

(a) (b)

Fig. 2.5.1: Bronchoscopic findings in a patient with esophageal atresia: (a) shows a tracheoesophageal fistula in the typical location proximal to the carina; and (b) shows an additional proximal fistula.

Furthermore, endoscopic placement and manipulation of a bronchial blocker is sometimes needed when a patient is too small for a double lumen tube and unilateral ventilation is required. During lung transplantation the anastomosis of the airways can be visualized to exclude distension or distortion before the pulmonary arteries and veins are anastomosed (Fig. 2.5.2).

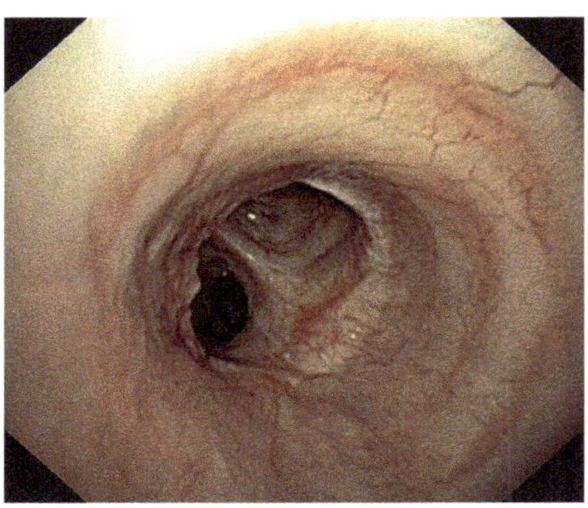

Fig. 2.5.2: Intraoperative view from the left main bronchus in a patient during lung transplantation showing an intact anastomosis with no relevant stenosis or dehiscence.

In Tab. 2.5.1 and 2.5.2 a list of different congenital or acquired airway abnormalities as well as functional pathologies is given. Congenital and acquired pathologies of the respiratory tract can look very similar. A subglottic stenosis for example can result from premature impaired development of the airways (online, Fig. 5) or a postnatal traumatic event (online, Fig. 11). It is therefore absolutely necessary to obtain detailed information regarding the child's complaints (e.g. beginning of symptoms, disease course, previous complaints, previous operations, etc.) and to perform a clinical examination prior to performing a diagnostic bronchoscopy to delineate the true diagnosis.

Tab. 2.5.1: Examples of congenital structural and functional anomalies of the airways.

Upper airways	Lower airways
Choanal atresia/hypoplasia	Subglottic stenosis (see online, Fig. 5)
Nasal masses	Subglottic hemangioma (see online, Fig. 6)
Congenital tumors of the upper airways	Tracheal stenosis
	Tracheo- and/or bronchomalacia (see online, Fig. 7b)
Pharyngeal collapse (see Fig. 2.5.1)	Laryngotracheo-esophageal cleft
Laryngomalacia (see online, Fig. 3)	Tracheobronchial branching anomalies (see online, Fig. 7a)
Laryngeal cleft	Tracheoesophageal fistula (see Fig. 2.5.1a+b)
Laryngeal cyst (see online, Fig. 4)	Bronchial agenesis, hypoplasia
Laryngeal web	Bronchial atresia
Laryngeal hypoplasia	Tracheobronchial hemangioma
Laryngeal atresia	Tracheal webs
vocal cord paralysis	Cartilaginous sleeves/esophageal remnants
	Congenital tracheal and/or bronchial tumors

Video showing laryngomalacia.
https://www.degruyter.com/view/supplement/9783110419825_Laryngomalacia.mp4

Video showing a subglottic hemangioma in a three month old infant.
https://www.degruyter.com/view/supplement/9783110419825_Subglottic_hemangioma.mp4

Video showing a congenital bronchial atresia of the lingula bronchus.
https://www.degruyter.com/view/supplement/9783110419825_Bronchial_atresia.mp4

Tab. 2.5.2: Examples of acquired structural and functional anomalies of the airways.

Upper airways	**Lower airways**
Foreign bodies (see Fig. 2.5.3)	Subglottic cysts
Nasal masses	Subglottic edema
Tumors	Subglottic stenosis, post-intubation stricture, granuloma (see Fig. 2.5.4)
Wegner granulomatosis	Bacterial/fungal tracheitis (see online, Fig. 12)
Adenoid/tonsillar hypertrophy	Secretion/mucous plugging
Pharyngeal and/or laryngeal edema (see online, Fig. 9)	Tumors (see online, Fig. 13)
Laryngeal papillomatosis (see online, Fig. 10)	Foreign bodies (see Fig. 2.5.5)
Vocal cord paralysis	Tracheobronchial malacia related to extra-luminal compression (see Fig. 2.5.6)
Vocal cord dysfunction	Follicular Bronchitis/Bronchiolitis
Laryngeal web (after intubation)	Tuberculosis
	Histoplasmosis
	Wegner granulomatosis
	Crohn's disease
	Sarcoidosis
	Stenosis insufficiency of brochial anastomosis (see online, Fig. 16)
	Endobronchial hemorrhage (see online, Fig. 17)
	Plastic bronchitis (see online, Fig. 18)
	Traumatic tracheal or bronchial perforation

Video showing laryngeal papillomatosis.
https://www.degruyter.com/view/supplement/9783110419825_Laryngeal_papillomatosis.mp4

Video showing severe invasive aspergillosis in a child after bone marrow transplantation.
https://www.degruyter.com/view/supplement/9783110419825_Invasive_aspergillosis.mp4

Video showing accumulation of bronchial secret in a child with primary ciliary dyskinesia and protracted bacterial infection.
https://www.degruyter.com/view/supplement/9783110419825_Protracted_bacterial_bronchitis.mp4

Video showing follicular bronchitis in a 4 years old boy with a common variable immunodeficiency.
https://www.degruyter.com/view/supplement/9783110419825_Follicular_bronchitis.mp4

Video showing tracheomalacia related to a dilated esophagus in a child with achalasia.
https://www.degruyter.com/view/supplement/9783110419825_Secondary_tracheomalacia_and_achalasia.mp4

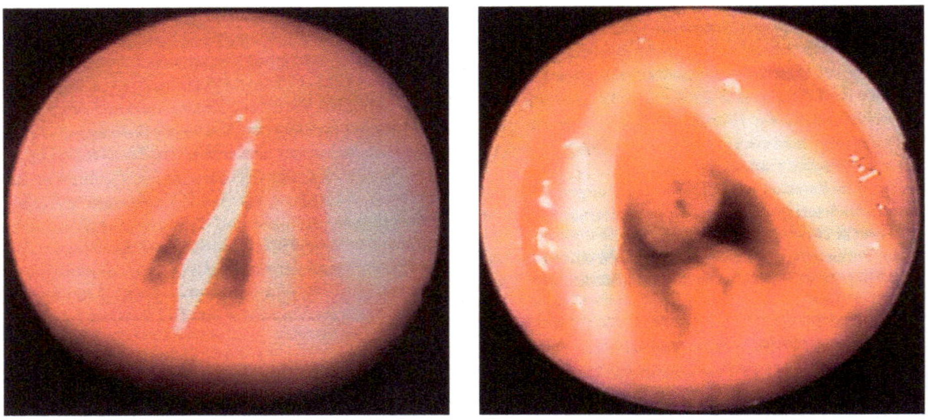

(a) (b)

Fig. 2.5.3: (a) Endoscopic view of the larynx showing the vocal cords (right and left) and a foreign body (in the middle). (b) same patient after removal of the foreign body with subglottic granulation tissue. The patient was referred with persistent cough and intermittent inspiratory stridor since 9 months of age.

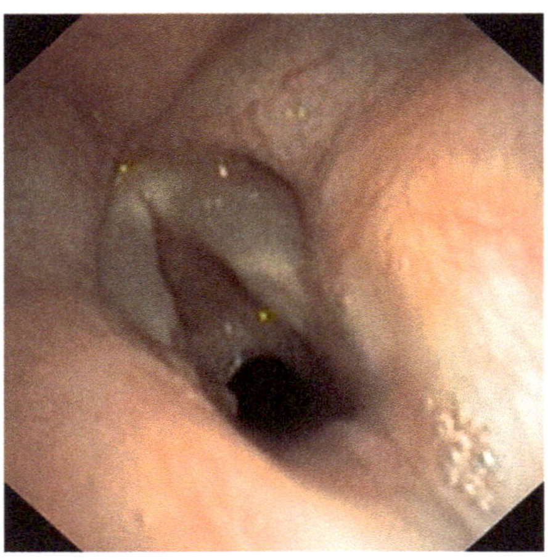

Fig. 2.5.4: Subglottic stenosis with a web-like appearance in a patient after protracted intubation and ventilation.

Video showing subglottic membranous stenosis after intubation.
https://www.degruyter.com/view/supplement/9783110419825_Subglottic_membranous_stenosis.mp4

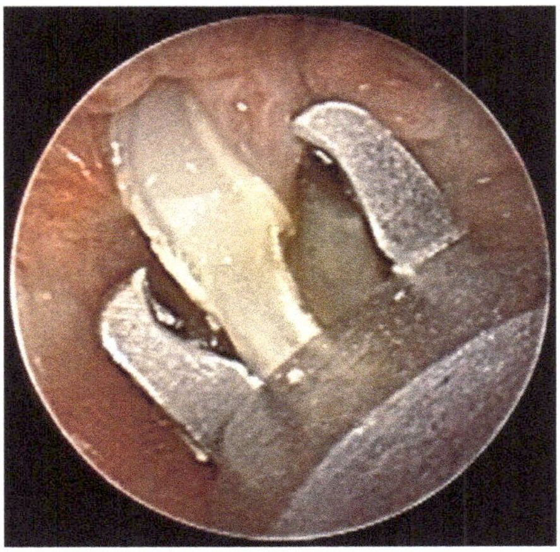

Fig. 2.5.5: Foreign body removal (aspirated tooth) from the right main bronchus. Of note is the extensive granulation tissue.

Video showing the removal of a foreign body (peanut) located in the right main bronchus.
https://www.degruyter.com/view/supplement/9783110419825_Removal_foreign_body.mp4

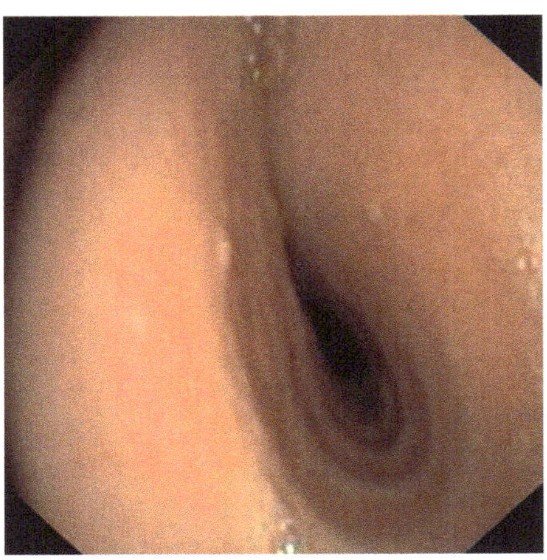

Fig. 2.5.6: Severe tracheomalacia in a 15-year-old boy with achalasia related to tracheal compression by a massive dilated esophagus.

Bronchoalveolar lavage (BAL)

Besides the visual evaluation of the respiratory tract, brochoalveolar lavage (BAL) is a very important diagnostic procedure used to recover cellular and non-cellular components from the bronchial and alveolar air spaces [28]. The cellular composition of BAL fluid (BALF) gives information not only regarding the microbial constituents of the lower airways, but also whether there is an inflammatory process involved. The differentiation of cellular components (e.g. neutrophilic granulocytes, lymphocytes, eosinophilic granulocytes) can give important hints for underlying diseases. In children with chronic wet cough, the detection of bacteria in significant amounts (which is normally defined as 100,000 colony-forming units per ml) together with a neutrophilic inflammation is diagnostic of a protracted bacterial bronchitis. An eosinophilic inflammation can be suggestive of asthma, allergic bronchopulmonary aspergillosis, Churg Strauss Syndrome or helminthic infections. In a patient with cystic lung lesions, CD1a positive cells are diagnostic for a pulmonary Langerhans cell histiocytosis, a diagnosis which otherwise can only be proven by lung biopsy. The detection of lipid laden macrophages is very sensitive but not specific for recurrent aspirations. Hemosiderin-laden macrophages are suggestive of pulmonary hemosiderosis. Also the analysis of non-cellular components is of great diagnostic importance, for example a BALF with milky appearance of increasing intensity in each fraction and with positive PAS staining is typical of alveolar proteinosis (online, Fig. 20b). As the middle lobe and the lingua are the smallest lobes of each lung, they provide superior fluid recovery and hence are the preferred sites for BAL. When a pathological process is presumed to be in a particular part of the lung, BAL should naturally be performed near that site. Usually three aliquots of pre-warmed (37°C) saline, each consisting of 1 ml/kg body weight (for children weighing up to 20 kg), or three 20-ml aliquots (for children weighing >20 kg) are used. Table 2.5.3 lists variables which routinely should be measured in BAL and provides information about specific diagnostic tests.

Tab. 2.5.3: Routine and optional variables measured in BALF.

Routine	**Comments**
Recovery	Acceptable quality if recovery is >40%
Numbers of cells per ml	Not performed in all centers. Normal range: 10–60 × 104/ml
Differential cell count	Macrophages, granulocytes, lymphocytes. Contamination with epithelial cells is an indicator of a poor quality BAL
Microbiological studies	Samples must be processed as soon as possible to avoid contamination
Hemosiderin staining	Hemosiderin-laden macrophages are suggestive of but not conclusive for alveolar hemorrhage
Lipid staining (e.g. Sudan)	Lipid-laden macrophages are suggestive of but not conclusive of aspiration

Tab. 2.5.3 (continued)

Routine	Comments
Periodic-acid-Schiff-staining (PAS)	PAS-positive non-cellular material is suggestive of but not conclusive of pulmonary alveolar proteinosis (e.g. may also be positive in glycogen storage diseases)
Optional	
Virological examinations	In some centers also used in routine diagnostics
Lymphocyte subsets	CD4/CD8-ratios when hypersensitivity pneumonitis or sarcoidosis is suspected (in children it is neither specific nor sensitive). More than 5% CD1a positive cells are diagnostic of Langerhans cell histiocytosis
Surfactant analysis	When inherited surfactant protein deficiencies (e.g. SPB-, SPC-, ABCA3-mutations) or other pulmonary alveolar proteinosis are suspected
Ziehl-Neelsen stain	When tuberculosis is suspected

Biopsies

There are two different bronchoscopic biopsy techniques which can be performed: endobronchial biopsy (EBB) and transbronchial biopsy (TBB). The rationale for EBB is to collect histological samples, typically with forceps under direct visualization, from the bronchial mucosa, masses invading the bronchial wall or masses present in the bronchial lumen (Fig 2.5.7).

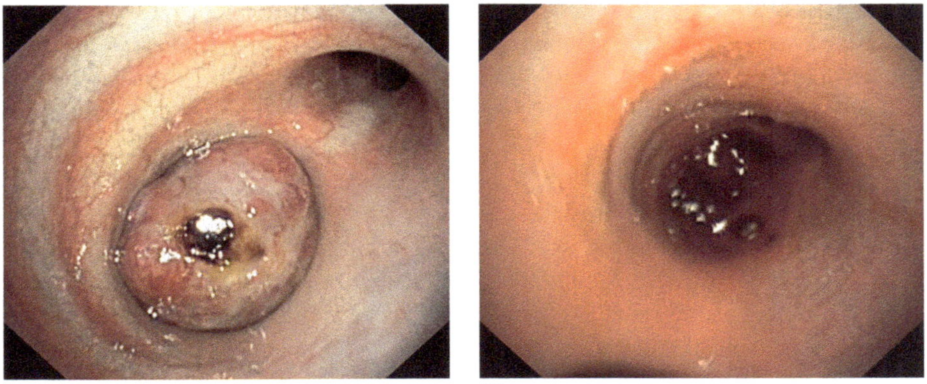

(a) (b)

Fig. 2.5.7: (a) Bronchoscopic view of a tumor in the right bronchus intermedius. (b) same patient after endoscopic biopsy with moderate bleedings. Histology revealed a typical carcinoid. The tumor as well as the middle lobe was resected, with creation of end to end anastomoses of the right main bronchus and the distal bronchus intermedius.

Video showing a biopsy of a endobronchial carcinoid.
https://www.degruyter.com/view/supplement/9783110419825_Biopsy_endobronchial_carcinoid.mp4

EBB can be performed with either a flexible or rigid bronchoscopic technique. An advantage of the rigid technique is that the tissue samples obtained can be bigger because the biopsy forceps used may be larger than those used with flexible bronchoscopes, especially in children. EBB is relatively safe with the main complications being endobronchial bleeding and in very rare cases, bronchial perforations [29]. Except for diagnostic biopsies from intraluminal masses or tumors, there is no convincing data supporting the clinical use of EBB in children. TBB are taken from the periphery of the lung, typically only from one side to avoid bilateral pneumothorax. In contrast to EBB, TBB is used to obtain peripheral lung tissue, including from broncheoli and alveoli, to look for pathologic processes of the terminal bronchial system and the interstitium. Usually TBB is performed under fluoroscopic guidance. A minimum of three (better five) samples of good quality from different lobes has to be obtained. A simple test for the quality of the probe is the "swimming test". When the biopsy pieces are "swimming" in formalin-or saline solution and do not sink to the bottom, it is very likely that air filled alveoli have been obtained. As the samples are very small, their diagnostic value tends to be limited. Therefore TBB is only routinely performed in lung transplanted children, either for surveillance investigations or when an acute cellular or humoral rejection is suspected. In children with suspected interstitial lung disease surgical biopsy, preferably with a minimally invasive technique, is strongly recommended.

The most common serious complications following TBB are bleeding and pneumothorax. Clinical significant bleedings have been reported in up to 6% of cases. Pneumothorax has been reported in up to 12%, but more often ranges between 1–3% of cases [30].

Foreign body aspiration/Interventional bronchoscopy

The main indication for interventional bronchoscopy in pediatric patients is the removal of aspirated foreign bodies (online, Fig. 16). Foreign body (FB) aspiration can cause acute respiratory distress in children and, if overlooked for a longer period, can lead to irreversible damage of the bronchi and/or lung parenchyma due to chronic inflammation and secondary infection. Therefore, early diagnosis and prompt extraction is very important. Although toddlers and preschool children are most affected, FB aspiration has to be considered in children of all age groups in case of any suggestive history or clinical findings. Boys are more affected than girls. Aspirated foreign bodies are more often logged in the right main or lower lobe bronchus then in the left main or lower lobe bronchus. When a FB-aspiration is directly observed by parents or caregivers diagnosis is quiet easy and further diagnostics like a chest X-ray are not necessary. In such cases bronchoscopy is strongly recommended even if the patient is symptom free and the physical examination does not reveal any pathological findings. Nevertheless, it has to be mentioned that about 30%–60% of all aspirations occur in unobserved moments thus making diagnosis more difficult in these cases. Information like a sudden evolving and persistent cough without evidence for infection, recurrent pneumonias at the same location or a persistent (unilateral) bronchial obstruction in a previously healthy child can then be very helpful. Clinical symptoms vary and depend on the size of the aspirated FB, its location in the airways and the time the FB remained in the bronchial system. Symptoms vary from complete obstruction with hypoxia and cardiorespiratory compromise to partial obstruction with coughing, wheezing, drooling, stridor and respiratory distress. FB located in the lower airway lead to pulmonary changes dependent on the type of impaction, including emphysema, collapse and consolidation of the bronchopulmonary segment which can be seen in chest X-ray. However in some circumstances chest X-ray can be normal. In these cases an additional expiratory scan can possibly be helpful. If the aspirated FB leads to a relevant impaction, a hyperinflation of the distal bronchopulmonary segments with consecutive mediastinal shift to the contralateral side can then be observed. Of note, a normal chest X-ray never rules out a FB aspiration. Therefore a bronchoscopy is always indicated in every patient with a typical history and/or a suggestive clinical presentation. Every FB-aspiration is an emergency and has to be treated urgently. Even if the child is in a stable condition, sudden occlusion of the airways in case of positional change of the aspirated foreign body can lead to life-threatening situations. Furthermore, formation of reactive granulation tissue can be very early and potentially lead to relevant complications during extraction. Flexible bronchoscopy has a diagnostic accuracy of near to 100% but a very limited therapeutic role. Therefore rigid bronchoscopy under general anesthesia is currently the gold standard treatment for aspirated FB. Complications for rigid bronchoscopy for aspirated FB aspiration are rare but potentially harmful; they include pneumothorax, laceration of the trachea and or bronchi, pneumomediastinum, edema of the mucus membrane, bleedings and severe respiratory failure. FB extraction should therefore only be performed by, or under the supervision of, medical staff experienced in the procedure.

Further Indications for interventional bronchoscopy in children primarily involve the restoration of airway patency. While the majority of such applications involve the use of a rigid bronchoscope, considerable therapeutic benefit can often be achieved with flexible instruments. Besides the removal of aspirated foreign bodies the removal of mucus plugs in children with atelectasis is a frequently indication. This goes often hand in hand with diagnostic bronchoscopy, as persistent atelectasis, especially of the middle lobe, is frequently caused by protracted bacterial infections and/or structural anomalies of the respiratory tract (e.g. bronchomalacia or airway stenosis). Due to ongoing technological improvements with increasingly more specialized equipment becoming available, there have been numerous interventional procedures devised in the last few decades. The number of these potential interventions continues to rise every year, but essentially is restricted to specialized centers and requires experienced, specially trained multidisciplinary teams to implement (Tab. 2.5.4).

Tab. 2.5.4: Indications for interventional bronchoscopy.

Endoscopic guided ETT placement
Endoscopic hemostasis in pulmonary hemorrhage
Removal of pseudomembranes obstructing the airways
Removal of bronchial casts (Fig. 18)
Dilatation of congenital or acquired airway stenosis
Stenting of malacic or compressed airways (Fig. 7c)
Resection or size reduction of intraluminal tumors of the respiratory tract (Fig. 13b)
Intralesional drug injection (e.g. larynx papillomatosis)
Whole lung lavage in patients with pulmonary alveolar proteinosis (Fig. 19)
Endobronchial laser therapy (e.g. webs, bulky granulomas, cysts, tuberculosis, hemangiomas)
Endoscopic bronchial occlusion

Hartmut Grasemann, Pierre Goussard

Comment

With great interest we read the excellent chapter "Bronchoscopy" by Dr. Nicolaus Schwerk. As nicely eluded to by the author, indications for bronchoscopy in children include diagnostic, therapeutic and interventional procedures as well as monitoring of disease. In general, bronchoscopy is associated with low morbidity and mortality if done under the necessary precautionary. With the availability of equipment that can be passed through the working channel of flexible scopes (e.g. grasping forceps, retrieval baskets and Wang transbronchial aspiration needles), more options for the use of flexible bronchoscopy in children are becoming available. These include removal of foreign bodies from the airways, which used to be an indication for rigid bronchoscopy only.

Video showing the removal of a foreign body using bronchoscopy.
https://www.degruyter.com/view/supplement/9783110419825_Bronchoscopy_2.mp4

Video showing the removal of a foreign body using bronchoscopy.
https://www.degruyter.com/view/supplement/9783110419825_Bronchoscopy_3.mp4

Ideally, interventional bronchoscopists should be trained in both rigid and flexible bronchoscopy as it may be necessary during a procedure to change from one method to the other. Video recording and archiving of bronchoscopy findings will allow for subsequent evaluations and comparison to findings on previous or future procedures.

The equipment needed to perform bronchoscopies including scopes of various sizes for the use in different age groups and multiple indications, proper maintenance of the damageable equipment, disinfection, as well as appropriate processing of obtained biopsy or lavage specimen samples is costly, which may limit the use in certain endemic geographic regions despite its potential benefits. For example, a recent study from South Africa suggested a potential role of flexible bronchoscopy for the rapid confirmation of suspected pulmonary tuberculosis in children, using nucleic acid amplification tests such as GeneXpert (Xpert) on bronchoalveolar lavage (BAL) samples [3]). Endobronchial biopsies (EBB) may be useful in children with bronchial involvement due to tuberculosis. EBB also can be diagnostic for Kaposi sarcoma in HIV-infected children. Similarly, in addition to CD4/CD8 counts in BAL fluid, in HIV-positive children too sick for an open lung biopsy, transbronchial biopsies (TBB) can be useful in the diagnosis of lymphocytic interstitial pneumonia (LIP), as well as in suspected pulmonary alveolar proteinosis (PAP).

One growing area in the use of flexible bronchoscopy is endobronchial ultrasound (EBUS) and transbronchial needle aspiration (TBNA). TBNA can be used in endoscopic lymph node decompression in children with life-threatening airway obstruction due to enlarge lymphnodes, which have herniated into the airway [32]. TBNA is also very helpful in making a tissue-based diagnosis in children with enlarged mediastinal lymph nodes. Sub-carinal lymph nodes can be biopsied without ultrasound guidance. This has been shown to be very effective and also safe, even in children less than 1 year of age [33]. TBNA can be done through the 2-mm working channel of a flexible scope (outer diameter as small as 4.0 mm). Onsite cytology can help differentiate tuberculosis and malignancies this way. Withd the smallest available ultrasonic bronchoscope size of 6.9-mm diameter, EBUS use is currently limited to older children.

Steve Cunningham

Comment

Modern bronchoscopy in children elucidates clinical problems and informs patient management safely and effectively. Schwerk's chapter demonstrates how this can be achieved. Principle within this chapter is the importance of dynamic direct visual assessment of the airway in understanding patient pathophysiology. Multidisciplinary interaction (pulmonology, thoracic, ENT, etc) during bronchoscopic evaluations can support integrated effective patient care management plans and common understanding between clinical teams.

Such interaction and understanding is important as different airway visualization techniques provide very different perspectives. What might appear to be normal airway dynamics to a rigid bronchoscopist may not appear normal to a flexible bronchoscopist and vice versa. In terms of approach, the most obvious differences that would be seen is the spontaneous breathing versus assisted breathing in a paralysed child, but even in spontaneously breathing child the airway dynamic effects of different approaches require to be appreciated: Suspended laryngoscopy may support the airway in an unphysiological manner; mask nasal approach is more physiological but the bronchoscope may enhance airway resistance (especially larger bronchoscopes) increasing traction malacia; laryngeal mask may distort the larynx and tracheal wall if poorly placed; endotracheal tube may inadvertently mask tracheomalacia by supporting the tracheal wall. It should be remembered too that the airway is subject to multiple progressive points of resistance – reduction of one or more proximal points of resistance (by for example an endotracheal tube) could reduce resistance in the lower airway on an area of bronchomalacia that has been particularly troublesome, leading to an under appreciation of the true problem. Collaborative working and an appreciation of different approaches can help minimize interdisciplinary differences in airway assessments in the same child.

One of the most common reasons for airway assessment in a young child is to assess a noise (stridor, wheeze, etc) emanating from the chest. Most important in this assessment is to “see” the noise. Visualization may require a range of diagnostic approaches under the same anesthetic with differing levels of anesthesia, but visualization should be the principle aim of any such investigation.

Experiential, collaborative working and adequate preparation of the patient to achieve the aims of a bronchoscopic procedure provide excellent patient care and support effective management planning. Schwerk’s chapter provides the structure for this and should be understood by all who would wish to care for children who require airway investigation and diagnostics.

Jaques De Blic

Comment

Since Gustav Killian who performed the first exploration with a rigid bronchoscope in 1897 and Chevalier Jackson who performed the first foreign body extraction with rigid bronchoscopy in 1905, bronchoscopy in children has become an inescapable tool in the evaluation of respiratory problems in children.

This chapter dedicated to pediatric bronchoscopy explores the differents aspects of the procedure. Some of them should be pointed out in particular. Kind of bronchoscopes (rigid or flexible) and size of the instrument need to be carefully chosen according to the weight and respiratory status of the child, the pathology to be explored and the procedure to be done. Flexible bronchoscopes are probably better for anatomical exploration, biopsies and bronchoalveolar lavage and rigid bronchoscopy for foreign body extraction and some other interventional procedures. However the use of basket forceps may avoid a rigid bronchoscopy [34] while exploration of the posterior membrane of the trachea and the search of a esotracheal fistula is probably best explored with rigid bronchoscope. Sedation is an important point that is underlined in this chapter. If there is no doubt whether rigid bronchoscopy should be performed under general anesthesia (ie deep sedation), flexible bronchoscopy may be done under conscious sedation or general anesthesia. The technique used depends on many factors including respiratory status, psychological and emotional status of the patient as well as underlying disease, type of procedure to be performed, drugs available and availability of anesthetist.

A detailed systematic inspection of the airways is the first step of the examination. Large series show that the most frequent indications for endoscopy are recurrent bronchopneumonia, persistent or recurrent pneumonia or atelectasis, severe recurrent or persistent wheezing [35]. In all these situations bronchoscopy is performed in search for an obstacle on the airways. The frequency of congenital and acquired abnomalities of the upper or lower airways is higher in children than in adults.

A special paragraph in this chapter is dedicated to bronchoalveolar lavage (BAL). BAL is probably the most common procedure performed during the bronchoscopy. The values of BAL in immunocompetent children are well detailed in this paragraph. Cytological analysis and staining are important when chronic interstitial pneumonitis is suspected. The other value of BAL is the detection of an infectious agent in the immunocompromized children, and it may be difficult to distinguish if the recovered agent such as cytomegalovirus or aspergillus fumigatus is responsible for the respiratory symptoms or just resident in the airways.

Except for foreign body extraction, bronchoscopy in children is still not popular among physicians out of hospital centers. This chapter should be read by all physicians in charge of children with respiratory diseases.

2.6 Further reading

[1] Li S1, Feng Z1, Wu L1, Huang Q1, Pan S2, Tang X3, Ma B4. Analysis of 11 trials comparing muscle-sparing with posterolateral thoracotomy. Thorac Cardiovasc Surg 2014 Jun;62(4):344–52.

[2] Rothenberg SS1, Pokorny WJ. Experience with a total muscle-sparing approach for thoracotomies in neonates, infants, and children. J Pediatr Surg 1992 Aug;27(8):1157–9; discussion 1159–60.

[3] Bleiziffer S, Schreiber C, Burgkart R, Regenfelder F, Kostolny M, Libera P, Holper K, Lange R. The influence of right anterolateral thoracotomy in prepubescent female patients on late breast development and on the incidence of scoliosis. J Thorac Cardiovasc Surg 2004 May;127(5):1474–80.

[4] Benedetti F1, Vighetti S, Ricco C, Amanzio M, Bergamasco L, Casadio C, Cianci R, Giobbe R, Oliaro A, Bergamasco B, Maggi G. Neurophysiologic assessment of nerve impairment in posterolateral and muscle-sparing thoracotomy. J Thorac Cardiovasc Surg 1998 Apr;115(4):841–7.

[5] Cherup LL, Siewers RD, Futrell JW. Breast and pectoral muscle maldevelopment after antero-lateral and posterolateral thoracotomies in children. Ann Thorac Surg 1986 May;41(5):492–7.
[6] Taguchi T1, Nagata K, Kinoshita Y, Ieiri S, Tajiri T, Teshiba R, Esumi G, Karashima Y, Hoka S, Masumoto K. The utility of muscle sparing axillar skin crease incision for pediatric thoracic surgery. Pediatr Surg Int 2012 Mar;28(3):239–44.
[7] Rostron A1, Dunning J. Does deflating the lungs and sawing from the xiphisternum reduce the chance of accidental pleurotomy during sternotomy? Interact Cardiovasc Thorac Surg 2005 Jun;4(3):272–4.
[8] Bigdelian H1, Sedighi M2. Evaluation of sternal closure with absorbable polydioxanone sutures in children. J Cardiovasc Thorac Res 2014;6(1):57–9.
[9] Christison-Lagay ER1, Darcy DG1, Stanelle EJ1, Dasilva S1, Avila E2, La Quaglia MP3. Trap-door" and "clamshell" surgical approaches for the management of pediatric tumors of the cervicothoracic junction and mediastinum. J Pediatr Surg 2014 Jan;49(1):172–6; discussion 176–7.
[10] Pimpalwar AP1, Kroeker TR, Ramachandran V. Cervicothoracic neuroblastoma arising from the stellate ganglion in children: the use of muscle and bone sparing transmanubrial transcostal approach. J Pediatr Surg 2008 Mar;43(3):E31–4.
[11] Jacobeus HC. The practical importance of thoracoscopy in surgery of the chest. Surg Gynecol Obstet 1921;4:289–96.
[12] Lawal TA, Gosemann JH, Kuebler JF, Glüer S, Ure BM. Thoracoscopy versus thoracotomy improves midterm musculoskeletal status and cosmesis in infants and children. Ann Thorac Surg 2009;87(1):224–8.
[13] Witt L, Osthaus WA, Schröder T, Teich N, Dingemann C, Kübler J, Böthig D, Sümpelmann R. Single-lung ventilation with carbon dioxide hemipneumothorax: hemodynamic and respiratory effects in piglets. Paediatr Anaesth 2012 Aug;22(8):793–8.
[14] McHoney M, Mackinlay G, Munro F, Capek A, Aldridge L. Effect of patient weight and anesthetic technique on CO2 excretion during thoracoscopy in children assessed by end-tidal CO2. J Laparoendosc Adv Surg Tech A 2008 Feb;18(1):147–51.
[15] Bishay M, Giacomello L, Retrosi G, et al. Decreased cerebral oxygen saturation during thoracoscopic repair of congenital diaphragmatic hernia and esophageal atresia in infants. J Pediatr Surg 2011;46(1):47–51.
[16] Bishay M, Giacomello L, Retrosi G, Thyoka M, Garriboli M, Brierley J, Harding L, Scuplak S, Cross KM, Curry JI, Kiely EM, De Coppi P, Eaton S, Pierro A. Hypercapnia and acidosis during open and thoracoscopic repair of congenital diaphragmatic hernia and esophageal atresia: results of a pilot randomized controlled trial. Ann Surg 2013 Dec;258(6):895–900.
[17] Metzelder ML, Ure BM. Fascial fixation of sleeved trocar prevents trocar dislocation and allows adjustment in pediatric laparoscopy. J Laparoendosc Adv Surg Tech A 2007 Apr;17(2):276.
[18] Reismann M, Gossner J, Glueer S, Schwerk N, Ure BM, Metzelder ML. Thoracoscopic resection of congenital pulmonary malformations in infants: is the feasibility related to the size of the lesion? World J Pediatr 2012 Aug;8(3):272–4.
[19] Metzelder ML, Kuebler JF, Shimotakahara A, Glueer S, Grigull L, Ure BM. Role of diagnostic and ablative minimally invasive surgery for pediatric malignancies. Cancer 2007 Jun 1;109(11):2343–8.
[20] Dingemann C, Zoeller C, Ure B. Thoracoscopic repair of oesophageal atresia: results of a selective approach. Eur J Pediatr Surg 2013 Feb;23(1):14–8.
[21] Dingemann C, Ure B, Dingemann J. Thoracoscopic procedures in pediatric surgery: what is the evidence? Eur J Pediatr Surg 2014 Feb;24(1):14–9.
[22] Lansdale N, Alam S, Losty PD, Jesudason EC. Neonatal endosurgical congenital diaphragmatic hernia repair: a systematic review and meta-analysis. Ann Surg 2010 Jul;252(1):20–6. doi:10.1097/SLA.0b013e3181dca0e8.

[23] Tsao K, Lally PA, Lally KP. Congenital Diaphragmatic Hernia Study Group. Minimally invasive repair of congenital diaphragmatic hernia. J Pediatr Surg 2011 Jun;46(6):1158–64. doi: 10.1016/j.jpedsurg.2011.03.050.
[24] Gander JW, Fisher JC, Gross ER, et al. Early recurrence of congenital diaphragmatic hernia is higher after thoracoscopic than open repair: a single institutional study. J Pediatr Surg 2011 Jul;46(7):1303–8. doi: 10.1016/j.jpedsurg.2010.11.048.
[25] Balfour-Lynn IM, Harcourt J. Bronchoscopic Equipment. In: Priftis KN, Anthracopoulos MB, Eber E, Koumbourlis AC, Wood RE., ed. Progress in Respiratory Research, Vol. 38, Paediatric Bronchoscopy. Karger 2010:12–21.
[26] Midulla F, de Blic J, Barbato A, Bush A, Eber E, Kotecha S, Haxby E, Moretti C, Pohunek P, Ratjen F; ERS Task Force. Flexible endoscopy of paediatric airways. Eur Respir J. 2003 Oct;22(4):698–708.
[27] De Blic J, Telion C. Sedation and anasthesia for bronchoscopy. In: Priftis KN, Anthracopoulos MB, Eber E, Koumbourlis AC, Wood RE., ed. Progress in Respiratory Research, Vol. 38, Paediatric Bronchoscopy. Karger 2010:22–29.
[28] de Blic J, Midulla F, Barbato A, Clement A, Dab I, Eber E, Green C, Grigg J, Kotecha S, Kurland G, Pohunek P, Ratjen F, Rossi G. Bronchoalveolar lavage in children. ERS Task Force on bronchoalveolar lavage in children. European Respiratory Society. Eur Respir J. 2000 Jan;15(1):217–31.
[29] Salva PS, Theroux C, Schwartz D. Safety of endobronchial biopsy in 170 children with chronic respiratory symptoms. Thorax. 2003 Dec;58(12):1058–60.
[30] Colin AA, Waltz DA. Special procedures. In: Priftis KN, Anthracopoulos MB, Eber E, Koumbourlis AC, Wood RE., ed. Progress in Respiratory Research, Vol. 38, Paediatric Bronchoscopy. Karger 2010:42–53.
[31] Walters E, Goussard P, Bosch C, Hesseling AC, Gie RP. GeneXpert MTB/RIF on bronchoalveolar lavage samples in children with suspected complicated intrathoracic tuberculosis: a pilot study. Pediatr Pulmonol. 2014 Nov;49(11):1133–7. doi: 10.1002/ppul.22970. Epub 2013 Dec 11.
[32] Goussard P, Gie RP, Janson JT, le Roux P, Kling S, Andronikou S, Roussouw GJ. Decompression of enlarged mediastinal lymph nodes due to mycobacterium tuberculosis causing severe airway obstruction in children. Ann Thorac Surg 2015 Apr;99(4):1157–63.
[33] Goussard P, Gie RP, Kling S, Nel ED, Louw M, Schubert PT, Rhode D, Vanker A, Andronikou S. The diagnostic value and safety of transbronchial needle aspiration biopsy in children with mediastinal lymphadenopathy. Pediatr Pulmonol 2010 Dec;45(12):1173–9.
[34] Tang LF, Xu YC, Wang YS, Wang CF, Zhu GH, Bao XE, Lu MP, Chen LX, Chen ZM. Airway foreign body removal by flexible bronchoscopy: experience with 1027 children during 2000–2008. World J Pediatr 2009 Aug;5(3):191–5.
[35] de Blic J, Marchac V, Scheinmann P. Complications of flexible bronchoscopy in children: prospective study of 1,328 procedures. Eur Respir J. 2002 Nov;20(5):1271–6.

3 Bronchopulmonary diseases

3.1 Introduction

Classification, diagnostic pathways and therapy recommendations relating to congenital malformations of the lung remain subjects of significant ongoing discussion. From the pediatric point of view, **Ernst Eber** summarizes the actual state of the debate, and his discussion is complemented with a surgical view provided by **Mark Davenport**. Particularly in terms of minimally invasive procedures, **Steven Rothenberg** contributes his outstanding experience in this topic.

Ernst Eber

3.2 Congenital thoracic malformations

The phrase "congenital thoracic malformation" (CTM) is an umbrella term for a number of developmental abnormalities, including pulmonary parenchymal lesions such as congenital cystic adenomatoid malformation (CCAM), extra- and intralobar bronchopulmonary sequestrations, and congenital lobar and segmental emphysemas as well as less frequent abnormalities such as bronchogenic and foregut duplication cysts [1, 2].

Over time, various classifications and nomenclatures have been proposed, based on the heterogeneous appearances of these malformations. The term "hybrid lesion" refers to a CTM with anatomical and/or histological overlap between a CCAM and a bronchopulmonary sequestration, e.g. a lesion with an abnormal blood supply and a histological appearance compatible with CCAM. Today it is assumed that CTMs share a common embryological origin and represent a spectrum of abnormalities of fetal lung development with significant overlap [1, 2]. It was proposed that airway obstruction *in utero* might result in defective lung development, with different patterns of lung malformation according to the level, timing and degree of the obstruction [3]. While there is histological evidence for peripheral bronchial atresia or stenosis to be associated with all types of CTMs, the mode and timing of these incidents are still unclear [4].

The European Surveillance of Congenital Anomalies (EUROCAT), a European network of population-based registries for the epidemiologic surveillance of congenital anomalies, consists of 43 registries in 23 countries and covers approximately 30% of the European birth population. During the last years, the estimated incidence of CCAMs was around 0.9/10,000 live births, or about one quarter of all CTMs [5].

In developed countries, >90% of fetal lung abnormalities are detected in antenatal screening programmes. Many of these lesions will have regressed and some even disappeared on postnatal ultrasound and chest X-ray examination. Nevertheless, all children with antenatally detected CTMs need postnatal evaluation including ultrasound with Doppler, chest X-ray and chest computed tomography (CT) scan with intravenous contrast or magnetic resonance imaging (MRI). These investigations shall characterize the malformation, its vasculature and whether a communication with the tracheobronchial tree is present. To rule out a foregut communication, an esophageal contrast study may be necessary. Further, all children should be evaluated for associated congenital disorders, in particular cardiac anomalies [1].

There is a lack of prospective studies on the natural history of antenatally detected CTMs. Thus, there is an urgent need for both a systematic approach to congenital lung malformations with separate clinical and pathological descriptions and structured prospective observations of the natural history of antenatally detected asymptomatic malformations, to be able to offer relevant counseling to parents in the future.

Further, more studies are needed to resolve the issue of lung growth and lung function both with surgical and non-surgical management. Clearly, the long-term respiratory outcome after surgery to some degree depends on the extent of lung resection. The potential for alveolar growth and hence the ability of children to replace lost lung parenchyma by compensatory lung growth is believed to decrease with age; however, the evidence is scanty and studies have produced conflicting results. To some extent, overexpansion of the residual lung contributes to compensation for volume loss [1, 2].

As regards management of CTMs, this chapter will focus on postnatal life. For reasons of reference, the terms CCAM, bronchopulmonary sequestration, congenital lobar and segmental emphysema, and bronchogenic and foregut duplication cyst will be used.

3.2.1 Congenital cystic adenomatoid malformation (CCAM)

A congenital cystic adenomatoid malformation (CCAM) is an abnormality of the terminal respiratory structures, containing no cartilage and consisting of cysts and solid airless tissue with bronchiolar elements. In the majority of cases, a single lobe is affected, with no particular preference for side and a predilection for the basal lobes. Bilateral lesions are uncommon and usually have a poor prognosis [1, 2].

The original Stocker classification distinguished three types (1, 2, and 3): In the "macrocystic type" (1) one or more large cysts predominate (this type may be hard to distinguish from lung cysts); the "microcystic type" (2) consists of numerous small cysts; and the "solid type" (3) is characterized by a mass of airless tissue. Subsequently, Stocker proposed a new name for these lesions – congenital pulmonary airway malformation (CPAM) and also the rarer types 0 and 4: type 0 is a tracheobronchial defect (also known as acinar dysplasia), characterized by firm small lungs with a bronchial airway; type 4 is an entirely alveolar defect at the lung periphery [6, 7].

Of the five types, only types 1, 2 and 4 are cystic, and only types 1, 2 and 3 are adenomatoid. Type 4 shows histological overlap with grade 1 pleuropulmonary blastoma, with the only distinguishing feature being a lack of blastema in CCAM type 4 [2]. Table 3.2.1 summarizes the characteristics of this classification.

Tab. 3.2.1: Classification of congenital pulmonary airway malformations according to Stocker [6, 7].

Type	Incidence	Cyst size	Histology
0	Rare		Complete failure of development beyond pseudoglandular stage (acinar dysplasia); lethal.
1	Common	Large cysts (>2 cm), can be multiple.	Pseudostratified ciliated columnar epithelium, intermixed with rows of mucous cells; possible malignant change (mucinous adenocarcinoma).
2	Common	Multiple small cysts, sponge-like.	Dilated bronchiole-like structures, intermixed with simplified alveolar parenchyma; occasionally striated muscle.
3	Rare	Solid	Bronchiolar structures separated by small air spaces with cuboidal lining, resembling late fetal lung.
4	Rare	Large cysts	Peripheral and thin-walled cysts, lined by alveolar or bronchiolar epithelial cells upon loose mesenchymal tissue; related to regressed and grade 1 pleuropulmonary blastoma.

Clinical features vary extensively. Antenatally, large lesions may compress the ipsilateral lung and via mediastinal shift also the contralateral lung, resulting in lung hypoplasia. Compression of the esophagus may cause polyhydramnios, and the resulting distension of the uterus may induce premature labor. Impairment of venous return and hydrops may lead to fetal or neonatal death. Antenatal assessment of large lesions comprises evaluation by fetal ultrasound, fetal echocardiogram, ultrafast MRI and fetal karyotype. However, *in utero* therapy is only required in a minority of highly selected fetuses. Proposed interventions include maternal steroid administration, puncture or shunting of macrocystic masses, alcohol embolization or lasering of a feeding vessel, lobectomy via hysterotomy for more solid masses and resection while on placental circulation. A pleural effusion may be treated with a pleuro-amniotic shunt. Fetal therapy requires the expertise of a highly skilled multidisciplinary team, and the evidence base for these interventions is relatively poor [1, 7].

However, the majority of fetuses have a good outcome, and an initially large lesion does not necessarily correlate with a poor prognosis; in fact, the growth pattern is unpredictable. Complete postnatal spontaneous resolution of a CCAM occurs very rarely. As diaphragmatic defects may be missed on ultrasound, CCAM and congenital diaphragmatic hernia sometimes are difficult to differentiate, not only antenatally but even in newborns. A correct diagnosis, prerequisite for providing appropriate management and parental counseling, may not be possible despite the use of serial ultrasound scans and MRI [1, 2].

Approximately 10% of neonates will have respiratory distress shortly after birth; they should undergo urgent CT to confirm the nature of the lesion and subsequent emergency surgery. In a recent review, the mortality rate during the neonatal period was suggested to be about 7% [8]. The majority are smaller lesions which are usually asymptomatic in early postnatal life (Fig. 3.2.1).

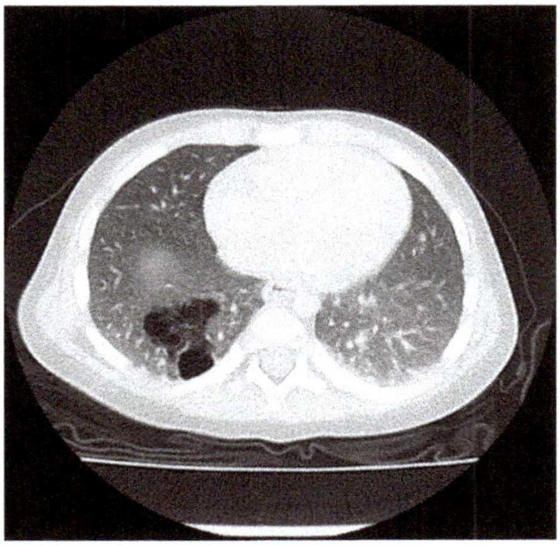

Fig. 3.2.1: Chest CT of a 10-month-old girl with a CCAM type 2 in the right lower lobe. The malformation was diagnosed antenatally, and the girl was asymptomatic.

If not detected antenatally, the diagnosis of smaller lesions may be delayed until school age, adolescence or even adulthood. However, many of them are diagnosed within the first two years of life, as they are prone to develop infection (pneumonia, lung abscess, empyema). Occasionally, they present later with hemoptysis, pneumothorax due to cyst rupture or high output cardiac failure (if there is a large systemic arterial blood supply) [1, 2, 7, 9].

In addition, there is a clear relationship between CCAM and malignant transformation although the risk of transformation and the overall prevalence are not known. Pleuropulmonary blastoma is a rare aggressive neoplasm with an unfavorable outcome; preschool children are typically affected. Some authors regard pleuropulmonary blastoma as the pulmonary dysontogenetic analog to Wilms' tumor in the kidney and neuroblastoma in the adrenal gland. Up to 40% of pleuropulmonary blastomas will show cysts, and with the histological overlap between CCAM type 4 and grade 1 pleuropulmonary blastoma there is potential diagnostic confusion [1, 2, 10, 11]. Bronchioloalveolar carcinoma has repeatedly been reported to arise in pre-existing CCAM type 1, and the mean age for this complication appears to be young adulthood. However, bronchioloalveolar carcinoma has also been described in pediatric cases with CCAM, strongly suggesting malignant transformation of underlying CCAM. Evidence suggests that CCAM is a pre-invasive lesion for mucinous bronchioloalveolar carcinoma, and it has been pointed out that lack of growth over many years cannot be entirely trusted as a criterion of benignity [1, 2].

Surgery is the accepted standard of care for symptomatic lesions, and is definitely indicated when a postnatal complication occurs or when antenatal treatment has already been performed [1, 9].

The main reasons for surgical management of asymptomatic lesions are (1) to prevent complications such as infection, bleeding, pneumothorax, sudden respiratory compromise and malignancy, (2) to reduce post-operative complications (compared to emergency surgery) and (3) to encourage compensatory lung growth (which may be better after early, rather than delayed, surgery). Based on the evidence available today, a weak recommendation can be given to resect asymptomatic cystic CTMs [1, 7, 9]. While a clear recommendation for the timing of surgery cannot be given at present, most surgeons opt for excision of the lesion during the first year of life, and many around the first birthday [1, 7]. Expert pathology review of the excised specimen is essential, and genetic analysis should be considered where appropriate. Of note, in a rather large series of antenatally detected, asymptomatic cystic malformations almost a quarter had histological evidence of infection whether they ultimately turned out to have CCAM, bronchopulmonary sequestration, or a hybrid lesion; almost 3% showed malignancy [12].

Surgery for asymptomatic lesions is controversial, but needs to be balanced against risks of radiation (serial imaging with CT scans with a not insubstantial risk of later cancer), general anesthesia (or sedation), equally important the potential loss to follow-up, and the risk of malignancy. As yet, MRI does not appear to be sufficiently detailed to replace CT in this field [1, 2, 7].

Whether surgery is performed or not, patients with CCAMs should be followed-up into adulthood with standardized protocols. A multi-disciplinary approach to the management of these lesions is of great importance.

3.2.2 Sequestration

The reported incidence of bronchopulmonary sequestrations ranges between 1% and 6% of all CTMs. Sequestrations are lesions predominantly comprising solid, nonfunctioning bronchopulmonary tissue, typically with no bronchial communication and aberrant blood supply via systemic arteries (from the lower thoracic or upper abdominal aorta or one of its major branches). They usually drain their venous blood normally into the left atrium; occasionally, venous drainage may also be abnormal to the right atrium, inferior caval vein or the azygos system. Depending on their appearances, sequestrations are commonly divided into intralobar and extralobar types. Intralobar sequestrations are lesions embedded in normal parenchyma, covered by visceral pleura in continuity with the normal lung. Extralobar sequestrations are invariably solid, have their own separate pleural covering maintaining complete anatomical separation of the mass from the rest of the lung, and are usually located beneath the left lower lobe. About two-thirds of all sequestrations are located in the posterior basal segment of the left lower lobe, and the lesions usually occupy a lung segment or less (Fig. 3.2.2).

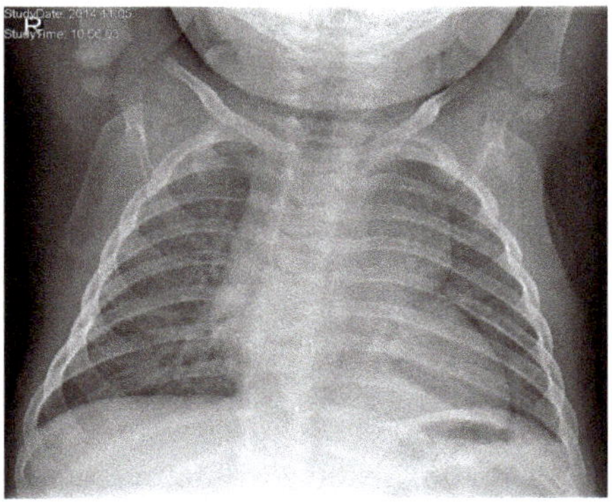

Fig. 3.2.2: Chest X-ray of a 6-month-old girl with an extralobar bronchopulmonary sequestration in the left lower lobe. The malformation was diagnosed antenatally, and the girl was asymptomatic.

In addition, a number of reports described ectopic (intra- or subdiaphragmatic) locations. Especially extralobar sequestrations may be found in association with diaphragmatic hernias or other malformations [1, 2, 7].

The lesions may contain cysts, and – as mentioned above – hybrid malformations with coexisting features of CCAM type 2 are seen in up to 60% of cases (Fig. 3.2.3a and b).

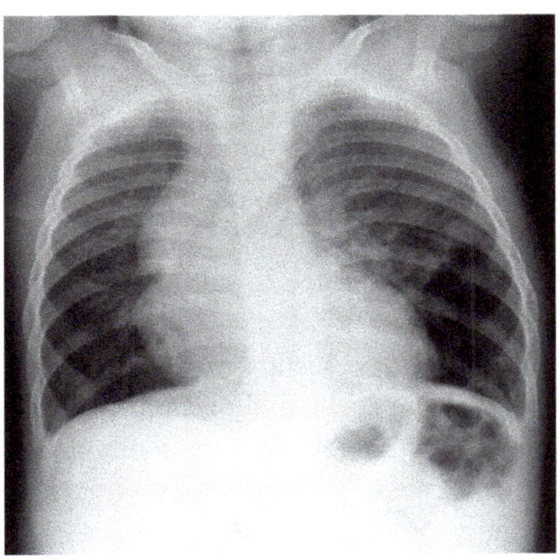

(a)

Fig. 3.2.3a: Chest X-ray of a 10-month-old girl with a hybrid lesion in the left lower lobe. The malformation caused a shift of the mediastinum to the right, and the girl presented with mild tachypnea.

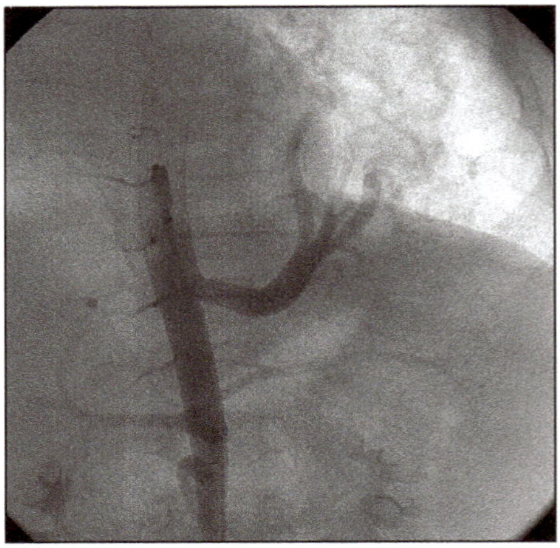

(b)

Fig. 3.2.3b: Angiography of a 10-month-old girl (same patient as in Fig. 3.2.3a) with a hybrid lesion in the left lower lobe, showing a large aberrant artery originating from the abdominal aorta.

In a large series of extralobar sequestrations, half (23/46) of the cases were associated with a coexistent CCAM, all of them type 2 lesions on histologic examination [1].

Antenatally, sequestrations present with increased echogenicity on ultrasound or increased signal intensity on MRI, similar to CCAM type 3 lesions. Differentiation between a bronchopulmonary sequestration and a CCAM is usually made on the basis of a separate blood supply; however, CCAMs can also have a separate blood supply. Antenatally, sequestrations appear to have a favorable outlook. A few will present with hydrothorax and pleural effusion, requiring *in utero* drainage. Many sequestrations show a decrease in size over time, and some even completely disappear on serial antenatal ultrasound scans. As for CCAMS, it is imperative to search for these malformations by CT or MRI angiography, even when they are undetectable on postnatal ultrasound and chest radiograph examinations [1, 2, 7]. Sequestrations have a variety of imaging appearances, including a consolidation, a mass or a cystic or multicystic lesion. Extralobar sequestrations are almost always airless, sharply defined and homogeneous.

In the majority of infants, a sequestration remains asymptomatic until infection develops. Recurrent localized pneumonitis, with fever and occasionally purulent sputum or hemoptysis, may develop at any age from infancy to adulthood, more frequently with increasing age and in patients with intralobar sequestrations. The malformation may also be found incidentally on a chest radiograph. The size of abnormal arteries and veins, and thus blood flow through the malformation may be considerable. As a consequence, a sequestration – functioning hemodynamically as a systemic arteriovenous malformation – may cause cardiovascular symptoms or even lead to cardiac failure. Bronchopulmonary sequestrations rarely have been linked with malignancy in adulthood (almost always but not exclusively intralobar sequestrations); speculatively, these tumors developed in hybrid lesions [1, 2].

As for CCAMs, surgery is the accepted standard of care for symptomatic sequestrations, and is indicated if antenatal treatment has already been performed or when a postnatal complication arises [1, 9].

Because the exact incidence of complications and the natural history of bronchopulmonary sequestrations are largely unknown, it is difficult to give an evidence-based argument for the treatment of antenatally diagnosed, asymptomatic sequestrations. Some authors believe that asymptomatic children with non-cystic sequestration may be followed up expectantly. Others advocate resection of all bronchopulmonary sequestrations because of the risks of complications (infection, hemorrhage and malignancy); in particular, resection of intra- and subdiaphragmatic bronchopulmonary sequestrations was suggested to rule out a tumor. As extralobar sequestrations appear to have a lower risk of developing complications than intralobar ones, their management is even more controversial [1, 9]. In any case, the risks of complications of the malformation itself must be weighed against the risks of surgical morbidity. Unfortunately, reasonable risk estimates are difficult to obtain from the literature. However, with the high frequency of hybrid lesions and the apparently low morbidity with modern surgical techniques, elective surgery might be the preferable strategy in children with an antenatally detected and postnatally verified lesion. In addition, the cost : benefit ratio of repeated CT scans with significant radiation exposure, as well as of office visits, needs to be considered.

As an alternative to surgery, embolization of the systemic feeding artery has been used in children with bronchopulmonary sequestrations [13, 14]. It was suggested that particularly infants with sequestrations who present with congestive heart failure might benefit from embolization alone or in combination with subsequent surgical resection. However, general anesthesia is also needed, embolization may not be as adequate as complete resection of the lesion, and long-term results are lacking. Thus, it appears that embolization cannot be recommended as sole treatment modality [1, 7, 14].

3.2.3 Congenital lobar and segmental emphysema

Congenital lobar emphysema (CLE) is characterized by hyperinflation of one or (rarely) more lobes, usually as a consequence of bronchial obstruction with a valve mechanism; localized malformations and/or deficiencies of bronchial cartilage, valvelike mucosal folds, and extrinsic bronchial compression all have been described as causes. Approximately half of the lesions are located in the left upper lobe; right upper lobe and middle lobe are less frequently affected. CLE often is associated with congenital heart disease [1, 2].

Recently, a sub-type of congenital parenchymal lung pathology, termed congenital segmental emphysema (CSE), has been described. CSE is characterized by postnatal evolution from an initially solid segmental appearance to a hyperlucent and hyperinflated segment. Other authors prefer the term "peripheral bronchial atresia" for the apparently same entity [15]. Bronchial atresia, the most likely underlying and often hidden pathology, is found within a spectrum of antenatally diagnosed lung lesions, such as CCAMs, bronchopulmonary sequestrations, hybrid lesions and CLEs. Further, CLE specimens may show both cystic adenomatoid and polyalveolar changes [4].

A polyalveolar lobe with an increased number of normally expanded alveoli per acinus may also cause radiologic "overinflation" and thus resemble CLE. The affected lobe, usually the left upper, is enlarged and air-filled, and clinically resembles CLE. The etiology is obscure but some authors speculate that the two morphological patterns classic hyperexpansion and polyalveolar lobe might be related to different outcomes of a putative lesion during lung development, depending on the timing of this lesion [1, 2].

Complications of CLE are mostly mechanical, and the lesion uncommonly causes symptoms outside the neonatal period; further, there is hardly any evidence for malignancy occurring in this lesion. CLE tends to compress the surrounding lung tissue and to displace the mediastinum, and thus to present early with respiratory distress (Fig. 3.2.4).

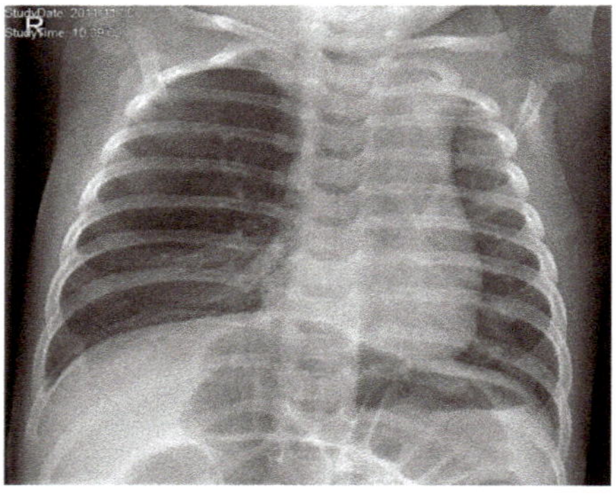

Fig. 3.2.4: Chest X-ray of a 3-month-old boy with congenital lobar emphysema of the right upper lobe. The malformation compressed the surrounding lung tissue and caused a shift of the mediastinum to the left, and the boy presented early with respiratory distress.

While the majority of patients present within the first weeks or months of life, a coincidental detection of the malformation may occur at any age. As the antenatal ultrasound appearance of CLE is relatively inconspicuous, this malformation is not readily diagnosed before birth. Postnatally, a chest radiograph and/or a chest CT scan are generally diagnostic. Flexible bronchoscopy may reveal the cause of bronchial obstruction [1, 2]. CLE may be misdiagnosed as pneumothorax, and patients with severe respiratory distress frequently undergo chest tube drainage.

For many years, surgical removal of the affected part of the lung (lobectomy or segmental lung resection) was the standard recommended treatment. More recently, several authors have advocated a conservative approach on the basis of CLE cases in whom symptoms gradually resolved (Fig. 3.2.5).

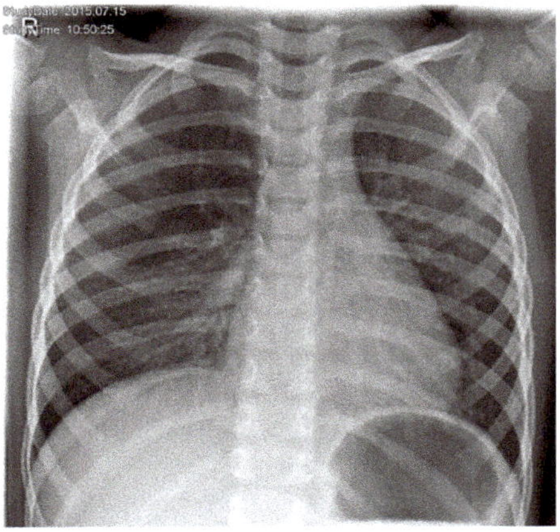

Fig. 3.2.5: Chest X-ray of a 4-year-old boy (same patient as in Fig. 3.2.4) with congenital lobar emphysema of the right upper lobe. Mild hyperinflation of the right upper lobe and no shift of the mediastinum; at this time, the boy was asymptomatic.

Thus, a number of pediatric pulmonologists now tend towards a trial of supportive treatment and observation instead of resorting to surgery immediately after diagnosis; surgical intervention may be reserved for children who do not improve or who present as newborns with very severe respiratory distress [1, 9, 16].

While conservative treatment in mildly to moderately symptomatic children with CLE appears to be appropriate, it calls for a close follow-up to ensure that there are no adverse outcomes with an expectant, non-surgical approach. In an old and small study, normal growth rate of functional lung tissue was reported for both children after surgical resection of CLE and children in whom CLE had been managed conservatively. Thus, it appears that growth of the remaining lung is not hampered by a non-resected cystic lesion, or space-occupying hyperinflated lobe. Since then, successful long-term expectant management has been repeatedly reported [16]. However, further data on long-term follow-up courses are clearly desirable, especially in the light of the finding that CLE specimens may show cystic adenomatoid changes [4].

3.2.4 Bronchogenic and foregut duplication cysts

Bronchogenic cysts originate from defective development of the large airways (trachea or bronchi) and share their origin with foregut duplication cysts; their prevalence is unknown. They are thick-walled (containing smooth muscle, and occasionally cartilage) cysts, and are lined by respiratory epithelium [2]. Bronchogenic cysts are usually single and sometimes quite large malformations; most of them are located in the paratracheal or carinal region thus presenting as mediastinal cysts, but intrapulmonary forms may also be seen (Figs. 3.2.6 and 3.2.7).

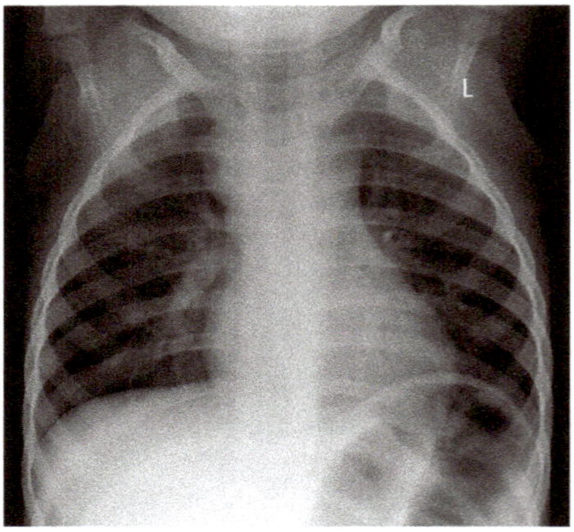

Fig. 3.2.6: Chest X-ray of a 1.5-year-old girl with a bronchogenic cyst projecting from the mediastinum. The typically rounded paratracheal mass with uniform density was found incidentally, and the girl was asymptomatic.

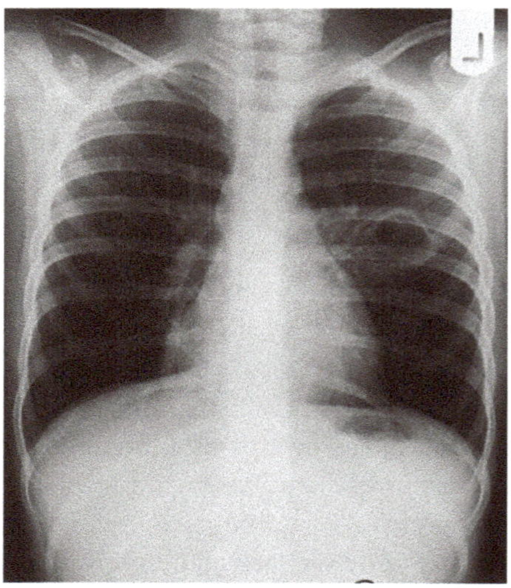

Fig. 3.2.7: Chest X-ray of a 7-year-old girl with an intrapulmonary bronchogenic cyst in the left lung. The lesion was found incidentally, and the girl was asymptomatic.

Foregut duplication cysts may be found in the posterior mediastinum. Apart from gut tissue, they may also contain neural elements and may be associated with vertebral malformations [1].

With wide-spread use of antenatal ultrasound, today these cysts are often detected before birth. Many cysts are asymptomatic and thus may be found incidentally on a chest radiograph. Bronchogenic cysts may be obstructive to neighboring structures (e.g. esophagus) and in case of airway compression may lead to cough, wheeze, dyspnea or even respiratory distress. Radiographic findings are variable, ranging from a rounded mass projecting from the mediastinum and with uniform density similar to that of the cardiac shadow to hyperinflation or atelectasis of a lobe or an entire lung. Air-fluid levels may be seen when the lesion communicates with the tracheobronchial tree. Chest CT or MRI usually permit to confirm the nature of the lesion [1].

Secondary infection of a cyst is a frequent complication and may cause acute distension with exacerbation of symptoms. In addition, peptic ulceration may develop in cysts containing gastric mucosa. As a serious complication, malignant transformation has been described leading to squamous cell carcinoma or bronchioloalveolar carcinoma from the lining epithelial cells to leiomyosarcoma from the wall, typically during adulthood [1, 2].

There is good evidence to recommend surgical resection of symptomatic bronchogenic cysts. In contrast, the evidence for conservative management of asymptomatic cysts is very limited. Both the high risk of developing typical cyst-related complications and the small risk of malignant transformation may justify removal of the lesion even in asymptomatic patients, as surgery can usually be performed without significant loss of functional lung tissue, and with virtually zero mortality and an acceptable rate of morbidity [1, 9, 17].

Steven Rothenberg

3.2.5 VATS in congenital thoracic malformations

There are numerous indications requiring pulmonary lobe resections in infants and children, but the majority are for the broad spectrum of bronchopulmonary malformations that present in early infancy and childhood. These include bronchogenic cysts, bronchopulmonary sequestrations, congenital pulmonary airway malformation (CPAM) and congenital lobar emphysema (CLE) [18]. These lesions may be detected by prenatal ultrasound, present as acute respiratory distress in the newborn period, or may remain undiagnosed and asymptomatic until later in life.

Treatment may vary somewhat depending on the time of diagnosis and the presentation, but in most cases complete lobar resection is the desired therapy. Minimally invasive techniques now allow these procedures to be done with much less pain and morbidity and avoid the long-term consequence of a thoracotomy in an infant or small child.

Thoracoscopic lobectomy can be one of the most technically demanding procedures performed by a pediatric surgeon. The ability to first correctly identify vital structures to both the affected lobe and those going to areas needing to be preserved, and then safely secure the large pulmonary vessels, and a general lack of adequate lung case volume for most pediatric surgical trainees make these procedures even more difficult to adopt. However, a strict adherence to certain principals and a full understanding of pulmonary anatomy can help in assuring that these procedures are done safely and correctly. The basics of a thoracoscopic approach (or VATS) [19] and the most important points are emphasized here.

Technique

The procedures are performed with the patient in a lateral decubitus position and in most cases single-lung ventilation, obtained by mainstem intubation of the contralateral side is desired. In cases where single-lung ventilation could not be achieved,

CO_2 insufflation alone is usually adequate to achieve lung collapse, but the anesthetist needs to take care not to increase inspiratory pressures and inflate the lung especially during critical aspect of the dissection. In general, bronchial blockers are not necessary, and often attempts to place them can take excessive time and are often unsuccessful or the blocker becomes dislodged during the procedure. Most infants and children with bronchopulmonary malformations tolerate single lung ventilation without any problem.

The room is set up to facilitate an anterior approach (Fig. 3.2.8a). This is used because there is more space from the anterior chest wall to the lung hilum, then from a posterior approach, as is typical with an open thoracotomy. The surgeon and assistant are at the patient's front with the monitor at the patient's back. The chest is first insufflated with CO_2 using a veress needle to help collapse the lung and avoid injury of the parenchyma with a trocar. Three trocars are used in almost all cases. The first port is placed between the posterior and mid axillary line in the fifth or sixth interspace. This placement allows determination of the position of the major fissure and evaluation of the lung parenchyma. The most common error is to place this port to far posterior. This forces the surgeon to look back on his instruments while working in the anterior portion of the fissure or the anterior hilum. This is extremely difficult as it forces the surgeon to work in a paradox (against the camera). The more anterior position avoids this and allows the surgeon to look down on his instruments for the majority of the procedure. The position of the fissure should dictate the placement of the other ports. The working ports are placed in the anterior axillary line above and below the camera port (Fig. 3.2.8b).

Three valved ports, ranging from 3 to 5 mm, are used in most cases. A fourth port can be added for retraction if necessary but is rarely needed. In the majority of cases

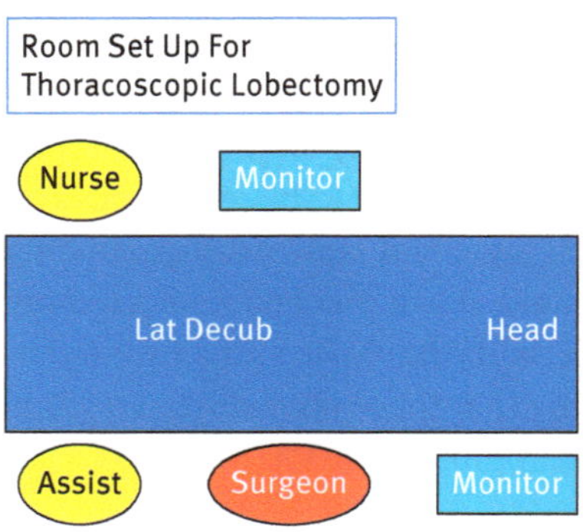

(a)

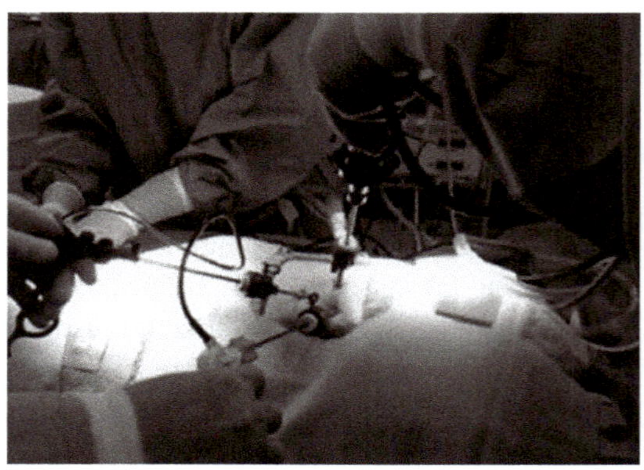
(b)

Fig. 3.2.8: (a) Room set up thoracoscopic lobectomy. (b) Trocar placement for a right-sided lobectomy. The camera port is in the mid-axillary line one interspace below and anterior to the tip of the scapula.

vessel sealing technology is used to handle the pulmonary vessels, especially in small infants. A bipolar sealing device in a 3-mm curved dissector design (JustRight Surgical, Louisville, Co.) is our preferred device. In larger patients (>20 Kg) the 5 mm Ligasure (Medtronic, Boulder, Co.) is used. These devices are preferred because it can be used to dissect out the vessels and obtain adequate vessel length. Two separate seals, a minimum of 3 to 5 mm apart are then created (Fig. 3.2.9a). If there is not adequate length of the vessel to achieve two separate seals, the surgeon can simply dissect into the lung parenchyma to get adequate length. The vessel is then partially divided with scissors between the seals to insure both seals are secure and there is no bleeding, before the vessel is completely divided and retracts (Fig. 3.2.9b). If there is any evidence of bleeding from the partially cut lumen the surgeon still has control and can regrasp and reseal the vessel. The same device and technique can also be used to seal and divide the lung parenchyma in cases of an incomplete fissure, resulting in an air and water tight seal of the lung.

Each lobe is approached relatively the same. The branches of pulmonary artery to the affected lobe are dissected out, sealed and divided first, often at the segmental level. In general the pulmonary vein is then similarly treated, and then lastly the bronchus. For the last few years, in lower lobectomies, the bronchus was divided prior to the vein

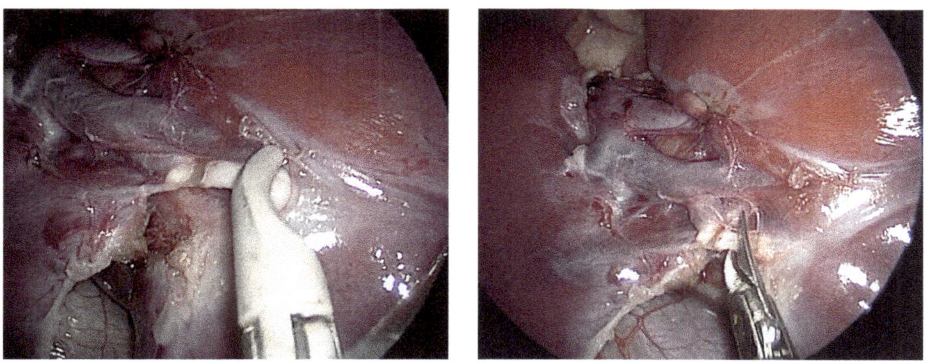

(a) (b)

Fig. 3.2.9: (a) Applying the distal seal to the segmental artery to the pulmonary artery with a 3-mm sealer. The proximal seal is already in place. (b) Cutting the vessel part way to insure both seals are competent before the vessel is completely divided.

because this yielded excellent exposure of the trunk of the inferior pulmonary vein, facilitating safe isolation and division. A chest tube is left in all cases of lobar resection.

In larger patients (generally those over 20 kg), an endoscopic stapler can also be used to secure some or all of the major pulmonary vessels. There is also now a 5-mm stapler (Justright Surgical) which can be used to take the main pulmonary vascular trunks in infants under 15 kg.

The bronchus to the affected lobe is dissected in a similar fashion to the artery and isolated. In infants under 10–15 kg, the 5-mm stapler is used to seal the bronchus (Fig. 3.2.10), if this is not available 5-mm clips or suture can be used. In larger patients a 12-mm endoscopic stapler was used.

If there are large space-occupying cysts, these are first “collapsed” using the vessel sealer. The cystic areas of the lung is grasped, and energy is applied. This causes the cyst to involute, creating more intrathoracic space and improving the surgeon’s ability to manipulate the lung and identify important structures.

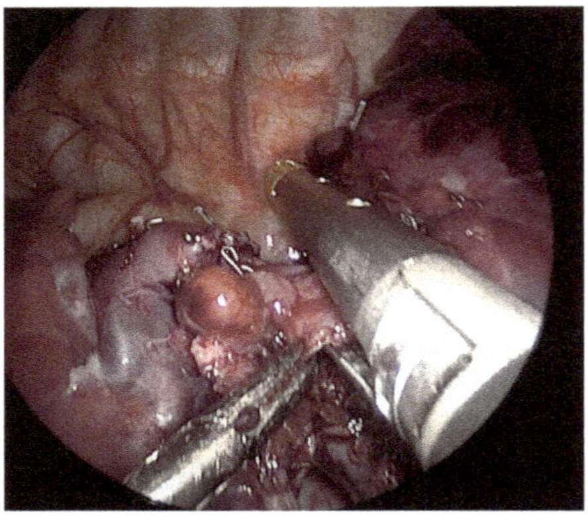

Fig. 3.2.10: Applying a 5-mm stapler to the bronchus of the left lower lobe in a 4-kg infant.

Discussion

Thoracoscopic lobectomy in children for congenital cystic lung disease is now an accepted and well-described technique [20–24]. Most authors agree on the relative merits of a thoracoscopic approach, including less pain, shorter hospital stay, and decreased long-term morbidity, including chest wall deformity, shoulder girdle weakness, and scoliosis [25]. Despite this general consensus, the adoption of this technique and surgeons’ comfort with the approach remain relatively low. We believe there are three main reasons for this. First, the average trainee in general surgery and pediatric surgery fellowship receives very little open or endoscopic thoracic training. Experience with lung biopsy, empyema, and mediastinal masses is usually adequate, but exposure to complex lung resections maybe limited. This lack of volume results in a decreased familiarity with pulmonary anatomy. Using a thoracoscopic approach further compounds this, as the surgeon can no longer put his or her hand in the chest cavity to palpate the structures and identify the anatomy.

One of the most difficult aspects of these cases is when the fissure is incomplete and the pulmonary vessels are not readily visible. We have found that using the tissue- sealing technology to dissect and divide the parenchyma of an incomplete fissure is the safest way to approach this. The fissure is approached layer by layer until the pulmonary artery is visualized. Using the vessel sealer results in limited bleeding and air leak.

The second issue has been standardizing an anterior approach. During an open thoracotomy the surgeon is generally positioned at the patient's back. For thoracoscopic lobectomies the surgeon and assistant are positioned at the patient's front. This is especially important in smaller patients, as there is more room from the chest wall to the mediastinum, where the pulmonary vessels arise. This added space was even more important early on because of the relatively large nature of the sealing and stapling technology available until recently. In many cases the jaws of the instruments barely fit into the thoracic cavity, and this could make the manipulation and firing the devices difficult. The new 3 mm sealer and 5 mm stapler have made this less of an issue but we still believ this approach is superior.

Understanding the anatomic relationships for each lobe using this anterior approach are critical to success. The three-dimensional relationships of the vessels and bronchi to each lobe, which cannot always be seen in the two- dimensional view of the scope are important to understand. It is often helpful to have a senior surgeon with significant thoracic experience available for consultation, even if they don't have significant thoracoscopic experience. The third major issue was standardizing the management of the pulmonary vessels.

Early in our experience we learned that thoracoscopic suture ligation of each individual vessel was difficult and time consuming. The small working space, difficulty in achieving traction and countertraction to obtain adequate vessel length while suturing, and the technical demands of tying a secure knot made this process laborious. We do not favor endoscopic clips for most vessels because of the risk of dislodging them during the extensive tissue manipulation necessary during a lobectomy.

Therefore, early on we adopted vessel sealing as a way to safely mange the pulmonary vessels [26]. The initial 5-mm sealing device used could manage a vessel up to 7 mm in diameter and was an adequate tissue dissector. The 3-mm sealing device now available can seal vessels up to 5 mm and works well as a dissector, especially in the smaller chest cavities of infants. It is more than adequate for most pulmonary vessels in children under 10 kg and for segmental branches in larger children. A key to using vessel-sealing technology effectively is to make proximal and distal seals on the vessel approximately 3–5 mm apart. Using scissors, a partial cut is made to determine that the seals are secure and that there is no bleeding once the lumen is entered. Once the vessel is partially divided and no bleeding is seen, the vessel can be completely divided. The benefit of the technique described is the opportunity to reseal the vessel before the vessel retracts and control is lost.

Because of the relatively large nature of the pulmonary vessels and the limited space in the chest cavity, it takes very little blood to obscure the operative field and force conversion to an open thoracotomy. For this reason, we have avoided any energy devices that seal and divide the vessel in one step, because if the seal fails the ability to salvage the situation is minimal. We have had only one conversion to open for bleeding since adopting this technique. That was a clear technical complication by the surgeon on a large sequestration vessel. A second vessel lying behind the first was not seen and was inadvertently cut while dividing the first vessel that was sealed.

For bronchus management we initially cut and then suture the bronchus using polydioxanone suture in smaller patients. This can be time consuming and technically demanding. We discovered that in most patients <10 kg the bronchus could be occluded using 5-mm endoscopic clips. If the lobar bronchus is too large, then distal dissection allows for a segmental bronchus to be taken. This decreases the size of the remaining main trunk. For example, the superior segment bronchus in a lower lobectomy can be occluded separately, and then the trunk to the basal segments can be taken with a second clip. In larger patients we used the 12-mm endoscopic linear staplers. However, because of the variations in anatomy and the close proximity of the bronchus to the other lobes, extreme care must be taken to avoid compromising the other bronchi. Therefore, if there is any question the bronchus to the target lobe should be divided sharply and sutured close. There is now new 5-mm stapling technology that better fits in the chest cavity of infants and children and should eliminate the use of clips and larger staplers in these smaller patients.

The benefits of thoracoscopic surgery are clear and have been well documented previously. We also favor earlier resection of prenatally diagnosed lesions before they become infected or the patients become symptomatic. We have documented our experience with infants <10 kg and showed that these procedures had shorter operative times, lower complication rates and shorter hospital stays [27]. In older infants, there can be significant adenopathy and inflammation in the fissures and around the pulmonary artery, making identification and safe division of these vessels much more difficult. These procedures are technically easier in infants at or near 5 kg despite the smaller working space as evidenced by the shorter operative times in this group when performed as compared with older patients. The length of stay (LOS) in this group is also shorter. Some are concerned with issues regarding hypercapnia, cerebral hypoxemia and hypoperfusion during anesthesia in these smaller infants. However, this has not been an issue in our experience or in large series reported from Stanford and The Children's Hospital of Philadelphia.

Many authors have clearly documented the issues involved with trying to operate on these lung lesions using thoracoscopy once the infant has already had a clinical chest infection. They document a higher complication rate in those patients who were diagnosed after a chest infection and underwent a thoracoscopic lobectomy compared with those diagnosed prenatally and operated on prior to any clinical infections. Garrett-Cox et al [28] found that 83% of patients converted to open surgery had a previous chest infection. These and other studies demonstrate that 30%–40% of patients with bronchopulmonary malformations will develop significant pulmonary infections during their lives; thus we prefer to remove these lesions before they become symptomatic to avoid a more complicated surgery.

The timing of surgery remains somewhat controversial, but there is little evidence to suggest that delayed resection improves outcome. In fact, because of the factors mentioned above, earlier resection would seem to be preferable. In our experience patients <5 kg had a shorter average operative time of 90 min and shorter LOS (<2 days). Several patients are operated on during the first week of life to avoid a return trip because the families had traveled significant distances to deliver at our maternal/fetal/neonatal center.

For those who argue for conservative nonoperative management of these lesions in asymptomatic patients, despite the high incidence of infection, we have seen two cases of unsuspected pulmonary blastoma[i]. We feel the risks of recurrent infection and possible malignancy outweigh the risks of intervention if a thoracoscopic approach is used in an institution with a large experience in these procedures.

Mark Davenport

Comment

This chapter offers an insight into a multiplicity of congenital intrathoracic pathology areas stretching from intrauterine life to adolescence from the perspective of the earliest years of the twenty-first century. There are things which have changed and some which have remained the same. There has been a fashion for an all-enveloping title for all these things – congenital thoracic malformation (CTM) or congenital pulmonary airway malformation (CPAM); indeed that they are all interlinked in some way [29]. While this gives the sense that there may be common progenitors there are enough dissimilarities within each pathological sector to retain clinical nomenclature – e.g. sequestrations (ICD 9th 748.5) are clinically, observationally, radiologically distinct from the cystic adenomatoid malformation (CCAM) (ICD 9th – 748.4) and this should still be the discerning clinician's focus.

A major therapeutic advance are maternal steroids (usually betamethasone) which can influence outcome in fetuses with significant CCAM (both macro and microcystic) with remarkable effect. The Philadelphia group recently reported an updated experience (n = 43) with both single shot and repeated steroid courses in fetuses with large macrocystic CCAM at risk of or actually with hydrops [30]. Over 80% showed a diminution in lesion size and as a consequence an increase in survival proportions and a clear decrease in the need for fetal lung resection.

The debate over resection or intervention for the asymptomatic lesion still carries on with verve and vigor, certainly within the UK and Europe if not the USA. Our original meta-analysis showed that about 3% of asymptomatic lesions would develop symptoms within infancy and that elective surgery was safer and less prone to complications than emergency surgery [8]. Having decided to remove a lung lesion then the next question will be how and it is clear that many surgeons have adopted thoracoscopic techniques to do this. In the USA, around 50% of lung resections are now minimally invasive (Fig. 3.2.11) [31]. However, as a large multi-institutional study recently showed it is still not easy, not quick and the actual benefits in terms of reducing hospital stay have not been proven [32].

One of the perceived advantages of early resection is to minimise the risk posed from neoplastic change. While the magnitude of this risk is still unknown there have been some developments in the understanding of causation. The commonest neoplasm, bronchioloalveolar carcinoma (BAC), exists in two forms either mucinous (mBAC) or non-mucinous (nmBAC) and the corresponding cells of origin appear to be a mucus-producing glandular cell and a type II pneumocyte or Club (formerly Clara) cell respectively [32]. The development of BAC in Type 1 CCAM has been associated with an underlying K-ras point mutation [33].

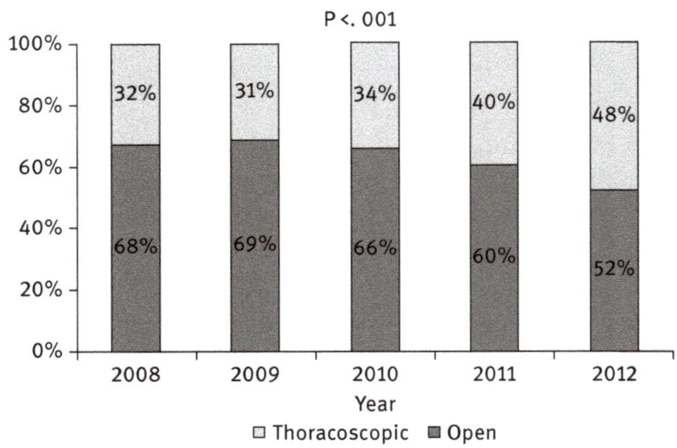

Fig. 3.2.11: Relative utilization of thoracoscopic resection of congenital cystic lung disease when compared to open resection increased with time in 1120 children ($P < .001$) [reproduced with permission from reference [4]].

3.3 Airway diseases

3.3.1 Introduction

Surgery of laryngotracheal disorders, particularly in newborns and infants, is extremely rare and extraordinary challenging. And while only a few specialists are known in this field, the contribution from **Konrad Hoetzenecker** and **Walter Klepetko** is as important as the invited comments from **Martin Elliot**. Performing tracheostomies is common practice in all age groups of pediatric medicine. The chapter written by

Martin Lacher and **Oliver Muensterer** cover this issue from indication to technical aspects and postoperative management.

Konrad Hoetzenecker, Walter Klepetko

3.3.2 Laryngotracheal reconstruction

Applied surgical anatomy of the pediatric laryngotracheal airway

A detailed anatomical understanding of the pediatric larynx and trachea is pivotal in laryngotracheal surgery. Although the basic anatomical structures are identical to the adult airway, there are important differences which have a considerable functional impact. The position of the larynx and the epiglottis is higher, making a simultaneous breathing and suckling possible. As a side effect, swallowing problems are rare in children, even after extensive resections and mobilization procedures.

Children are clinically more susceptible to airway compromise than adults. The pediatric airway is only a few millimeters in diameter, therefore stenosis or dynamic obstructions can dramatically reduce the airway cross-section [34]. This is especially relevant in the glottic region, where the mucosa, due to its lax structure, is more prone to edema formation compared to adults.

Blood supply is similar to adults and limited to small anastomoses fed by the thyroid arteries and the bronchial arteries. The main blood supply comes from vessels running in the trachoesophageal groove. Therefore, only minimal dissection should be performed in this area in order to avoid compromise of the perfusion of the anastomosis/reconstruction.

Preoperative evaluation

A precise preoperative evaluation is essential before planning a surgical correction of airway problems in children. After documentation of the complete medical history and coexisting malformations or comorbidities children should undergo transnasal flexible laryngoscopy. Respiration, vocal cord function, swallowing and vocalization must be tested and documented. However, transnasal laryngoscopy requires a cooperative child and toddlers often refuse the procedure. In addition, an endoscopic evaluation under general anesthesia has to be performed in every patient before the operation. The extent of the lesion, its height related to the vocal cords, position of a pre-existing tracheostomy and the overall length of the airway must be measured. Lesions should be classified according to the modified Myer-Cotton grading (Tab. 3.3.1), which was developed to correlate the type of stenosis and comorbidities with patients' outcome [35]. By variation of the depth of anesthesia, dynamic obstructions can be detected. In some cases additional imaging methods (eg. CT scans) can be useful. However, for laryngotracheal stenosis their value usually is limited.

Tab. 3.3.1: Modified Myer-Cotton grade. It combines the grade of airway stenosis, its extension towards the glottis and patients' comorbidities. SGS = subglottis stenosis.

Myer-Cottongrade	Isolated SGS (a)	Isolated SGS + comobidities (b)	Isolated SGS + glottis involvement (c)	Isolated SGS + glottis involvement + comobidities (d)
I 0–50%	Ia	Ib	Ic	Id
II 51–70%	IIa	IIb	IIc	IId
III 71–99%	IIIa	IIIb	IIIc	IIId
IV No lumen	IVa	IVb	IVc	IVd

Laryngotracheal stenosis

Laryngotracheal stenosis is the prevailing airway problem in children. The etiology of the disease is in most cases preterm delivery and the requirement for intubation. Larynogotracheal stenosis is a sequela of a poor tube management mainly caused by a tube too big in diameter [36]. This results in a combined damage of the glottis and the subglottic airway, eventually with an additional ankylosis of the arythenoid joints. Currently, few guidelines for neonatal intubation are available, but it is generally agreed that the smallest possible tube, which can provide an adequate ventilation, should be used. During intubation the slightest resistance when advancing the tube should lead to the use of a smaller tube. Cuffed tubes should be avoided when long-time ventilation is required, since localized tracheomalacia can develop at the site of the cuff. Most children will at some point of time need a tracheostomy.

There are two different techniques to correct pediatric laryngotracheal stenoses: tracheoplasty and extended partial cricotracheal resection.

Tracheoplasty

The technique of tracheoplasty has been developed in the 1970s [37]. The basic consideration behind this correction technique is an enlargement of the narrowed airway diameter by an interposition of cartilage grafts. Most of the time the grafts will be harvested from the costal arch, however grafts from the upper wing of the thyroid or resected tracheal rings can also be used. Tracheoplasty should only be applied in mild to moderate laryngotracheal stenosis. The mucosal lining has to be intact and there should not be any evidence of ongoing scar proliferations. In the latter, tracheoplasty usually owns poor results with a high likelihood of restenosis. Therefore, these patients should be corrected using the technique of extended partial cricotracheal resection.

Surgical steps: After complete exposure of the laryngotracheal skeleton, a complete anterior laryngeal split is performed. Care should be taken to exactly stay in

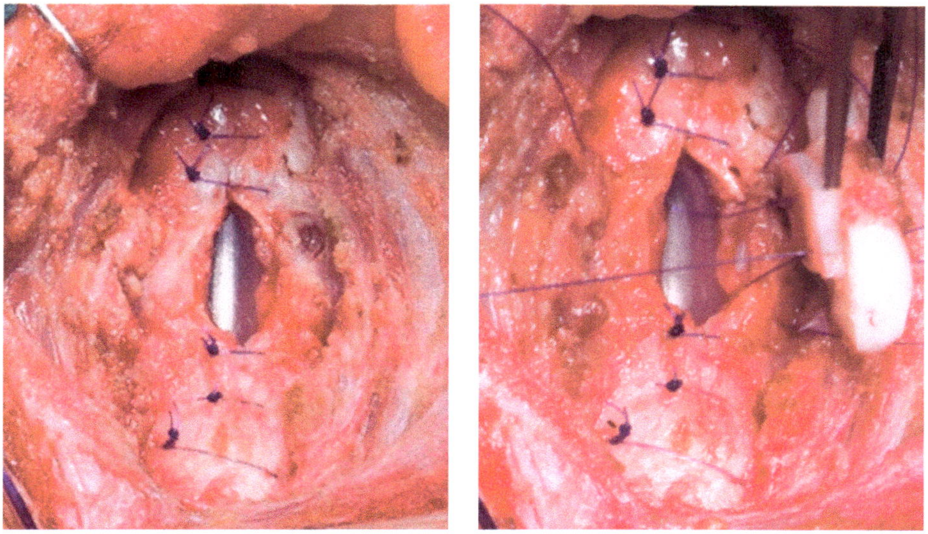

Fig. 3.3.1: Last surgical steps of a tracheoplasty. After inserting an LT-Mold and closing the anterior laryngeal fissure the remaining airway defect is coverd by a boat-shaped cartilage graft.

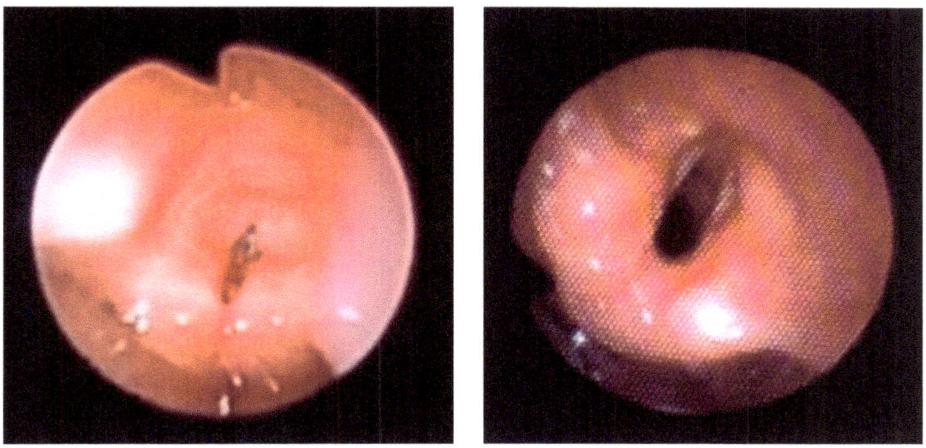

Fig. 3.3.2: Preoperative endoscopic findings and the postoperative result after tracheoplasty. A significant lumen enlargement was achieved.

the midline in order to avoid any damage to the vocal cords. Then the cricoid plate is completely split in the midline. The two halfes of the plate are carefully lifted from adjacent fibers to the hypopharyx in order to create a space for the insertion of the cartilage graft. A graft is harvested from the rib cage and tailored with two steps laterally. This leads to a stable interposition between the split cricoid plate. The size of the cartilage graft must be chosen carefully. A graft, which is dimensioned too small will result in an insufficient lumen enlargement. A graft, which is too broad will lead to poor functional results with breathy voice and swallowing problems. The dorsal cartilage is secured with four 6-0 absorbable sutures. Since the pediatric airway skeleton is still elastic an internal splinting is needed in order to stabilize the newly reconstructed airway. The LT-Mold, developed in Lausanne is the best currently available device. It is made of soft silicone and mimics the anatomical shape of the pediatric airway. Thus, the formation of granulation tissue is significantly reduced. The LT-Mold is positioned intralaryngeally and fixed to the thyroid with two deep stiches through the prosthesis. The remaining anterior airway defect, which has been created due to the lumen enlargement, is then covered by a second boat-shaped cartilage graft.

Extended partial cricotracheal resection

The technique of extended partial cricotracheal resection combines a posterior cartilage graft enlargement with a wide anterior resection. It is more complex, compared to the technique of tracheoplasty and should be reserved to complex stenoses with extensive scarring. Although good results can be achieved even in very small children (<10 kg) [38], usually a minimal weight of 7 kg is recommended for correction to allow a precise reconstruction.

Surgical steps: The laryngotracheal airway is exposed and the trachea is divided from the cricoid. Care should be taken to avoid injury to the recurrent nerves and the vessels running in the tracheoesophageal groove. In the next step the cricoid arch is removed and a complete anterior laryngeal split is performed. This leads to a wide exposure of the posterior scars. All scar formations on the anterior surface of the cricoid plate have to be completely removed in order to avoid restenosis. Next the cricoid plate is divided in the midline and a rib cartilage is interposed (similar to the tracheoplasty). The height of an existing tracheostomy is important and the further surgical steps have to be planned accordingly. A distally placed tracheostomy can be kept but the skin insertion has to be relocated at the end of surgery. If the tracheostomy was placed high it has to be included in the resection at the time of the operation and a second tracheostomy will be placed below the reconstruction. For the thyrotracheal anastomsosis the distal trachea is trimmed in a way that a large dorsal mucosal flap and a V-shaping of the anterior aspect is created. The dorsal mucosal flap is used to fully cover the cartilage graft and the cricoid plate, in that way adapting healthy mucosa to healthy mucosa. A running 6-0 suture is used to equally distribute tension on the flap and to adjust incongruence. An LT-Mold is placed intralaryngeally and the rest of the thyrotracheal anastomosis is performed using single 4-0 or 5-0 PDS stiches.

Subglottic stenosis

Isolated subglottic stenosis without the involvement of the glottic airway is less frequently seen in children compared to the adult population. A stenosis at the height of

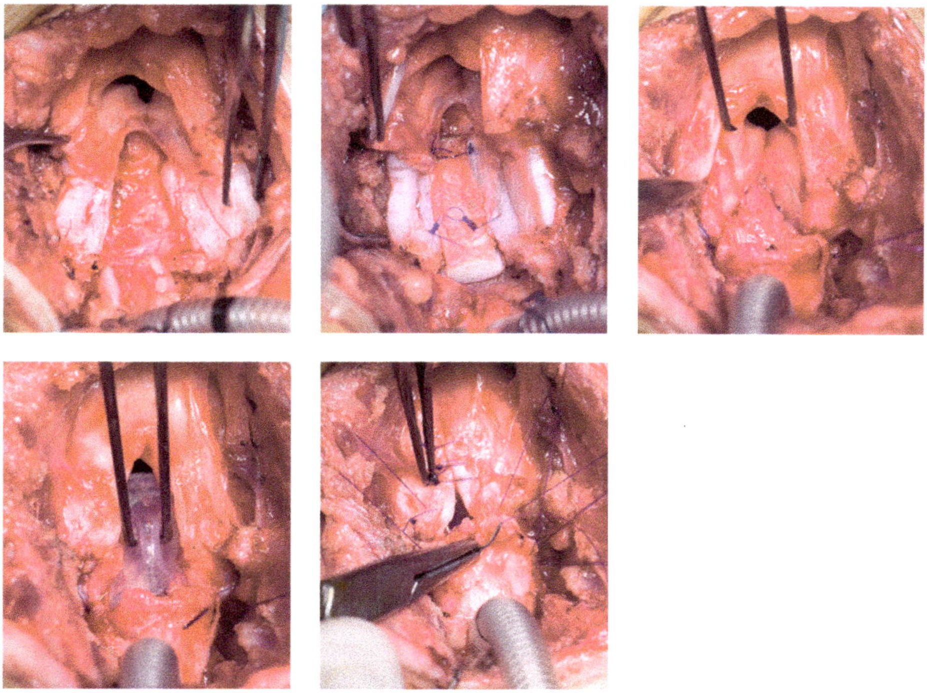

Fig. 3.3.3: Surgical steps of an extended partial cricotracheal resection. A rib cartilage is grafted between the split cricoid plate. It is covered by a mucosal flap. After placing an LT-Mold the thyrotracheal anastomosis is completed. *(obtain permission – Oxford University Press, Eur J Cardiothorac Surg. 2015 Aug 7)*

the cricoid plate can either be the result of a longtime intubation or a poorly placed tracheostomy. Since the cricoid is the only ring-shaped cartilage, an oversized orotracheal tube can lead to pressure caused necrosis of the mucosa, in that way starting a cascade of uncontrolled inflammation and scar formation. In some cases a high placed tracheostomy (at the level of the first tracheal cartilage ring) can lead to a proximal erosion of the cricoid, especially in kyphotic individuals. This results in the development of an anterior subglottic stenosis.

Surgical steps: The repair of isolated subglottic stenosis in children is similar to the techniques used in adults. For anterior stenosis a classical Grillo technique can be used, resecting the anterior cricoid arch and performing a thyrotrachael end-to-end anastomosis. Care should be taken to equally adjust incongruency of the airway lumen between the upper and lower part of the anastomosis. Sometimes a reduction plasty of the distal trachea might be necessary to overcome this problem. If an extensive cicatrization is present on the cricoid plate a complete mucosectomy is necessary. The denudated cricoid plate subsequently has to be covered with a mucosal flap of the distal trachea. In some cases a partial anterior split with an interposition of the anteriorly V-shaped distal trachea might be necessary in order to obtain a sufficient lumen enlargement. These extended subglottic reconstructions are often associated with a swelling of the vocal cords, since resection margins come close to the vocal folds. If a glottis swelling occurs a small tracheostomy has to be placed below the anastomosis in order to secure the airway. In most cases the tracheostomy can be abandoned within the first postoperative days when the swelling has resolved.

Tracheal stenosis/malacia

Stenosis and malacia restricted to the trachea should be grouped into short-segment and long-segment lesions according to available techniques of repair.

Short-segment lesions:
In contrast to larynogtracheal stenosis, which can be typically found in very small children, pure short-segment tracheal stenosis are more frequent in older children. The main etiology is (comparable to adults) an improper cuff-management during intubation or airway damage caused by the cuff or the tip of a tracheostomy canula. Most of the time the damage is located in the cervical trachea and involves only a short segment. Thus, correction is relatively simple with a resection of the affected segment and an end-to-end anastomosis. When the stenosis is located in the intrathoracic part of the airway the surgical approach to the trachea is either through a right posterolateral thoracotomy or a median sternotomy.

Short-segment tracheomalacia is nearly always associated with vascular abnormalities (vascular rings). A combined treatment of the vascular malformation together with the airway damage is necessary. However, it is still controversial how to approach the tracheomalacia [39]. An aortopexy can offer good results in patients with low-grade malacia. In more severe malacia a resection of the diseased tracheal segment has to be performed. The placement of airway stents should be avoided since stents will lead to the formation of granulation, airway inflammation and subsequent multilevel stenosis, which are very hard to repair.

Long-segment lesions:
Long-segment tracheal stenosis are congenital disorders and generally associated with complete tracheal rings. Since the stenosis often affects more than 50% of the tracheal length, a resection and end-to-end anastomosis is not possible. Slide-tracheoplasty is the established technique which uses the stenotic part for reconstruction and offers excellent long-term success [40]. The stenotic trachea is horizontally transected in its mid, the upper part is longitudinally incised posteriorly and the lower part anteriorly. Both segments are then slid together. In this way the length of the trachea is diminished by 50% but the cross-sectional area is increased four-fold.

This technique has also been used to correct congenital stenosis extending to the bronchial system [41].

Postoperative follow-up and outcome

Postoperative care is a key factor for success in pediatric airway surgery. Adequate resection/reconstruction is only one step in the treatment of these complex patients. After pediatric laryngotracheal surgery an LT-Mold is needed in most children in order to support the airway reconstruction. The LT-Mold prosthesis is kept in situ for 6 to 8 weeks depending on the complexity of the reconstruction. The mold can be removed microlaryngoscopically and, subsequently, children can be weaned from the tracheostomy. Swallowing rehabilitation only plays a minor role since postoperative aspiration is hardly seen, even in cases of extensive reconstruction. Interestingly, the reconstructed airway does not lose its capacity to grow. This has been repeatedly shown by different groups [42, 43].

Outcomes after laryngotracheal surgery are excellent in highly experienced centers. Successful decanulation after partial extended cricotracheal resection can be achieved in more than 90% of all patients [44]. The reason for unsuccessful weaning from the canula are in most cases severe coexisting neurological comorbidities. After laryngotracheal reconstruction overall cannulation rates range from 80% to 100% in low-grade (Myer-Cotton II) stenosis [45]. Results of LTR for high grade stenosis are poorer with only 50% to 80% percent decanulation rates. Accordingly, Myer-Cotton IV stenosis should be repaired by extended partial cricotracheal resections, as mentioned above. Overall survival after correction of long-segment congenital stenosis, by a slide tracheoplasty is reported to be as high as 88% in the largest reported series summarizing a 17-year experience of a high volume center [41].

Conclusion

The management of pediatric airway problems is complex and requires a dedicated team. Outstanding expertise of thoracic surgeons, phoniatricians, logopedics and pediatricians is necessary in order to achieve good long-term results. A centralization of these highly demanding patients should be considered in order to offer patients and their parents optimal treatment.

Martin Lacher, Oliver Muensterer

3.3.3 Tracheostomy

Abstract: Tracheostomy is usually performed because of significant upper airway compromise, a need for better tracheobronchial toilet, for prolonged positive pressure, or ventilatory support. The major indications include airway obstruction, long-term respiratory support and facilitation of secretion clearance. Tracheostomy is associated with a significant impact on the psychosocial development of the child. Therefore any alternative treatment option prior to proceeding with tracheostomy should be evaluated. In contrast to adults, tracheostomy is carried out in an open fashion. Percutaneous dilatational tracheostomy is not as suitable for children because the airway is small and often unstable. Complications during the procedure include damage to surrounding structures, hemorrhage, or pneumothorax/pneumomediastinum. The most common long-term complications are partial obstruction of the cannula and accidental decannulation. Therefore extensive education of the caregivers along with preparation of a safe home environment is essential for a successful transition to home care. When the initial indication for a tracheostomy no longer exists the child can be decannulated. This process includes confirmation of airway patency, weaning/capping and closure of the tracheocutaneous fistula. The latter usually happens spontaneously, surgical closure is necessary in only <10% of cases. If congenital high airway obstruction is diagnosed prenatally, tracheostomy during ex utero intrapartum therapy (EXIT) is a special indication. Rarely, a pediatric surgeon may be required to emergently obtain an airway at the bedside via incisional or needle cricothyroidotomy in an infant who is too unstable for transport to the operating room. Despite the morbidity of the procedure tracheostomy nowadays is a routine surgical procedure which can be performed safely in experienced institutions.

Introduction

The trachea is a conduit between the upper airway and the tracheobronchial tree, which delivers moist warm air to the lungs, and expels carbon dioxide and sputum into the surrounding atmosphere. The intention of a tracheostomy is to provide a child with a secure, functional access for gas exchange. It is usually performed because of significant upper airway compromise, a need for better tracheobronchial toilet, for prolonged positive pressure or ventilatory support. A tracheostomy may be a temporary or long-term, in some cases life-long intervention.

Technically speaking, the term tracheostomy refers to the surgical creation of a percutaneous opening into the trachea, whereas the term tracheotomy describes an incision of the trachea. However, many practitioners use these terms interchangeably.

This chapter discusses the indications for and technical considerations of tracheostomy in children.

Indications for tracheostomy

The three major indications for long-term tracheostomy in children are:
- Airway obstruction
- Congenital anomalies (e.g. subglottic stenosis, laryngeal web)

- Trauma (e.g. birth trauma, child abuse, accidents)
- Tumors (e.g. hemangiomas, lymphatic malformations, papillomatosis, cervical teratoma)
- Functional obstruction (e.g. vocal cord palsy)
- Laryngomalacia/Tracheomalacia
- External compression of the trachea
- Infectious or allergic processes leading to swelling (e.g. epiglottitis, diphtheria)
- Long-term respiratory support
- Pulmonary pathology (e.g. bronchopulmonary dysplasia)
- Hypoventilation syndromes (e.g. Ondine's curse, central hypoventilation)
- Facilitation of secretion clearance (pulmonary toilet)
- Neurologic injury or disease (e.g. cerebral palsy, spinal muscular atrophy)
- Chronic aspiration

Over the recent years, the incidence of and the indications for pediatric tracheostomy has changed. Several decades ago, tracheostomy was performed primarily as a life-saving intervention to secure an airway in children with life-threatening airway obstruction due to infectious disorders [46]. Since then, vaccination programs and anesthetic skills have dramatically reduced the number of emergency tracheostomies performed for acute upper airway obstruction. Today, the indication for tracheostomy is generally ruled by the anticipation of long-term (cardio-) respiratory compromise due to persistent ventilatory insufficiency, or by the presence of a fixed obstruction of the upper airway that is unlikely to resolve in the near future [47]. A recently published study revealed that among ventilated children in Canada, the prevalence of tracheostomy was less than 1.5% [48]. Compared to the current practice in adults, tracheostomy in children is generally less frequently indicated, usually placed late in the course of a chronic illness, and performed surgically rather than percutaneously [49].

Preoperative work-up and planning

The majority of children undergo the procedure as very young infants. Apart from its morbidity, tracheostomy is associated with a significant impact on the psychosocial development of the child. Therefore any alternative treatment option prior to proceeding with tracheostomy should be evaluated.

If the skin of the patient's neck is infected by bacteria or fungi, this should be treated before any operation is performed unless emergency tracheostomy is indicated. Children who are planned to undergo congenital heart surgery, and in whom tracheostomy placement is anticipated in the future, may be best managed by completing the cardiac surgery before tracheostomy is performed. Otherwise, the risk of cardiac infection may be increased as the sternal incision is close to the tracheostomy site. Tracheostomy following cardiac surgery, however, does not seem to be a risk factor for mediastinitis by itself [50]. Most of the children who are scheduled for tracheostomy already have an endotracheal tube in place. For certain indications (e.g. immature airway) the severity of laryngotracheomalacia with dynamic airway collapse may be assessed by direct laryngoscopy and/ or bronchoscopy via facemask. It is important to note that direct laryngoscopy requires removal of the endotracheal tube, which should only be performed under controlled conditions and with the potential of surgical intervention if the airway is lost during the maneuver.

Pediatric tracheostomy is usually performed electively with secure airways (e.g. for prolonged intubation). Therefore it is reasonable to check the hematocrit, platelet count and coagulation factors preoperatively so that adequate correction can be made. In case of an emergency, the decision to perform an emergent tracheostomy is not affected by any lab values.

The selection of the appropriate tube type and size is one of the key elements of preoperative planning and depends on the dimension of the child's airway and the clinical indication [51]. Most pediatric tracheostomy tubes are cuffless, however, in large children and adolescents cuffed tracheostomy tubes are sometimes used either. Low-pressure cuffs should be the preferred devices used in children.

A suitable tube should be small enough to allow the child to phonate by being able to force air around the tube, yet big enough to prevent a significant insufflation leak which may cause hypoventilation [52, 53]. However, if the tube is too large or a cuffed tracheostomy is overinflated for a prolonged period of time, it may injure the tracheal mucosa by chronic focal pressure, leading to vascular compromise, ulceration and ultimately, fibrous stenosis. The correct diameter can be estimated on the basis of the patient's endotracheal tube size, which corresponds to its inner diameter.

The length of the tracheostomy cannula is another important variable, especially in neonates and infants to allow adequate air entry, easy suctioning and clearance of secretions. If the tube is too short, it may lead to accidental decannulation or formation of a false tract. A tube that is too long may erode the carina or ventilate a single main bronchus only, most likely the right. This may lead to left mainstem bronchial occlusion and atelectasis. As selecting the correct length is important, tracheostomy tubes are usually available in two lengths, short or long.

The following pediatric tracheostomy tube sizes, determined on the basis of patient age and weight, were recommended by Wetmore [54]:
- Premature neonates or babies who weigh less than 1000 g–2.5 mm
- Babies who weigh 1000–2500 g–3 mm
- Neonates aged 0–6 months – 3–3.5 mm
- Infants aged 6 months to 1 year – 3.5–4 mm
- Infants aged 1–2 years – 4–5 mm

- For children older than 2 years the following formula for size estimation has been proposed by the American Heart Association [55]:
- Cuffed tubes: (age [years] + 16)/4
- Uncuffed tubes: (age [years] + 12)/4

As the child grows, a progressively larger tracheostomy tube is required. Early signs of the need for a bigger tube are nocturnal dips in oxygen saturation or low-pressure ventilator alarms. To prevent this, the tube size should be increased as a planned procedure at least every two years [56].

Technique

The majorities of tracheostomies are elective procedures and therefore conducted under general anesthesia. Most children will have already been endotracheally intubated and may require more prolonged and/or more effective form of secure airway. Tracheostomies should be performed using the conventional dissection technique. In contrast to adults, percutaneous dilatational tracheostomy is not as suitable for children because the airway is small and often unstable: The trachea is soft, compressible, and very mobile. Anatomic landmarks can be difficult to palpate and a displaced tube may not be easily replaced.

Although several techniques of performing a tracheostomy exist, they follow a basic guideline: The trachea's outer wall is exposed. An incision is made through two of the tracheal cartilaginous rings and a tracheostomy tube inserted into the windpipe.

Regardless of the surgical technique used, the anesthetist should decrease the amount of inspired oxygen in the patient gas mix to the lowest fraction possible to prevent a surgical fire in the operating field [57].

Position of patient

Once the patient is anesthetized, the infant is positioned supine, sufficiently toward the foot of the operating table so that the surgeon can easily access the infant's neck and the anesthetist can reach and manipulate the endotracheal tube when necessary. A roll should be placed under the shoulders to extend the neck (Fig. 3.3.4). The

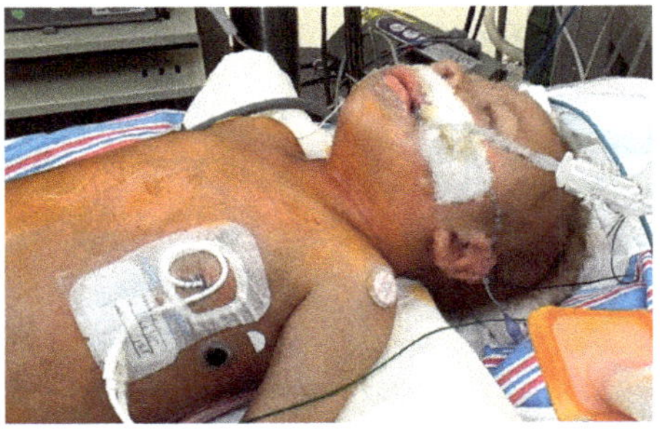

Fig. 3.3.4: Position of an infant for tracheostomy placement. The shoulders are elevated on a roll; the head is hyperextended on the neck and supported by a doughnut-form support.

occiput is stabilized by a head ring and the table is tilted into a minimal head-up position. After proper positioning, the entire neck from the lower lip to below the nipples is prepped and draped. Care must be taken that the superior most surgical drape allows easy access to the patient by the anesthetist. Any tape of the endotracheal tube should be loosened beforehand so that the anesthetist can easily remove the tube at the appropriate time. Care must be taken not to dislodge the endotracheal tube prematurely.

Incision and dissection to expose the trachea

Once prepped and draped, the surgeon should carefully palpate and mark the anatomic landmarks for the incision. These include the infant's hyoid bone, thyroid notch and cricoid cartilage. The cricoid is often difficult to palpate, especially in neonates. It may be helpful to ask the anesthetist to jiggle the endotracheal tube from above to assist with the location of the trachea.

Once the landmarks are identified, an adequate horizontal skin incision is made midway between the cricoid and the suprasternal notch and deepened through fat and platysma (Fig. 3.3.5). The skin incision should be large enough to accommodate the endotracheal tube and allow safe dissection of the trachea. Alternatively, the incision may be made in the lower neck crease, about the width of one finger

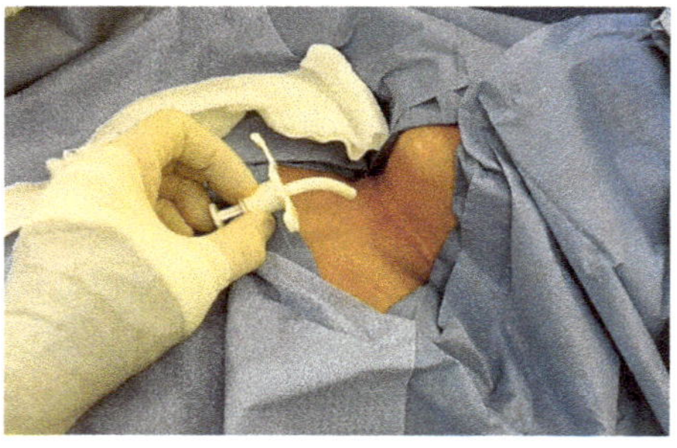

Fig. 3.3.5: An adequate skin incision is made midway between the cricoid and the suprasternal notch and deepened through fat and platysma, large enough to facilitate easy exposure of the trachea and accommodate the tracheostomy tube with a small gap.

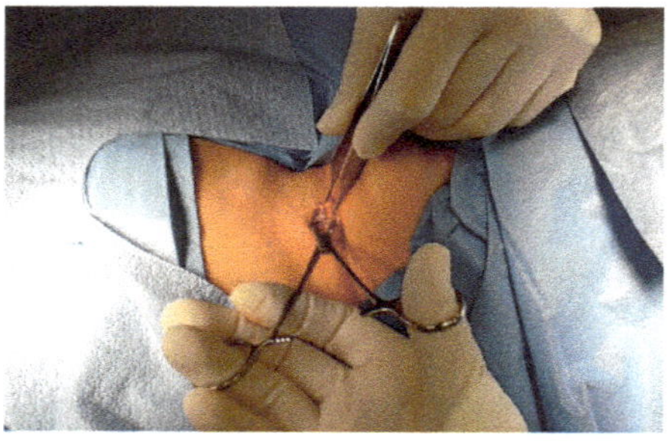

Fig. 3.3.6: The precervical fascia is opened, and the strap muscles are divided longitudinally.

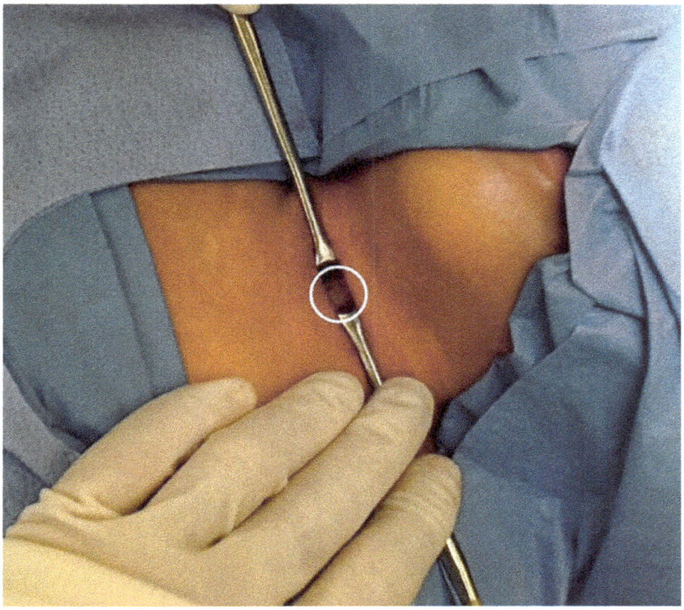

Fig. 3.3.7: Two retractors are placed deep to the muscle edges of the strap muscles and gently retract laterally to better expose the trachea below (trachea visible in the center of white circle).

above the jugular notch. However, it should not be too low to avoid dissecting in the mediastinum.

Next, the anterior cervical fascia is opened vertically in the midline. The incision is then deepened until the deep cervical fascia overlying the sternohyoid and sternothyroid strap muscle is encountered. Branches of the anterior jugular vein are cauterized and divided with the bipolar diathermy. Once the strap muscles are separated by blunt dissection (Fig. 3.3.6), two retractors are placed deep to the muscle edges and gently retract laterally to better expose the trachea below (Fig. 3.3.7).

Rarely, the isthmus of the thyroid gland, which has a variable size and relationship to the trachea, must be divided for proper tracheostomy positioning. If this is necessary, the use of bipolar diathermy is sufficient in small children. In adolescents with a bulky isthmus, the division over suture ligations is preferable.

Opening the trachea and insertion of the cannula

Before making the incision in the trachea, the correctly sized tracheostomy cannula should be opened and available on the operating table. Its outer diameter is visually compared to the exposed trachea and the appropriate size is reconfirmed.

To limit bleeding after accessing the lumen of the trachea, the delicate pretracheal fascia can be lightly scored with electrocautery to coagulate any tiny vessels on the surface of the trachea in the midline.

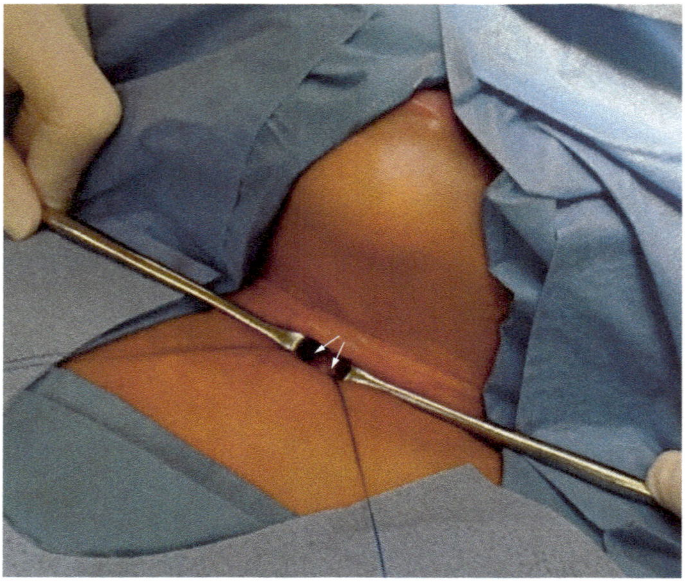

Fig. 3.3.8: Traction sutures of fine polypropylene are placed around the third tracheal ring to stabilize the trachea before incision (arrows).

Before opening the trachea, two polypropylene stay sutures are placed on either side of the trachea, each one incorporating one or two tracheal rings (Fig. 3.3.8). During the operation, these sutures help to distract the tracheal incision for ease of placement of the tracheostomy cannula and also secure the airway in case of bleeding, dislodgement, or loss of retraction.

The anesthetist prepares the endotracheal tube for removal. Suction should be available to prevent blood or secretions interfere with the surgeon's view or enter the trachea. Using a No. 11 scalpel blade, a vertical incision is made in the trachea through the third, fourth and fifth tracheal rings along the score mark (Fig. 3.3.9) preserving the first tracheal ring. In neonates and infants, where distances are small, it is preferable to leave the second ring intact as well.

The surgeon asks the anesthetist to withdraw the endotracheal tube gently to clear the tracheotomy incision. A tracheostomy cannula, which should be lubricated with a water-soluble surgical lubricant, is then inserted into the tracheal opening perpendicularly to the tracheostomy and subsequently directed and rotated caudally toward the carina. A sterile anesthetic connector is fitted to the adapter and its end passed out of the surgical field to the anesthetist (Fig. 3.3.10).

Once that is achieved, the anesthetist should administer several deep breaths to the patient to prove that the infant can be ventilated adequately through the new airway, indicating that the cannula is in proper place. Equal chest rise should be observed during this maneuver. In case of unilateral right-sided

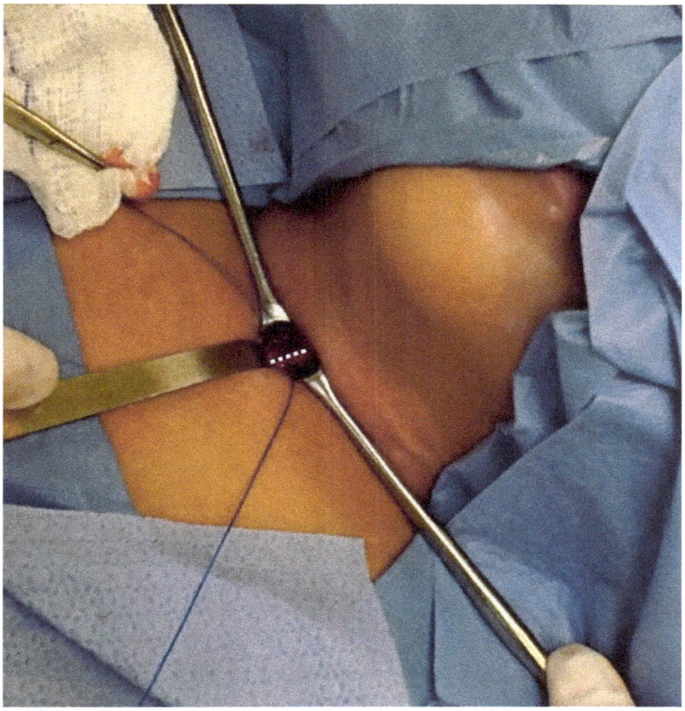

Fig. 3.3.9: The trachea is opened through a midline vertical incision across two to three tracheal rings (dotted line). The incision must be long enough to avoid excess tube pressure against the cartilages. A tight tube can result in pressure deformity and reabsorption of cartilage.

chest rise, the tracheostomy tube may be too long and should be exchanged for a shorter one.

Particularly in neonates, even a cannula of the correct diameter may ultimately be too long with its tip resting on the carina. In such cases, several pieces of gauze may be used to bolster the gap between the skin level and the tracheostomy collar, thus pulling the tip of the cannula away from the carina.

While the assistant holds the tracheostomy tube in place, the skin edges may be secured with sutures on each side of the tube (Fig. 3.3.11). Special care has to be taken to leave a gap of the skin around the tube to avoid postoperative surgical emphysema by allowing air to escape. Finally, the lateral wings of the cannula body need to be secured to the patient. The roll underneath the patients' shoulders is then removed and an umbilical or hook-and-loop tape placed around the neck. This tape is passed through the holes in the end of the wings and then tied tightly with the neck in flexed position, which may prevent tube dislodgement.

The two Polypropylene stay sutures that were placed in the anterior tracheal wall are now tied at their ends, left 6–8 cm in length, and taped securely to the anterior

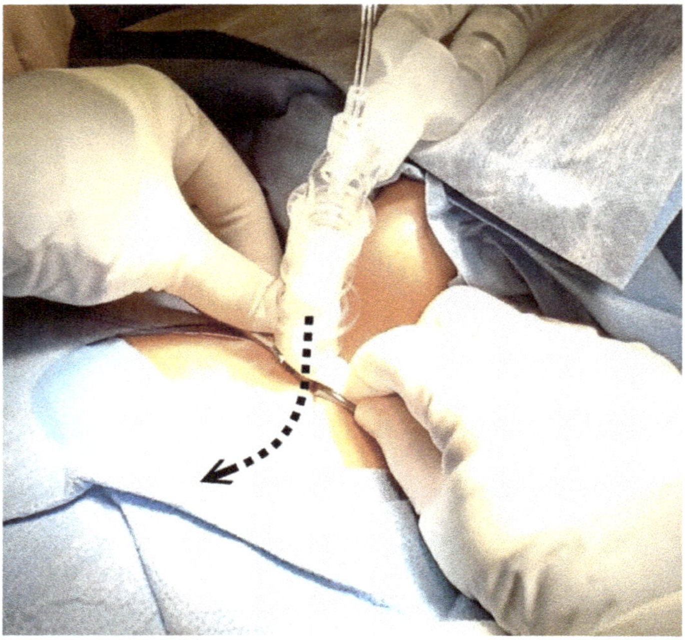

Fig. 3.3.10: Tube insertion into the trachea is accomplished by having the anesthetist pull back the endotracheal tube to the cephalad margin of the new stoma, inserting a tracheal suction catheter downwards into the trachea through the newly established opening, and then advancing the tracheostomy tube over the catheter into the trachea caudally (direction of the black interrupted arrow). This method is safer than using the tube obturator, the short tip of which sometimes slips out of the stoma and allows the tracheostomy tube to pass anterior to the trachea and into the mediastinum through a false tract.

chest wall. In this location they can be easily found and pulled apart to identify the tracheal incision if needed in an emergency to reinsertion of the cannula (Fig. 3.3.12).

All infants with a fresh tracheostomy should be transferred to the intensive care unit (ICU) for close observation.

Video showing a tracheostomy surgery (Quelle: „Anna Junge, http://medjunge.de/“). https://www.degruyter.com/view/supplement/9783110419825_Tracheostomy.mp4

Early postoperative care

Most surgeons order a chest X-ray in the recovery room or ICU to verify that the tip of the cannula is sufficiently clear of the carina (Fig. 3.3.13). However, the utility of

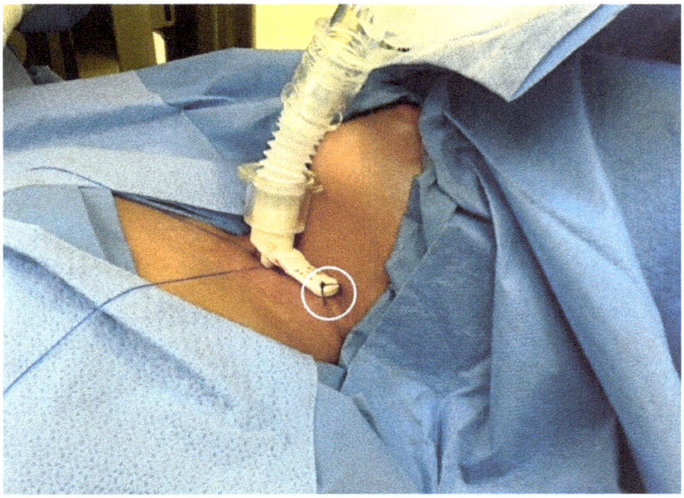

Fig. 3.3.11: The wings of the tracheostomy tube are bilaterally sutured to the lateral cervical skin to prevent acute dislodgement of the fresh tracheostomy using 2-0 silk sutures (circle). These sutures will be cut at the time of the first cannula change.

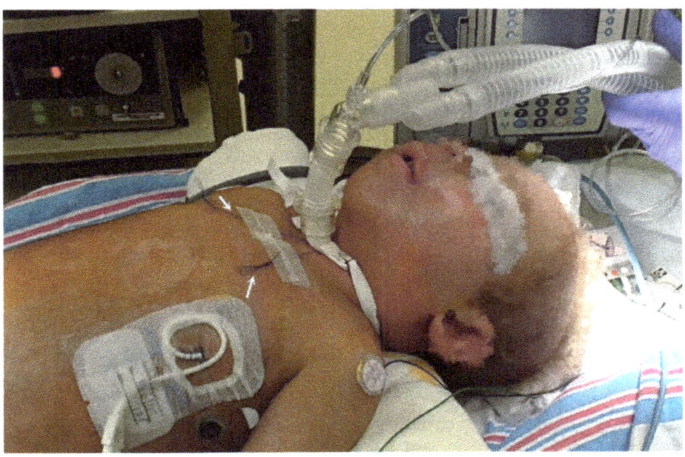

Fig. 3.3.12: The two Polypropylene stay sutures that were placed laterally at the site of tracheotomy are tied in loose loops and taped securely to the anterior chest wall (white arrows). The sutures are left in place until the first tracheostomy change as a precaution against accidental postoperative decannulation. In this location, they can be easily found and pulled apart to identify the tracheal incision in case they are needed in an emergency reinsertion of the cannula.

routine postoperative chest radiography in pediatric tracheostomy has recently been questioned. Some authors suggest to reserve a postoperative chest radiography for cases with suspicion of a complication on the basis of intraoperative findings or clinical parameters [58].

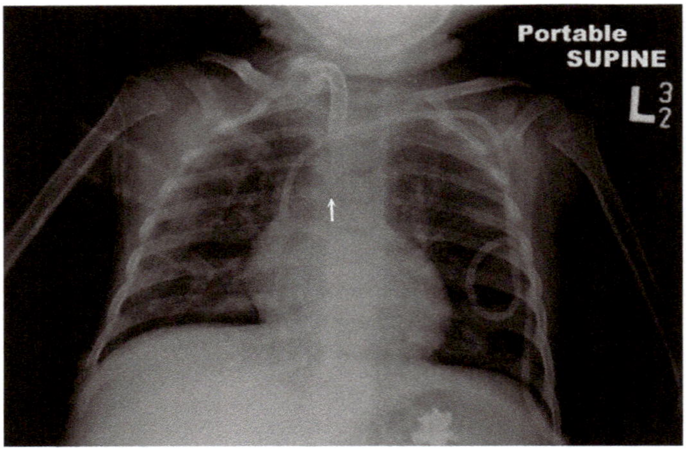

Fig. 3.3.13: A postoperative plain chest radiograph is ordered either on the operating table or in the recovery room to verify good placement of the tracheostomy. Ideally, the tip of the cannula should be located in the mid-trachea, half way between the insertion site and the carina (white arrow).

A spare tracheostomy cannula of the same model and size as the one placed primarily in the patient must be available at the bedside at all times. The tracheostomy tube should be kept clear of secretions by frequent intermittent suctioning, particularly in the immediate postoperative period. Moreover, adequate humidification of the inspired gas should be provided.

During the first postoperative week, the site of the tracheostomy has to be cleaned at least once a day. The fresh cannula should be left in place for at least 10 days. Thereafter, with appropriate tract formation, the tracheostomy tube can be changed safely for the first time. The sutures to the edges of the tracheal incision should be left in place until the first tracheostomy change. All tracheostomy exchanges are an opportunity to instruct the parents or caregivers on the procedure. Ideally, the parents will be able to change the tracheostomy with confidence and competence at the time of discharge. Once it is evident that the tracheostomy tube can be replaced with ease it is safe to remove the sutures at the edges of tracheal incision.

Home instruction and care

Extensive education of the parents or caregivers along with preparation of a safe home environment is essential for a smooth and successful transition to home care. Prior to the child's discharge, all caregivers must undergo a structured and detailed training program to become competent in long-term tracheostomy management. This training includes the acquisition of skills in tube exchange, suctioning, cleaning, dressing, fixation, as well as humidification of inspired air, and application of medications. Parents and all caregivers have to become familiar with equipment for continuous or intermittent positive pressure ventilation as well as using a bag valve mask device for manual ventilation in conjunction with suctioning. Last but not least, the family or caretakers must be instructed and certified in emergency management and cardiopulmonary resuscitation [53]. They must know how to troubleshoot the entire system in case of problems, including the technical devices, and the cannula attachments [59, 60].

The first cannula change should be should be performed on the surgical ward and take advantage of the opportunity to further instruct and reassure the parents. Until the family becomes familiar and comfortable with the management of the cannula and new devices, home nursing visits should be arranged. The presence of a nurse at home is absolutely mandatory for the first scheduled tracheostomy change outside of the hospital after discharge.

Complications

Different series have reported complication rates ranging from 30%–86% [61–63]. The incidence of complications is related to the initial indication for the tracheostomy [64]. Moreover, higher complication rates occur in pre-term infants and are associated with gestational age, low birth weight and medical condition of the child.

During procedure

- Damage to surrounding structures, e.g. esophagus, recurrent laryngeal nerve, brachiocephalic vein
- Hemorrhage
- Pneumothorax/Pneumomediastinum

Accidental injuries to the surrounding structures should be rare if the surgeon is familiar with the anatomy of the infant's neck. Correspondingly, damage to the vagus nerves, the recurrent laryngeal nerves, the esophagus or brachiocephalic vessels has not been described in recent pediatric series [61–63].

Hemorrhage may occur at the time of surgery and is generally controlled easily with electrocautery or vessel ligation. Rarely, especially in neonates, the thyroid gland is located near the incision site on the anterior trachea and is inadvertently divided or lacerated. In such cases, bleeding can usually be controlled with sutures or electrocautery.

Under rare circumstances, a false passage may be created during the introduction of the tube, and subsequent positive pressure ventilation will result in a pneumothorax or pneumomediastinum [58, 63].

Immediate post-op

- Surgical emphysema
- Bleeding if case of innominate or inferior thyroid artery laceration
- Obstruction (e.g. clot, mucus)
- Dislodgement

Surgical emphysema

Among the most prominent early complications are air-tracking issues, such as pneumothorax, pneumomediastinum and subcutaneous emphysema. However, in a recent study on 421 pediatric tracheostomies, these complications occurred in only 0.7% of all cases [58]. In this series no significant relationships were found between the incidence of air-tracking complication and surgical specialty, patient age or circumstances of the procedure (elective, urgent/emergent) [58].

Bleeding

Compared to intraoperative bleeding, late hemorrhage is often more problematic and can be more serious. The first step of management is to assess whether the hemorrhage is coming from the tracheal lumen or from the lateral tissues at the site of the incision. This is accomplished by suctioning the cannula and inspecting the wound carefully. If the source of bleeding is a small skin vessel, it usually can be controlled with simple suture ligation or sometimes even with infiltration of 1% Lidocaine containing 1:100 000 epinephrine.

A rare type of hemorrhage during the early postoperative course is profuse bleeding from one of the great vessels, such as the innominate vein or artery. This can occur from erosion of the vessels when a deep and tight-fitting tracheostomy tube compresses the vessels against the manubrium or clavicle. After surgical tracheostomy, the frequency of this severe complication is reported to be 0.1%–1% with a peak incidence at 7–14 days post procedure. It is usually fatal unless immediate treatment is instituted [65, 66].

Obstruction, e.g. clot, mucus

The cannula can be blocked by mucus, blood clots, or pressure of the airway walls. Blockage can be prevented by frequent suctioning, air humidification and selecting an appropriately sized tracheostomy tube.

Dislodgement

At all times, and especially in the immediate postoperative period, the cannula can become dislodged. As described earlier, there are different techniques for securing the cannula in place in order to avoid this complication. Even so, despite all best efforts, the neck tie may pull loose, and sutures may tear, allowing the cannula to dislodge. If dislodgement occurs, it must be noticed immediately. Therefore, it is recommended to transfer all infants to the intensive care unit after the procedure for close observation. Replacing the cannula in this situation should be performed by someone familiar with cannula insertion. Ideally, a surgeon is available to replace the cannula and resecure the device. As explained earlier in the chapter, the stay sutures on either side of the trachea should be taped to facilitateaccess and retraction in order to expose the tracheal lumen. Usually it is not necessary to use instruments to insert the cannula.

However, if no proper exposure can be achieved, two small right-angled retractors are sufficient to complete the job.

Late post-op & homecare

- Obstruction and dislodgement of tube
- Granulation tissue
- Infection/wound breakdown
- Erosion of the tracheostomy tube
- Fibrosis, scarring, stenosis of the trachea

The most common complications of home care include partial obstruction of the cannula and accidental decannulation. Therefore, the importance of proper education and training of parents and caretakers in tracheostomy management, particularly in suctioning, cleaning and changing the cannula, can't be emphasized enough [67–69].

In the long term, persistent granulation tissue may develop at the tracheostomy site as a result of chronic irritation of the tip of the tracheostomy tube against the tracheal wall or from the repeated suctioning of the trachea. The incidence is reported around 10%. Granulation tissue can be exophytic at the level of the skin, or intraluminal. Exophytic granulation tissue at the skin should be cauterized with silver nitrate. This can be initiated during outpatient visits and carried out by the caretakers every month if needed. In case of granulation tissue located within the trachea at the stoma site, it can be left alone in most of the cases until decannulation. In contrast, the formation of granulation tissue at the tip of the cannula can create a 'ball-valve' effect with air trapping leading to obstructive symptoms or bleeding. This can be confirmed by introducing a flexible bronchoscope through the cannula to visualize the tracheal lumen beyond the tip of the tube. Many authors suggest to remove intraluminal granulation tissue with laser treatments, which are applied via flexible fiber [70].

Infection is an unusual complication and should be treated with the appropriate antimicrobials according to culture results. A superficial wound dehiscence is usually treated conservatively.

The presence of a tracheostomy increases mortality as well as morbidity. In a retrospective observational cohort analysis of 228 children enrolled in a university-affiliated home mechanical ventilation program Edwards et al. reported that tracheostomy-related deaths were responsible for 19% of all deaths in this patient population. Complications included obstruction of the tube, bleeding from tracheal granulomas and misplacement of the tracheostomy tube into a false track [71]. However, other studies report on death-rates directly attributable to tracheostomy complications of only 0.7% [61]. Downes and Pilmer compared the incidence of life-threatening tracheostomy-related accidents in children during home ventilation to those cared for in the hospital in the early 1980s [72]. In this study, the frequency was found to be eight times greater among those cared for at home (2.3/10,000 patient days) versus the pediatric ICU (0.3/10,000 patient days).

Special considerations

Ex uterointrapartumtherapy (EXIT)

When congenital high airway obstruction is diagnosed prenatally, management may include tracheostomy during ex utero intrapartum therapy (EXIT). In such cases, the baby is delivered via controlled C-section with the placental circulation and the umbilical cord intact while an airway is secured. If this cannot be achieved by transpharyngeal endotracheal intubation, tracheostomy must be considered as a life-saving procedure.

EXIT procedures have been initially described as an approach to secure the newborn's airway after prenatal tracheal occlusion for treatment of lung hypoplasia in the setting of congenital diaphragmatic hernia [73]. Within the last two decades,the indications for an EXIT procedure have been expanded to secure the fetal airway before complete delivery whenever severe compromise of the neonatal airway is anticipated (e.g. extrinsic or intrinsic obstructive malformations of the lung, large neck masses and intrathoracic lesions) [74]. Outcomes for fetuses with those lesions have dramatically improved due to the introduction and the advancement of this technique [75]. Using EXIT it is possible to secure the fetal airway and even safely perform surgery on the fetus while uteroplacental blood flow is preserved [74].

In most centers, EXIT is not a routinely performed surgical procedure. An experienced interdisciplinary team (anesthesiology, gynecology, neonatology and pediatric surgery), extensive, meticulous planning and close intra-operative monitoring (fetal pulse oximetry, echocardiography, i.v. access) is required [72].

Tracheostomy during EXIT-to-airway is frequently needed when conventional transpharyngealendotracheal intubation failed, especially in patients with fetal neck masses or other causes of fetal airway obstruction such as tracheal atresia or other congenital high airway obstruction [75]. In particular, prenatal diagnosis of an underdeveloped chin, micrognathia and possibly polyhydramnios as present in patients with Pierre-Robins-Sequence (triad of micrognathia, glossoptosis and U-shaped palatal cleft) [76] should be a red flag for the team that is preparing an EXIT procedure and possibly, tracheostomy (Figs. 3.3.14 and 3.3.15). The tracheostomy itself is performed in the previously described technique.

Emergency needle cricothyroidotomy

Rarely, a pediatric surgeon may be required to emergently obtain an airway in an infant who is too unstable for transport to the operating room, and in whom the airway is acutely compromised in a way that precludes securing it noninvasively. In this situation, a bedside needle cricothyroidotomy may at least temporarily allow for adequate gas exchange until a more definitive airway can be obtained [77].

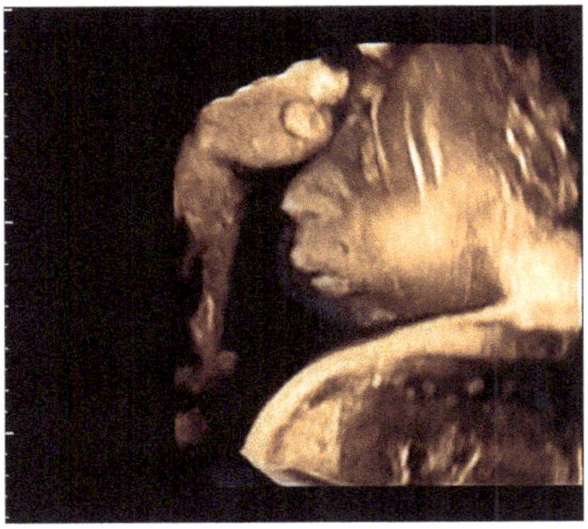

Fig. 3.3.14: Prenatal ultrasound of a fetus, gestational age: 30+5 weeks, with micrognathia (photo: courtesy of Hasbargen U, MD, PhD. Department of Gynecology and Obstetrics, Ludwig-Maximilians-University, Munich, Germany).

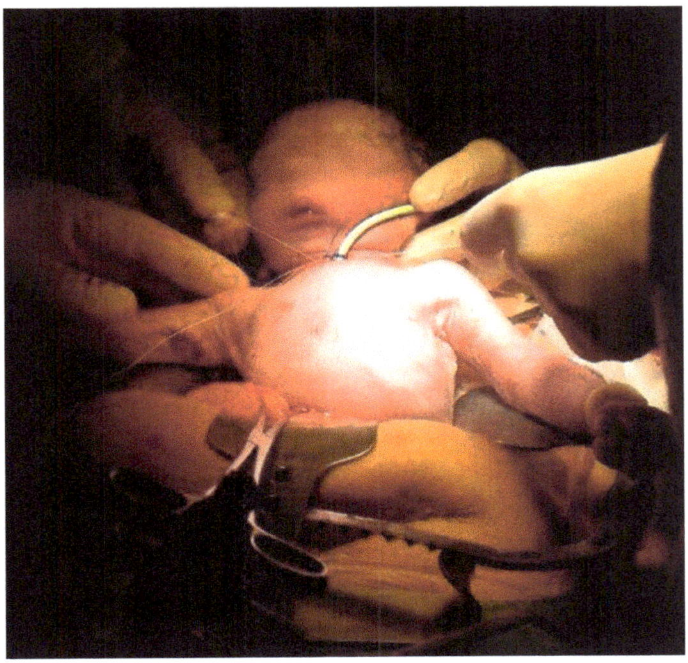

Fig. 3.3.15: Intraoperative impression of a tracheotomy procedure during EXIT. The fetus remains partly *in utero* and connected to the uteroplacental blood flow until the airway is secure. (photo: courtesy of Hasbargen U, MD, PhD. Department of Gynecology and Obstetrics, Ludwig-Maximilians-University, Munich, Germany).

Needle cricothyroidotomy is technically easier and quicker to perform on children than surgical, incisional cricothyroidotomy. It is indicated as a life-saving rescue procedure when an airway cannot be obtained and maintained by conventional means (bag-mask, endotracheal intubation, laryngeal mask, etc.).

The equipment required includes a 16 or 18 g intravenous over-the needle catheter, a 5-ml syringe, the adapter hub of a 3.0-mm endotracheal tube, an oxygen tube that can connect the source (wall outlet or oxygen tank), and a bag-valve device that will attach to a standard endotracheal tube.

The patient is positioned supine on a shoulder roll and the neck is extended. Sedation or local anesthesia is given as indicated. The anterior neck is prepped and draped in a sterile fashion. Right-hand dominant surgeons should stand on the patient's left. In this case, the left hand palpates the cricothyroid membrane with the index fingertip and stabilizes the trachea in the midline between the thumb and middle finger. The dominant right hand is used to insert the over-the-needle catheter with a connected 5-ml syringe through the cricothyroid membrane percutaneously, and advance it at a 45° angle inferiorly. The plunger of the syringe is slighly withdrawn to create a vacuum while the catheter needle is advanced. Once the needle enters the trachea, the practitioner will notice air entry into the syringe (filling the syringe with a few ml of saline before the maneuver can help by demonstrating bubbles upon entry). Once intratracheal position is verified, the catheter is advanced over the needle into the trachea, and the needle is withdrawn. The catheter is hubbed down to the skin, correct placement is confirmed by again aspirating air through the catheter, and it is secured in place using tape.

Subsequently, the 3.0-mm endotracheal tube adapter hub is connected to the intravenous catheter (this particular size hub will fit into the Luer-lock connector of the catheter). The oxygen tubing is connected via a bag-valve device [78]. A continuous flow of 8–15 l/min of 100% oxygen is titrated to achieve adequate oxygenation without pulmonary overdistension. In principle, the needle cricothyroidotomy provides influx of oxygen into the lungs, while efflux relies on passive flow through the patient's incompletely obstructed natural airways. If the patient's chest becomes hyperinflated, the inflow should be cycled to allow at least partial expiration through the catheter. Alternatively, a jet ventilator may be connected for jet ventilation if personnel with appropriate experience are available. Complications of needle cricothyroidotomy include bleeding, infection, aspiration, mechanical obstruction of the catheter, barotrauma including pneumothorax and damage to the surrounding structures.

Decannulation

When the initial indication for a tracheostomy no longer exists decannulation should be considered. Although this procedure is usually anticipated well in advance, certain criteria have to be met prior to removal of the tracheostomy tube:

- The original upper-airway obstruction is resolved
- Airway secretions are controlled
- Mechanical ventilation is no longer needed.

The timing for decannulation depends mostly on the indication for the tracheostomy in the first place. Children with subglottic stenosis may have their tube removed at the time of their laryngoplasty, which may be any time between 4–6 months and 2 years postoperatively, sometimes even later. If the reason for tracheostomy was severe tracheomalacia, it would be unusual to attempt decannulation within the first year of age. Instead, the infant should undergo repetitive bronchoscopic examination to assess whether malacia is still present and free of any potential obstructing lesions such as granulation tissue. For this purpose, the patient should not be paralyzed and the anesthesia should be light.

At some point the airway will be mature enough and the airway remains patent, so decannulation can be attempted.

Practical steps of the procedure

There is no single best way of tracheal decannulation. In each child, the approach should be tailored to the individual's condition [79].

Based on practice rather than evidence, the process of decannulation consists of the following four steps:

- Confirmation of airway patency
- Weaning and capping
- Removal of tracheostomy tube
- Closure of the tracheocutaneous fistula (spontaneous or surgically).

Weaning

There are various methods for this process. The most common one includes the usage of a Passy-Muir Speaking Valve (PMV). The PMV requires the child to exhale through the nose/mouth while still allowing inhalation via the tracheostomy tube. By doing this, the child breathes only partially through the tracheostomy which helps the treating surgeon/pulmonologist determine whether the patient is ready to be decannulated. Another technique of weaning from a tracheostomy tube is **down-sizing;** which means that the current tracheostomy tube **size** is exchanged for a smaller size. Consequently, the resistance to breathing through the tracheostomy increases, usually requiring more respiration activity through the nose and mouth.Both techniques may be conducted in combination during the weaning process.

Capping

Capping is another important step in the decannulation process. A "cap" is placed over the external tracheostomy tube opening and closes off the airflow via the tube, therefore allowing respiration exclusively through the natural upper airway. The first time the cap is trialed, the surgeon is present to closely assess the child's tolerance of breathing through the nose and mouth. After this initial capping, trials may be started using a particular schedule (e.g. when awake) or fulltime for a period of a few to several days.

If there are any signs of respiratory distress or if the child is unable to cough and clear secretions, the cap should always be removed immediately. Moreover, the child's tracheostomy tube should always remain uncapped during sleep at home as signs of airway distress may be too subtle to be recognized by family or home care nurses. An overnight capping trial should only be conducted in an ICU setting.

If a child is tolerating around-the-clock capping well, this indicates that the tracheostomy tube is no longer needed and decannulation can be planned.

The third step consists of removal the tracheostomy tube. After successful overnight capping the tube is removed the following day and the stoma is covered with a small occlusive dressing. Most surgeons keep these patients in the hospital for 24 to 48 hours, or longer if there is any concern, to assure that the tracheostomy is no longer needed.

The forth step usually happens spontaneously: the remaining tracheocutaneous (TC) fistula which is kept covered with a small bandage will start to close over the next few days to weeks. In a minority of patients (<10%), the fistula has to be surgically closed. This option would be considered if the tract is still open 1 year after decannulation in a young child. In an infant or adolescent with a larger airway, surgical closure may be conducted sooner. Usually, this minor procedure includes excising the stoma and placing a simple stitch or two in the anterior trachea.

Conclusion and future directions:
The prevalence of tracheostomy has decreased in recent years. Nowadays only 1%–2% of ventilated children require this procedure. Although it can be performed safely in experienced institutions, tracheostomy may be associated with significant morbidity and, although rare, mortality. Moreover, it continues to have a significant impact on the psychosocial development of the child. Therefore any alternative treatment option prior to proceeding with tracheostomy should be evaluated.

3.4 Further reading

[1] Eber E. Antenatal diagnosis of congenital thoracic malformations: early surgery, late surgery, or no surgery? Semin Respir Crit Care Med 2007;28:355–66.
[2] Davenport M, Eber E. Long term respiratory outcomes of congenital thoracic malformations. Semin Fetal Neonatal Med 2012;17:99–104.
[3] Langston C. New concepts in the pathology of congenital lung malformations. Semin Pediatr Surg 2003;12:17–37.
[4] Kunisaki SM, Fauza DO, Nemes LP, et al. Bronchial atresia: the hidden pathology within a spectrum of prenatally diagnosed lung masses. J Pediatr Surg 2006;41:61–5.
[5] EUROCAT: European Surveillance of Congenital Anomalies. www.eurocat-network.eu/
[6] Stocker JT. Congenital pulmonary airway malformation: a new name and expanded classification of congenital cystic adenomatoid malformation of the lung. Histopathology 2002;41(Suppl. 2):424–31.

[7] Kotecha S, Barbato A, Bush A, et al. Antenatal and postnatal management of congenital cystic adenomatoid malformation. Paediatr Respir Rev 2012;13:162–70.

[8] Stanton M, Njere I, Ade-Ajayi N, Patel S, Davenport M. Systematic review and meta-analysis of the postnatal management of congenital cystic lung lesions. J Pediatr Surg 2009;44:1027–33.

[9] Baird R, Puligandla PS, Laberge JM. Congenital lung malformations: informing best practice. Semin Pediatr Surg 2014;23:270–7.

[10] Priest JR, Williams GM, Hill DA, Dehner LP, Jaffé A. Pulmonary cysts in early childhood and the risk of malignancy. Pediatr Pulmonol 2009;44:14–30.

[11] Nasr A, Himidan S, Pastor AC, Taylor G, Kim PC. Is congenital cystic adenomatoid malformation a premalignant lesion for pleuropulmonary blastoma? J Pediatr Surg 2010;45:1086–9.

[12] Durell J, Thakkar H, Gould S, Fowler D, Lakhoo K. Pathology of asymptomatic, prenatally diagnosed cystic lung malformations. J Pediatr Surg 2015; Nov 4. [Epub ahead of print]

[13] Brown SC, De Laat M, Proesmans M, et al. Treatment strategies for pulmonary sequestration in childhood: resection, embolization, observation? Acta Cardiol 2012;67:629–34.

[14] Cho MJ, Kim DY, Kim SC, Kim KS, Kim EA, Lee BS. Embolization versus surgical resection of pulmonary sequestration: clinical experiences with a thoracoscopic approach. J Pediatr Surg 2012;47:2228–33.

[15] Paramalingam S, Parkinson E, Sellars M, Diaz-Cano S, Nicolaides KH, Davenport M. Congenital segmental emphysema: an evolving lesion. Eur J Pediatr Surg 2010;20:78–81.

[16] Özçelik U, Göçmen A, Kiper N, Doğru D, Dilber E, Yalçin EG. Congenital lobar emphysema: evaluation and long-term follow-up of thirty cases at a single center. Pediatr Pulmonol 2003;35:384–91.

[17] Kirmani B, Kirmani B, Sogliani F. Should asymptomatic bronchogenic cysts in adults be treated conservatively or with surgery? Interact Cardiovasc Thorac Surg 2010;11:649–59.

[18] Rothenberg SS, Cromblehome TM. Congenital lung malformations. In: Ziegler M, Azizkhan R, Weber T, von Allmen D, eds. Operative Pediatric Surgery, 2nd ed. New York: McGraw Hill, 2014, pp. 407–422.

[19] Rothenberg SS. Thoracoscopic pulmonary resection. Semin Pediatr Surg 2007;16:231–237.

[20] Rothenberg SS. First decades experience with thoraco- scopic lobectomy in infants and children. J Pediatr Surg 2008;43:40–45.

[21] Diamond IR, Herrera P, Langer JC, Kim PC. Thoracoscopic versus open resection of congenital lung lesions: A case matched study. J Pediatr Surg 2007;42:1057–1061.

[22] Vu LT, Farmer DL, Nobuhara KK, Miniati D, Lee H. Thoracoscopic versus open resection for congenital cystic adenomatoid malformations of the lung. J Pediatr Surg 2008;43:35–39.

[23] Albanese CT, Sydorak RM, Tsao K, et al. Thoracoscopic lobectomy of prenatally diagnosed lung lesions. J Pediatr Surg 2003;38:553–555.

[24] Lawal TA, Gosemann JH, Kuebler JF, Gluer S, Urer BM. Thoracoscopy versus thoracotomy improves midterm musculoskeletal status and cosmesis in infants and children. Ann Thorac Surg 2009;87:224–228.

[25] Rothenberg SS, Kuenzler K, Middlesworth W, Kay S, Yoder S, Shipman K, Rodriguez R, Stolar C. Thoracoscopic lobectomy in infants <10kg with prenatally diagnosed cystic lung disease. J Laparoendosc Adv Surg Tech A 2011;21:181–184.

[26] Laje P, Pearson EG, Simpao AF, Rehman MA, Sinclair T, Hedrick HL, Adzick NS, Flake AW. The first 100 infant thoracoscopic lobectomies: Observations through the learning curve and comparison to open lobectomy. J Pediatr Surg 2015 Nov;50(11):1811–6.

[27] Fingeret A, Garcia A, Borczuk AC, Rothenberg SS, Aspelund G. Thoracoscopic lobectomy for type I pleuropulmonary blastoma in an infant. Pediatr Surg Int 2014;30:239–242.

[28] Garrett-Cox R, MacKinlay G, Munro F, Aslam A. Early experience of pediatric thoracoscopic lobectomy in the UK. J Laparoendosc Adv Surg Tech A 2008;18(3):457–459.

[29] Langston C. New concepts in the pathology of congenital lung malformations. Semin Pediatr Surg 2003;12:17–37.
[30] Peranteau WH, Boelig MM, Khalek N, et al. Effect of single and multiple courses of maternal betamethasone on prenatal congenital lung lesion growth and fetal survival. J Pediatr Surg 2016 Jan;51(1):28–32.
[31] Polites SF, Habermann EB, Zarroug AE, et al. Thoracoscopic Vs open resection of congenital cystic lung disease- utilization and outcomes in 1120 children in the United States. J Pediatr Surg 2016 DOI: http://dx.doi.org/10.1016/j.jpedsurg.2015.12.004 Published online: January 12 2016.
[32] Singh R, Davenport M. The argument for operative approach to asymptomatic lung lesions. Semin Pediatr Surg 2015;24:187–95.
[33] Kim MY, Kang CH, Park SH. Multifocal synchronous mucinous adenocarcinomas arising in congenital pulmonary airway malformation: a case report with molecular study. Histopathology. 2014 Dec;65(6):926–32.
[34] Adewale L. Anatomy and assessment of the pediatric airway. Paediatr Anaesth 2009; 19 Suppl 1:1–8.
[35] Monnier P, Ikonomidis C, Jaquet Y, George M. Proposal of a new classification for optimising outcome assessment following partial cricotracheal resections in severe pediatric subglottic stenosis. Int J Pediatr Otorhinolaryngol 2009;73:1217–21.
[36] Dankle SK, Schuller DE, McClead RE. Risk factors for neonatal acquired subglottic stenosis. Ann Otol Rhinol Laryngol 1986;95:626–30.
[37] Cotton R. Management of subglottic stenosis in infancy and childhood. Review of a consecutive series of cases managed by surgical reconstruction. Ann Otol Rhinol Laryngol 1978;87:649–57.
[38] Ikonomidis C, George M, Jaquet Y, Monnier P. Partial cricotracheal resection in children weighing less than 10 kilograms. Otolaryngol Head Neck Surg 2010;142:41–7.
[39] Pillai JB, Smith J, Hasan A, Spencer D. Review of pediatric airway malacia and its management, with emphasis on stenting. Eur J Cardiothorac Surg 2005;27:35–44.
[40] Koopman JP, Bogers AJ, Witsenburg M et al. Slide tracheoplasty for congenital tracheal stenosis. J Pediatr Surg 2004;39:19–23.
[41] Butler CR, Speggiorin S, Rijnberg FM et al. Outcomes of slide tracheoplasty in 101 children: a 17-year single-center experience. J Thorac Cardiovasc Surg 2014;147:1783–89.
[42] Sunwoo WS, Cha W, Song CM et al. Tracheal growth after airway stenosis surgery: serial radiographic comparative study. Acta Otolaryngol 2012; 132 Suppl 1:S124–9.
[43] Jaquet Y, Lang F, Pilloud R et al. Partial cricotracheal resection for pediatric subglottic stenosis: long-term outcome in 57 patients. J Thorac Cardiovasc Surg 2005;130:726–32.
[44] George M, Ikonomidis C, Jaquet Y, Monnier P. Partial cricotracheal resection in children: potential pitfalls and avoidance of complications. Otolaryngol Head Neck Surg 2009; 141:225–31.
[45] Hartnick CJ, Hartley BE, Lacy PD et al. Surgery for pediatric subglottic stenosis: disease-specific outcomes. Ann Otol Rhinol Laryngol 2001;110:1109–13.
[46] Aberdeen E, Downes JJ. Artificial airways in children.Surg Clin North Am 1974 Oct;54(5):1155–70.
[47] Gallagher TQ, Hartnick CJ. Pediatric tracheotomy. Adv Otorhinolaryngol 2012;73:26–30.
[48] Principi T, Morrison GC, Matsui DM, et al. Elective tracheostomy in mechanically ventilated children in Canada. Intensive Care Med 2008 Aug;34(8):1498–1502.
[49] Wood D, McShane P, Davis P. Tracheostomy in children admitted to paediatric intensive care. Arch Dis Child 2012 Oct;97(10):866–69.
[50] Hoskote A, Cohen G, Goldman A, Shekerdemian L. Tracheostomy in infants and children after cardiothoracic surgery: indications, associated risk factors, and timing. J Thorac Cardiovasc Surg 2005 Oct;130(4):1086–93.

[51] McMurray JS, Holinger LD. Otolaryngic manifestations in children presenting with apparent life-threatening events. Otolaryngol Head Neck Surg 1997 Jun;116(6 Pt 1):575–9.
[52] Make BJ, Hill NS, Goldberg AI, et al. Mechanical ventilation beyond the intensive care unit. Report of a consensus conference of the American College of Chest Physicians. Chest 1998 May;113(5 Suppl):289S–344S.
[53] Sherman JM, Davis S, bamonte-Petrick S, et al. Care of the child with a chronic tracheostomy. This official statement of the American Thoracic Society was adopted by the ATS Board of Directors, July 1999. Am J Respir Crit Care Med 2000 Jan;161(1):297–308.
[54] Wetmore RF. Pediatric Otolaryngology. Tracheotomy. Philadelphia: Saunders, 2003.
[55] 2005 American Heart Association Guidelines for Cardiopulmonary Resuscitation and Emergency Cardiovascular Care; Part 12: Pediatric Advanced Life Support. http://circ.ahajournals.org/content/112/24_suppl/IV-167.full.
[56] Hofer CK, Ganter M, Tucci M, Klaghofer R, Zollinger A. How reliable is length-based determination of body weight and tracheal tube size in the paediatric age group? The Broselow tape reconsidered. Br J Anaesth 2002 Feb;88(2):283–5.
[57] Smith LP, Roy S. Operating room fires in otolaryngology: risk factors and prevention. Am J Otolaryngol 2011 Mar;32(2):109–14.
[58] Genther DJ, Thorne MC. Utility of routine postoperative chest radiography in pediatric tracheostomy. Int J Pediatr Otorhinolaryngol 2010 Dec;74(12):1397–400.
[59] Joseph RA. Tracheostomy in infants: parent education for home care. Neonatal Netw 2011 Jul;30(4):231–42.
[60] Oberwaldner B, Eber E. Tracheostomy care in the home. Paediatr Respir Rev 2006 Sep;7(3):185–90.
[61] Carr MM, Poje CP, Kingston L, Kielma D, Heard C. Complications in pediatric tracheostomies. Laryngoscope 2001 Nov;111(11 Pt 1):1925–28.
[62] Rocha EP, Dias MD, Szajmbok FE, Fontes B, Poggetti RS, Birolini D. Tracheostomy in children: there is a place for acceptable risk. J Trauma 2000 Sep;49(3):483–5.
[63] Donnelly MJ, Lacey PD, Maguire AJ. A twenty year (1971–1990) review of tracheostomies in a major paediatric hospital. Int J Pediatr Otorhinolaryngol 1996 Mar;35(1):1–9.
[64] Halfpenny W, McGurk M. Analysis of tracheostomy-associated morbidity after operations for head and neck cancer. Br J Oral Maxillofac Surg 2000 Oct;38(5):509–12.
[65] Schaefer OP, Irwin RS. Tracheoarterial fistula: an unusual complication of tracheostomy. J Intensive Care Med 1995 Mar;10(2):64–75.
[66] Allan JS, Wright CD. Tracheoinnominate fistula: diagnosis and management. Chest Surg Clin N Am 2003 May;13(2):331–41.
[67] Messineo A, Giusti F, Narne S, Mognato G, Antoniello L, Guglielmi M. The safety of home tracheostomy care for children. J Pediatr Surg 1995 Aug;30(8):1246–8.
[68] Caussade S, Paz F, Ramirez M, et al. [Clinical experience in home care of children with tracheostomy]. Rev Med Chil 2000 Nov;128(11):1221–6.
[69] Reiter K, Pernath N, Pagel P, et al. Risk factors for morbidity and mortality in pediatric home mechanical ventilation. Clin Pediatr (Phila) 2011 Mar;50(3):237–43.
[70] Epstein SK. Late complications of tracheostomy. Respir Care 2005 Apr;50(4):542–9.
[71] Edwards JD, Kun SS, Keens TG. Outcomes and causes of death in children on home mechanical ventilation via tracheostomy: an institutional and literature review. J Pediatr 2010 Dec;157(6):955–9.
[72] Downes JJ, Pilmer SL. Chronic respiratory failure–controversies in management. Crit Care Med 1993 Sep;21(9 Suppl):S363-4.
[73] Mychaliska GB, Bealer JF, Graf JL, Rosen MA, Adzick NS, Harrison MR. Operating on placental support: the ex utero intrapartum treatment procedure. J Pediatr Surg 1997 Feb;32(2):227–30.

[74] Moldenhauer JS. Ex Utero Intrapartum Therapy. SeminPediatrSurg 2013 Feb;22(1):44–49.
[75] Dighe MK, Peterson SE, Dubinsky TJ, Perkins J, Cheng E. EXIT procedure: technique and indications with prenatal imaging parameters for assessment of airway patency. Radiographics 2011 Mar;31(2):511–26.
[76] Robin P. A fall of the base of the tongue considered as a new cause of nasopharyngeal respiratory impairment: Pierre Robin sequence, a translation. 1923. Plast Reconstr Surg 1994 May;93(6):1301–3.
[77] Mace SE, Khan N. Needle cricothyrotomy. Emerg Med Clin North Am 2008 Nov;26(4): 1085–101, xi.
[78] Yealy DM, Plewa MC, Stewart RD. An evaluation of cannulae and oxygen sources for pediatric jet ventilation. Am J Emerg Med 1991 Jan;9(1):20–3.
[79] Gray RF, Todd NW, Jacobs IN. Tracheostomy decannulation in children: approaches and techniques. Laryngoscope 1998 Jan;108(1 Pt 1):8–12.

Clemens Aigner, Walter Klepetko

4 Lung transplantation

4.1 Introduction

The performance of pediatric lung transplantation remains the domain of a few highly specialized centers. Written by the experts **Clemens Aigner and Walter Klepetko**, and supported by **Axel Haverich**, this chapter presents a state-of-the-art position.

4.2 General considerations

Lung transplantation is an established therapy for virtually all non-malignant end-stage lung diseases. Lung transplantation in children presents some unique challenges that are not directly comparable to adult lung transplantation. This article focuses on the perioperative surgical aspects of the procedure. Differences in the immune system, tolerance mechanisms, psychosocial and long term care are equally important, however, they are beyond the scope of this chapter. The first pediatric lung transplantation was performed in a 16-year-old boy in 1987 in Toronto [1]. Pediatric lung transplantation is a relatively rare procedure with around 120 procedures reported annually to the registry of the International Society for Heart and Lung Transplantation by 45 centers [2]. Even large centers perform only 10–20 procedures per year. Ideally this complex treatment should be performed in dedicated centers of expertise only. Survival after pediatric lung transplantation has improved over recent years mainly due to improvements in candidate selection, immunosuppression and refinements in the surgical technique and perioperative management.

4.3 Indications

Children in need of lung transplantation represent a specific spectrum of indications. Almost 80% of the children are older than 11 years at the time of their transplant. In the case of a progressive lung disease on maximal medical therapy with a short life expectancy and a poor quality of life a referral for lung transplantation is indicated.

Cystic fibrosis (CF), pulmonary arterial hypertension, congenital heart disease and surfactant protein B deficiency are the most common indications in infant transplantation with substantial variations in different age groups (Tab. 4.3.1)[3].

Tab. 4.3.1: Common indications for pediatric lung transplatation (ISHLT registry report 2013).

Age group	Indication	% in age group
<1 year	spB Deficiency	20.4%
	CHD	14.8%
	iPAH	13.0%
	Fibrosis	13.0%
1–5 years	iPAH	21.8%
	IPF	12.6%
	Fibrosis (other)	11.5%
	OB	9.2%
	CHD	8.0%
6–10 years	CF	50.5%
	OB	10.7%
	iPAH	10.2%
	Fibrosis (other)	7.7%
>11 years	CF	69.1%
	iPAH	7.9%
	OB	4.6%

The spectrum of indications and ideal timing for referral are outlined in Tab. 4.3.2. In the recent guidelines of the International Society for Heart and Lung Transplantation (ISHLT) specific recommendations for the selection of pediatric recipients are mentioned for the first time [4].

Tab. 4.3.2: Indications and timing for referral.

Disease	Timing of referral
CF	FEV < 30%, rapid decline, increasing frequency of hospitalization and exacerbations, recurrent hemoptysis and/or pneumothorax
IPAH	WHO class III/IV, evidence of right heart failure, inadaequate reponse to medical therapy
Eisenmenger syndrome	Progressive pulmonary arterial hypertension, impaired exercise tolerance
Interstitial lung disease	Histologic evidence amd progressing functional decline
Bronchopulmonary dysplasia	Respiraotry failure, progressive pulmonary arterial hypertension
Pulmonary vascular disorders	Evidence in histology and right heart catheterization
Surfactant dysfunction	Progressive or treatment refractory respiratory failure, progressive pulmonary arterial hypertension

There are relatively few absolute contraindications to lung transplantation, which is comparable to the adult population. However, there is a long list of relative contraindications, which may vary from center to center. In the CF population, chronic infection with specific pulmonary pathogens such as the burkholderia cepacia complex may be a contraindication. In adolescent recipients, non-compliance is the main reason for chronic graft dysfunction. Thus, this needs to be addressed during the pretransplant workup. Untreatable extrapulmonary organ dysfunction usually is a contraindication for lung transplantation unless combined organ transplantation is possible. Combined lung-liver transplantation is a typical example in CF patients.

Pediatric patients requiring mechanical ventilation and extracorporeal life support still represent a high risk group for transplantation, however recent results by a number of experienced centers show very favorable outcomes in this group based on a careful patient selection.

4.4 Allocation and size matching

The average waiting time for a suitable donor lung varies significantly in different countries, however, particularly for smaller children longer waiting times can be expected thus referral and listing should be early enough. Allocation algorithms vary substantially between different countries. The lung allocation score (LAS), which has been used in the United States since 2005, was also introduced in some European countries and allocates organs based on an algorithm to calculate waiting list mortality and expected one year survival post-transplant [5, 6]. Children below the age of 12 years automatically receive the highest possible LAS score in the Eurotransplant area. In the United States there is an ongoing discussion about the allocation of lungs of donors aged > 12 years towards recipients < 12 years. Size matching is crucial and frequently limits the organ availability for pediatric recipients. Therefore several strategies have been developed to overcome this aspect of donor organ shortage and to be able to utilize oversized donors. These aspects will be discussed in detail in the chapter on surgical technique. Donor and recipient height, gender, and total lung capacity (TLC) are the most important parameters used for size matching. Depending on the underlying disease the real TLC may differ significantly from the predicted TLC of the recipient, which has to be taken into account accordingly [7].

4.5 Surgical technique and lobar transplantation

The technique of pediatric lung transplantation is basically comparable to adult transplantation. While the general principles of the operation are equal in all centers, differences in technical details can be observed. This chapter describes the Vienna technique. Intubation is usually performed with a left-sided double lumen tube to allow unilateral ventilation. In very small children a standard tube with the use of a bronchus blocker is an alternative. The choice, which lung is transplanted first, depends on donor as well as recipient issues. The preoperative recipient V/Q scan is an important tool in this decision process. Usually the functionally worse side is transplanted first. In case of a quality difference between the donor lungs, e.g. due to traumatic alterations or other minor impairments, the better lung will be transplanted first. The implantation in bilateral procedures is performed in a sequential technique.

Pneumonectomy is performed in standard fashion with stapling of the pulmonary artery and pulmonary veins. The bronchus is prepared centrally and opened with a scalpel. Two polydioxanone stay sutures are placed at the angles between the cartilaginous and the membranous portion. Thereafter the lung is removed from the chest cavity and the vessels are prepared intrapericardially. Meticulous hemostasis has to be performed before beginning with the implantation.

The donor lung is then unpacked and the vessels are prepared and shortened (Fig. 4.5.1). The pulmonary artery has to be carefully inspected for any intraluminal embolism. The bronchus is shortened with not more than one cartilage ring remaining after the separation of the upper lobe bronchus and careful preservation of the peribronchial tissue. This is equally important for the area adjacent to the anastomosis as well as the bronchus intermedius on the right side, which is particularly prone to ischemic alterations. A bacteriological swab is taken and any residual mucus is removed from the bronchial system. Thereafter the implantation is performed with permanent topical cooling of the donor lung with ice slush. The first step is the bronchial anastomosis, which is performed using a double-armed polydioxanone suture, starting at one end of the cartilaginous part, going over the membranous portion in a single running suture technique and then using the same single running suture for the anterior cartilaginous part. In case of a bronchial size mismatch the imbalance is adjusted over the whole circumference. Usually the anastomosis is not covered with any additional tissue. Some centers still use interrupted suture techniques on the cartilagineous part of the bronchus.

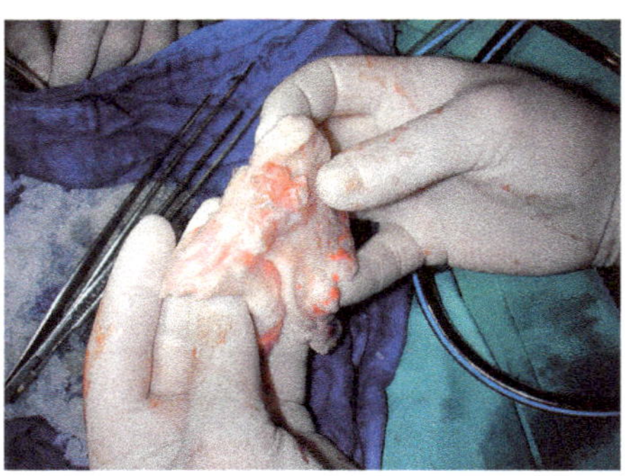

Fig. 4.5.1: Pediatric donor lung prior to implantation.

Thereafter the left atrium is clamped intrapericardially with a Satinsky clamp. A close surveillance of the hemodynamic situation is warranted at this point. The left atrium is opened and anastomosed at a level where myocardial muscle tissue is present, since at the level of the veins the tissue is too fragile to allow for a safe anastomosis. Usually a prolene running suture is used. An everting suture technique providing direct adaptation of donor and recipient endothelium is preferable to minimize the risk of thrombosis. The suture is secured with a clamp but at this stage not yet knotted. The next step is clamping and opening the pulmonary artery. The anastomosis is once more performed in a running technique.

After administering the initial dose of immunosuppression, retro- and antegrade flushing is performed to flush out the preservation solution and de-air the vasculature. Thereafter the sutures of the artery and atrium are knotted. Protective ventilation without any manual recruitment maneuvers is started at this stage. Finally hemostasis is performed with special attention to the donor pulmonary ligament and pericardium, which can be a source of substantial bleeding. After completing the implantation of the first lung the recipient pneumonectomy and implantation of the donor lung is performed in an identical way on the contralateral side.

At the end of the operation 24 French drainages are placed in the costodiaphragmatic sinus and towards the apex and the incision is closed. It is beneficial to insert an additional small drain, which can be left in place to avoid basal fluid collection without compromising mobilization of the patient after the standard chest drains are removed.

In order to increase the donor pool for pediatric recipients, methods of downsizing donor organs are important to be able to accept oversized donors [8]. In case of a minor size mismatch of up to 20%, TLC non-anatomical simple wedge resections are an effective tool to tailor the donor lung. The most accessible target areas for these resections are the middle lobe on the right side and the lingula on the left side. In case of a more pronounced size discrepancy, lobar transplantation becomes an option. The division of the lobes is performed at the backtable immediately prior to the implantation to allow the most accurate size matching. The parenchyma of the donor lung is subdivided by standard stapler devices after identification of the artery in the interlobar fissure. The arterial branches are ligated, the veins and the bronchus are divided and after complete excision of the lobar carina, the lobes are separated and the implantation is performed in standard fashion. Polydioxanone 5/0 is used for the bronchial anastomosis. Lobar transplantations can be performed using all combinations of lobes, with the exception of a right upper lobe in combination with the middle lobe, which should be avoided since it requires leaving a bronchial stump, which is at high risk for dehiscence.

4.6 Living donation

Living donor lobar transplantation is an alternative for pediatric recipients if a cadaveric donor organ cannot be expected to be available in due time. Only few centers have accumulated large experience with this approach. Two adults, either parents or close relatives donate a lower lobe each to perform a bilateral lobar transplantation. In the US this approach has virtually disappeared after introduction of the lung allocation score [9]. The center in Kyoto has accumulated a large experience and developed several technical details including right and left inverted lobar transplantation and sparing the native upper lobe in recipients [10–12]. In Vienna, 5 cases of living donor lobar lung transplantation have been performed so far. Recipient outcome is comparable and in some series even superior to recipients of brain dead donor organs. No donor mortality has been described.

4.7 Extracorporeal support

There is a great variability in the use of extracorporeal support in lung transplantation. Extracorporeal life support as bridge to transplantation is increasingly used in selected patients and satisfying outcomes are demonstrated by many single center reports [13]. Patients with cystic fibrosis and pulmonary arterial hypertension are the most frequently bridged patient groups demonstrating the importance of this approach in the pediatric patient population [14, 15]. The concept of awake bridging recently has received great interest since it allows some degree of mobilization and physiotherapy and avoids the negative effects of long-term sedation. However, this approach requires a fully compliant patient and applicability has to be judged very carefully in the pediatric setting.

The pulmonary vasculature of children is not yet fully developed. In our experience recipients of pediatric organs are at an increased risk for the development of reperfusion edema and primary graft dysfunction. During a bilateral sequential procedure the first implanted lung is exposed to the entire cardiac output during the implantation of the second lung. To avoid a volume overflow the intraoperative use of extracorporeal support during the procedure is mandatory. For this purpose extracorporeal membrane oxygenation (ECMO) has replaced cardiopulmonary bypass as the routine device in many centers [16–18]. Advantages include a decreased systemic inflammatory response, the avoidance of full heparinization and – if necessary – the possibility to directly prolong the support into the postoperative period. For the intraoperative use central cannulation provides better drainage compared to a peripheral approach and is the preferred approach.

Postoperative ECMO support can be indicated for the treatment of severe primary graft dysfunction or as a planned prolongation in patients with pulmonary arterial hypertension and consecutive hemodynamic impairments. The use of adequately sized cannulas depending on the vessel diameter is required. While in adult lung recipients postoperative ECMO support is routinely performed through a femoro-femoral approach, in very small children it can be beneficial to leave the central cannulation to avoid problem with small femoral vessels.

4.8 Outcome

The most comprehensive outcome report on pediatric lung transplantation is the annual ISHLT registry report [2]. Median survival for patients receiving transplants between 1990 and 2013 was 53 years. In the pediatric population long-term outcome is independent of the age group. There is a significant survival benefit of bilateral transplantation compared to single lung transplantation with a median survival of 5.6 vs. 2.2 years (Fig. 4.8.1).

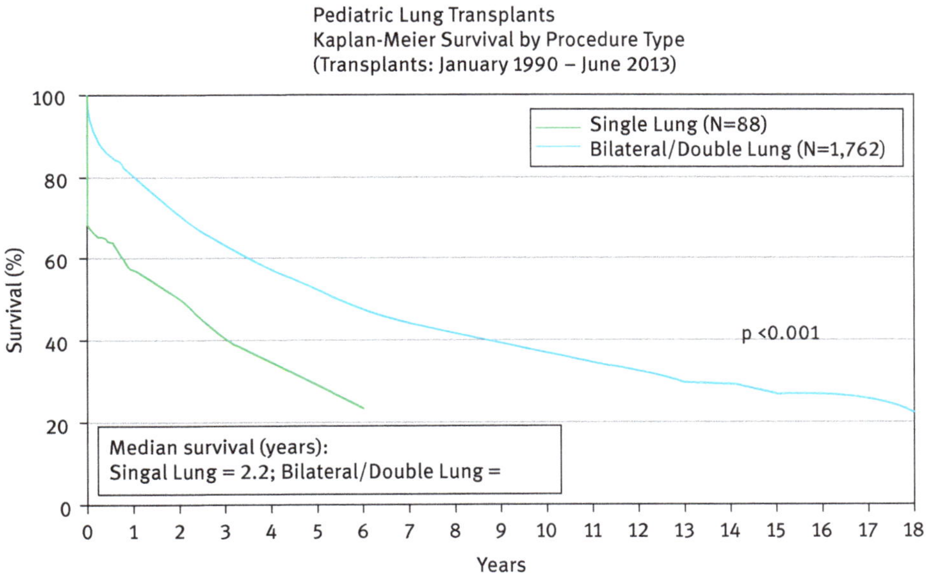

Fig. 4.8.1: ISHLT registry pediatric lung transplantation, survival single vs. double lung transplantation.

Our own experience with pediatric lung transplantation in Vienna has been published three year ago and currently in 2015 consists of 82 primary pediatric lung transplant procedures and 14 pediatric retransplantations [19]. Main indications were CF (63%), IPH (12%) and Eisenmenger (6%). The leading indication for retransplantation was CLAD in 80% of cases. In 95% of the cases bilateral procedures were performed, single lung transplantation and combined heart-lung transplantation were performed each in 2.5% of the cases. Five year survival significantly improved with increasing experience and reached 71.16% in the recent decade (Fig. 4.8.2). Freedom from chronic lung allograft dysfunction 5 years after transplantation was 72%. In our experience results in pediatric recipients are comparable to the adult population in the recent decade.

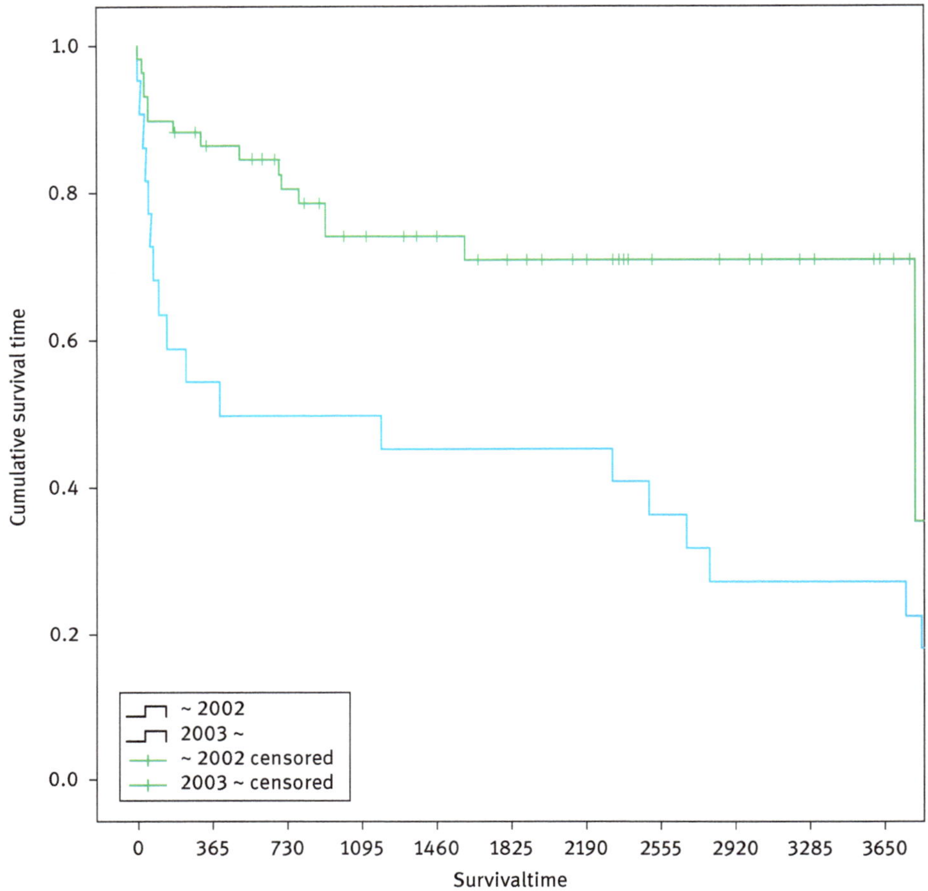

Fig. 4.8.2: Vienna pediatric lung transplantation, survival comparison 1989–2002 versus 2003–2014 (p = 0,002). One year survival 54.5% vs. 86.6%; 5 year survival 45.5% vs. 71.1%; 10 year survival 27.3% vs. 71.1%.

4.9 Retransplantation

Retransplantation in the pediatric setting is obviously very rare with only five to eight procedures reported annually since 2000. Outcome after pediatric retransplantation is worse compared to primary transplantation with a 1 year survival of 56.88% and a 5 year survival of 33.9%, however, these results have significantly improved in the past years and 5 year survival rates of more than 40% have been reported by single centers [20] and in patients undergoing retransplantation more than 12 months after primary transplantation. Mirroring the situation in adult recipients, survival rates for retransplantation later than 12 months after the primary procedure are significantly better compared to early retransplantation less than a year after primary lung transplantation [21]. In our own experience retransplantation for chronic lung allograft dysfunction successfully prolongs patient survival with 62.3% 5 year survival after the first retransplant procedure. Due to continuous improvements in outcome, more patients are presenting for retransplantation and a growing number of experienced centers have started to perform pediatric retransplantation. Lobar and size reduced lung transplantations are important options in paediatric retransplantation equal to the primary procedure [22].

4.10 Summary

Lung transplantation in children is a rare, however well established procedure providing equal outcomes to adult lung transplantation. Due to the complex management of these patients it should be performed in dedicated centers of excellence only to provide the best possible outcome.

Axel Haverich

Comment

Lung transplantation in children remains a challenge in many aspects. Notwithstanding translating adult surgery to a smaller individual, significant characteristics of pediatric organ transplantation in general have to be recognized. Surgery starts with the indication. In their chapter on 'Indication for ped-LTx', Aigner and Klepetko rightly focus on the characteristics of various lung diseases in different age groups with respect to indication for surgery. In our experience at Hannover Medical School, lung dysplasia represents an important indication in the very young age group, as listed in Tab. 4.3.2, data from the ISHLT. Here, psycho-social inflictions become overt, probably more so than in other indications since the patients may have never left the hospital after their birth.

Like in heart, kidney and liver transplantation, organ donation remains one impeding factor of broader application of lung transplantation in children. Accordingly, both downsizing larger donor organs and living-related concepts have been adapted from liver transplantation in children. The surgical technique in lung transplantation is correctly described by the authors. Long-term results, however, remain significantly inferior in lung transplants than after pediatric liver transplantation, which highlights the enormous importance of the lung as an organ directly communicating with the outside world.

This fact seems to play an even more important role in children than in adults, which may hint at bronchiogenic infections as a potentially precipitating factor of chronic allograft dysfunction. However, while ventricular assist devices do only play a bridging role in HTx, ECMO has been shown to exhibit a rescue function after the operative procedure, as well. The Vienna group has to be complimented for their initial introduction of this therapeutic concept, especially in patients, adults and pediatric, undergoing lung replacement for PHT. Altogether, this chapter comprises a fine review of our current knowledge in pediatric lung transplantation. Its increased clinical application should stimulate reading, not only by pediatric surgeons.

4.11 Further reading

[1] Mendeloff EN. The history of pediatric heart and lung transplantation. Pediatr Transplant. 2002 Aug;6(4):270–9.

[2] Goldfarb SB, Benden C, Edwards LB, Kucheryavaya AY, Dipchand AI, Levvey BJ, Lund LH, Meiser B, Rossano JW, Yusen RD, Stehlik J. The Registry of the International Society for Heart and Lung Transplantation: Eighteenth Official Pediatric Lung and Heart-Lung Transplantation Report-2015; Focus Theme: Early Graft Failure. J Heart Lung Transplant. 2015 Oct;34(10):1255–63.

[3] Kirkby S, Hayes D Jr. Pediatric lung transplantation: indications and outcomes. J Thorac Dis. 2014 Aug;6(8):1024–31.

[4] Weill D, Benden C, Corris PA, Dark JH, Davis RD, Keshavjee S, Lederer DJ, Mulligan MJ, Patterson GA, Singer LG, Snell GI, Verleden GM, Zamora MR, Glanville AR. A consensus document for the selection of lung transplant candidates: 2014 — an update from the Pulmonary Transplantation Council of the International Society for Heart and Lung Transplantation. J Heart Lung Transplant. 2015 Jan;34(1):1–15.

[5] Eberlein M, Garrity ER, Orens JB. Lung allocation in the United States. Clin Chest Med. 2011 Jun;32(2):213–22.

[6] Gottlieb J, Greer M, Sommerwerck U, Deuse T, Witt C, Schramm R, Hagl C, Strueber M, Smits JM. Introduction of the lung allocation score in Germany. Am J Transplant. 2014 Jun;14(6):1318–27.

[7] Aigner C, Jaksch P, Taghavi S, Wisser W, Marta G, Winkler G, Dekan G, Wolner E, Klepetko W. Donor total lung capacity predicts recipient total lung capacity after size-reduced lung transplantation. J Heart Lung Transplant. 2005 Dec;24(12):2098–102.

[8] Slama A, Ghanim B, Klikovits T, Scheed A, Hoda MA, Hoetzenecker K, Jaksch P, Matilla J, Taghavi S, Klepetko W, Aigner C. Lobar lung transplantation – is it comparable with standard lung transplantation? Transpl Int. 2014 Sep;27(9):909–16.

[9] Yusen RD, Hong BA, Messersmith EE, Gillespie BW, Lopez BM, Brown KL, Odim J, Merion RM, Barr ML; RELIVE Study Group. Morbidity and mortality of live lung donation: results from the RELIVE study. Am J Transplant. 2014 Aug;14(8):1846–52.

[10] Date H, Sato M, Aoyama A, Yamada T, Mizota T, Kinoshita H, Handa T, Tanizawa K, Chin K, Minakata K, Chen F. Living-donor lobar lung transplantation provides similar survival to cadaveric lung transplantation even for very ill patients. Eur J Cardiothorac Surg. 2015 Jun;47(6):967–72.

[11] Chen F, Miyamoto E, Takemoto M, Minakata K, Yamada T, Sato M, Aoyama A, Date H. Right and left inverted lobar lung transplantation. Am J Transplant. 2015 Jun;15(6):1716–21.

[12] Aoyama A, Chen F, Minakata K, Yamazaki K, Yamada T, Sato M, Date H. Sparing Native Upper Lobes in Living-Donor Lobar Lung Transplantation: Five Cases From a Single Center. Am J Transplant. 2015 Dec;15(12):3202–7.

[13] Lang G, Taghavi S, Aigner C, Rényi-Vámos F, Jaksch P, Augustin V, Nagayama K, Ghanim B, Klepetko W. Primary lung transplantation after bridge with extracorporeal membrane oxygenation: a plea for a shift in our paradigms for indications. Transplantation. 2012 Apr 15;93(7):729–36.

[14] Schmidt F, Sasse M, Boehne M, Mueller C, Bertram H, Kuehn C, Warnecke G, Ono M, Seidemann K, Jack T, Koeditz H. Concept of "awake venovenous extracorporeal membrane oxygenation" in pediatric patients awaiting lung transplantation. Pediatr Transplant. 2013 May;17(3):224–30.
[15] Hayes D Jr, McConnell PI, Tobias JD, Whitson BA, Preston TJ, Yates AR, Galantowicz M. Survival in children on extracorporeal membrane oxygenation at the time of lung transplantation. Pediatr Transplant. 2015 Feb;19(1):87–93.
[16] Aigner C, Wisser W, Taghavi S, Lang G, Jaksch P, Czyzewski D, Klepetko W. Institutional experience with extracorporeal membrane oxygenation in lung transplantation. Eur J Cardiothorac Surg. 2007 Mar;31(3):468–73.
[17] Machuca TN, Collaud S, Mercier O, Cheung M, Cunningham V, Kim SJ, Azad S, Singer L, Yasufuku K, de Perrot M, Pierre A, McRae K, Waddell TK, Keshavjee S, Cypel M. Outcomes of intraoperative extracorporeal membrane oxygenation versus cardiopulmonary bypass for lung transplantation. J Thorac Cardiovasc Surg. 2015 Apr;149(4):1152–7.
[18] Ius F, Sommer W, Tudorache I, Avsar M, Siemeni T, Salman J, Molitoris U, Gras C, Juettner B, Puntigam J, Optenhoefel J, Greer M, Schwerk N, Gottlieb J, Welte T, Hoeper MM, Haverich A, Kuehn C, Warnecke G. Five-year experience with intraoperative extracorporeal membrane oxygenation in lung transplantation: Indications and midterm results. J Heart Lung Transplant. 2015 (Epub ahead of print).
[19] Gruber S, Eiwegger T, Nachbaur E, Tiringer K, Aigner C, Jaksch P, Keplinger M, Klepetko W, Lang G, Taghavi S, Graf A, Eichler I, Frischer T, Szépfalusi Z. Lung transplantation in children and young adults: a 20-year single-centre experience. Eur Respir J. 2012 Aug;40(2):462–9.
[20] Müller C, Görler H, Ballmann M, Gottlieb J, Simon AR, Strüber M, Hansen G. Pulmonary retransplantation in paediatric patients: a justified therapeutic option? A single-centre experience. Eur J Cardiothorac Surg. 2011 Feb;39(2):201–5.
[21] Scully BB, Zafar F, Schecter MG, Rossano JW, Mallory GB Jr, Heinle JS, Morales DL. Lung retransplantation in children: appropriate when selectively applied. Ann Thorac Surg. 2011 Feb;91(2):574–9.
[22] Aigner C. Retransplantation. Curr Opin Organ Transplant. 2015 Oct;20(5):521–6.

Jochen Hubertus and Dietrich von Schweinitz

5 Tumors in childhood and adolescence

5.1 Introduction

The indescribable benefit in pediatric oncology is that the diagnosis and treatment of each particular tumor are strictly performed in adherence to protocols that are regularly updated by national and international cooperative and interdisciplinary societies. This chapter, which was compiled by **Jochen Hubertus** and **Dietrich v. Schweinitz**, describes pulmonary, mediastinal and thoracic wall tumors and highlights some of the essential aspects of the most recent protocols developed by the SIOP (International Society of Pediatric Oncology).

5.2 Primary lung tumors in childhood and adolescence

5.2.1 General considerations

Primary lung tumors are extremely rare entities in children and adolescents. In most cases, diagnosis is difficult owing to the non-specificity of the symptoms and rarity of the disease. The overall incidence of primary, malignant, pediatric lung tumors is estimated to be 0.5 per 1,000,000 children and adolescents younger than 19 years of age, comprising only 0.2% of all pediatric malignancies [1]. In contrast, the incidence of benign lung tumors is 5 times higher, and that of metastatic lung lesions originating from Wilms tumors, osteosarcomas, Ewing sarcomas or rhabdomyosarcomas is 60 times higher [2]. Neville et al. reported an equal sex ratio, as observed in other studies [1]. The median age at diagnosis is 16 years, and the incidence increases with age; 65% of patients are between 15 and 19 years of age [1].

Unspecific symptoms are specific for primary lung tumors in this cohort. They include cough, wheezing, hemoptysis, and recurrent pneumonia [3]. Owing to this unspecific appearance and the rarity of the disease, patients are treated for respiratory infections first, and diagnosis is often delayed for up to 1 year [4, 5]. Despite this delay, the prognosis of these lesions is good to excellent for most entities [1]. The exceptions are malignancies commonly appearing later in life, including squamous cell carcinoma (SCC), adenocarcinoma and small cell lung carcinoma (SCLC). One third of these tumors would have already metastasized at time of diagnosis, and the prognosis of these patients decreases to 28% [1].

As previously described, both benign and malignant tumors are observed, while metastatic diseases are the most clinically relevant. The most common malignant histology of primary pulmonary tumors is carcinoid tumors (51.3%–63%), followed by mucoepidermoid carcinoma (9%–18%), SCC (4.5%–9%), adenocarcinoma (6.5%–8%), broncheoalveolar carcinoma (2%), SCLC (1%), pulmonary blastoma (4.5%) and others (3.9%) [1, 3].

Benign tumors include inflammatory myofibroblastic tumors (42%), arteriovenous malformations (29%), hemangiomas (11%), lymphatic/venous malformations (11%), papillomas (5%), leiomyomas (1%), mucus gland tumors (1%) and others (1%) [2, 6].

Treatment is sometimes complicated by the rarity of the tumors and their delayed diagnosis. As such, no standardized treatment protocols exist, and therapy is guided by personalized strategies. In this context, surgery plays a crucial role because complete resection of the tumor is usually feasible and essential to cure the patient. Negative predictive factors related to surgery are tumor size (>5 cm) and positive lymph nodes [3]. Another negative predictor is histology. In particular, SCC, adenocarcinoma and SCLC have poor outcomes. The different entities and their specific characteristics will be described in detail hereafter.

5.2.2 Bronchial carcinoid tumor

Bronchial carcinoid tumors account for 51.3%–63% of primary lung tumors in children and adolescents [1, 3], with an incidence of 0.25 per 1,000,000 children and adolescents younger than 19 years of age [1]. They belong to the so-called neuroendocrine tumors that can arise in almost every part of the body. Most of the well-differentiated neuroendocrine tumors are located in the intestine, while 25% originate from neuroendocrine cells in the bronchi, known as enterochromaffin cells or Kulchitsky cells [7]. More than 90% of carcinoid tumors are considered low-grade malignant tumors (<2 mitoses/10 high-power fields [HPF], nuclear pleomorphism and absence of necrosis) [7, 8]. In general, neuroendocrine bronchial tumors range from low-grade (typical bronchial carcinomas, Grade 1) to intermediate-grade (atypical bronchial carcinoids, Grade 2) to high-grade (large cell neuroendocrine carcinoma and SCLC, Grade 3) malignancies [7]. The molecular biology and cytogenetics of carcinoid tumors are still under investigation. In contrast to other carcinoid tumors, the bronchial ones do not seem to be associated with multiple endocrine neoplasia type 1 (MEN-1), an autosomal dominant genetic disorder otherwise associated with tumors of multiple endocrine organs. Sporadic neuroendocrine/carcinoid tumors have been linked to loss of heterozygosity at the *MEN1* locus (chromosome 11q13) [9]. Deletions of chromosome 11q were identified in 66% of atypical and 47% of typical carcinoid tumors. The 11q deletion was rarely identified in poorly differentiated neuroendocrine lung cancers [10].

5.2.2.1 Typical and atypical bronchial carcinoids (Grade 1/2)

Clinical presentation

Since both types of bronchial carcinoids are always located centrally in the bronchial tree, they become conspicuous, with symptoms of central obstruction, cough, hemoptysis, asthma-like symptoms or recurrent pneumonia. These symptoms are unspecific, but their recurrence in a child with obstructive pneumonia localized in the same lobe, persistent cough or wheezing that is not responsive to the usual therapy should alert the physician and suggest diagnostic procedures such as chest X-ray and bronchoscopy [8]. Carcinoid syndrome, which presents with flushing, diarrhea, palpitations and asthma-like symptoms, is caused by serotonin release from the tumor. Unlike in the gut, classic carcinoid syndrome is rare in bronchial carcinoids and is generally associated with metastatic disease [8, 11].

Diagnosis and imaging

Upon encountering the persistent symptoms described above, physicians should be aware of bronchial carcinoids as a rare, but important differential diagnosis. As a first diagnostic step, a chest radiograph is required. Additionally, endoscopy plays a central role in the diagnosis and initial management of carcinoids. A bronchial biopsy should be taken whenever possible. The macroscopic appearance of a bronchial carcinoid is a smooth, pink–reddish or yellow endobronchial mass often covered by intact mucosa [8]. Despite harvesting a biopsy for histological confirmation of the diagnosis, debulking of the obstructing mass with or without a laser is also feasible. The physician should be aware of the risk of a major hemorrhage, and careful endoscopic assessment should only be performed in specialized centers with great experience.

Laboratory parameters include chromogranin A, neuron-specific enolase (NSE), and serotonin. Urinary tests with 24-hour urinary excretion of 5-hydroxyindolacetic acid are also indicated [12]. Computed tomography (CT) of the chest with intravenous contrast enables the visualization of extra-bronchial components to distinguish tumors from atelectasis and staging of the disease. An ultrasound study of the upper abdomen is also recommended. An octreotide scintigraphy scan is useful in the case of disseminated disease or Cushing's syndrome for staging; it can also be useful during follow-up to detect local recurrence or distant metastasis. Due to the high grade of differentiation of typical bronchial carcinoids and its low metabolic activity, the role of fluorodeoxyglucose–positron emission tomography (F18-FDG-PET) scanning is more uncertain [8]. In fact, gallium-68 (Ga-68-) DOTA-PET seem to be the PET tracers of choice in the initial evaluation of patients with suspected bronchial carcinoids (Fig. 5.2.1). In this setting, Ga-68-somatostatin analogue PET/CT could be performed primarily and, if negative, F-18-FDG PET/CT could be performed subsequently [13].

Treatment

Surgery represents the treatment of choice for pulmonary carcinoids, achieving long-term survival in cases of radical resection in both adults and children [14]. Since most tumors are low-grade, lung-sparing surgery is feasible in almost all cases and should be performed whenever possible. In addition, resection can be performed with free margins of only 1–2 mm without an increase in the local recurrence rate. Oncological

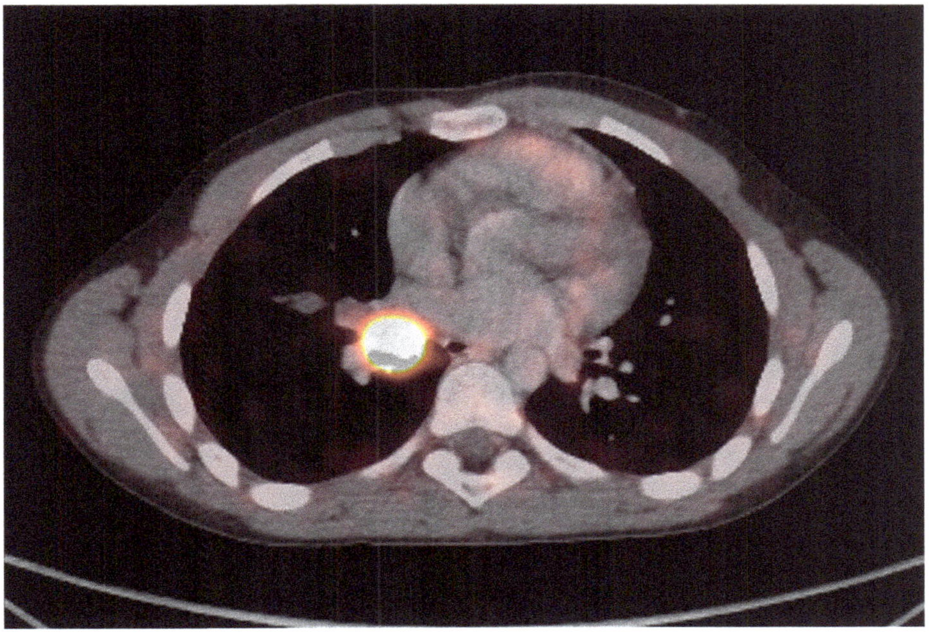

Fig. 5.2.1: PET/CT scan of an typical carcinoid of the right lower bronchus.

results are similar to those of pneumonectomy, but the quality of life and orthopedic outcomes are better after lung-sparing surgery [14], compromising bronchoplasty, wedge resection or sleeve resection (Fig. 5.2.2).

Lymph-node dissection should always be performed during tumor resection. However, whether a radical lymph-node dissection is necessary for bronchial carcinoid treatment or whether lymph-node sampling might be enough remains controversial.

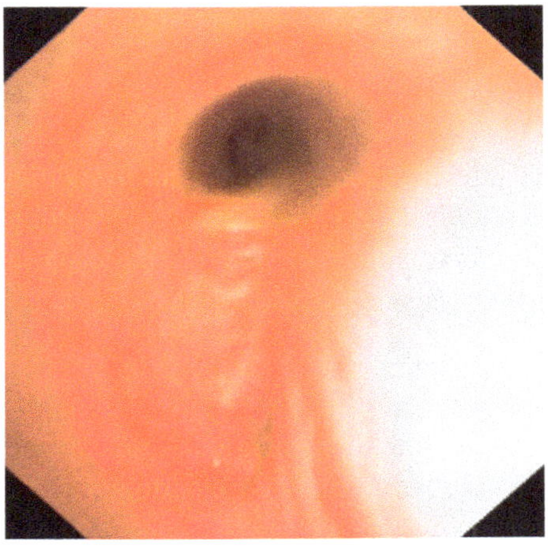

Fig. 5.2.2: Bronchoscopic view after resection of the carcinoid.

The prognostic relevance of lymph-node involvement in adult bronchial carcinoid has been described [15], but this is not yet established for children.

Currently, there is no consensus on adjuvant therapy in pulmonary carcinoids after complete resection. Indeed, both prognostic studies and trials in the adjuvant setting are lacking. Only patients with atypical carcinoids with positive lymph nodes, especially if there is a high proliferative index, should be considered for adjuvant therapy and on an individual patient basis in the context of a multidisciplinary tumor board meeting. Clinical trials are needed in this setting [16].

Prognosis

Even if the prognosis is excellent after complete tumor resection (20-year disease-free survival of 94% [8]), long-term follow-up is strongly recommended because late, local recurrences have been described.

5.2.3 Mucoepidermoid carcinoma of the bronchus

Mucoepidermoid carcinoma, as defined by the World Health Organization, is a combination of mucus-secreting, squamous and intermediate cell types. These three cell types can be organized into different patterns including glands, tubules, cysts, nests and solid areas. The relative frequency of these three cell types in a given case varies considerably and serves as one of the histologic criteria for grading this tumor. It is not uncommon in adults, but it is rare in children, even if the true incidence is unclear. The majority of the literature consists of case reports or small series. Mucoepidermoid carcinoma of the lung, however, is rare, with a reported frequency of 0.1% to 0.2% of all primary lung tumors. Usually, mucoepidermoid carcinomas arise in the parotid and submandibular salivary glands and in the minor salivary glands of the oral cavity and perimaxillary region. Mucoepidermoid carcinoma of the bronchus occurs in patients with a wide range of ages (from 3 to 78 years), and both sexes are affected equally [17].

Clinical presentation

Since mucoepidermoid carcinomas arise from salivary glands of the main bronchial tree, the clinical symptoms are unspecific and manifest as central airway obstruction with cough, hemoptysis, bronchitis, wheezing, fever and chest pain [18]. Owing to these unspecific symptoms, diagnosis is delayed in most cases.

Diagnosis and imaging

Mucoepidermoid carcinomas typically arise from bronchial mucous glands in the main stem bronchus or in the proximal portion of lobar bronchi as an endobronchial polypoid growth. Similar to the recommendations for bronchial carcinoids, every therapy refractory finding of obstructive pneumonia should lead to further investigations, starting with a chest radiograph and a bronchoscopy. However, since the tumor is covered by normal respiratory epithelium, bronchial lavage and brushing are seldom diagnostic, and forceps biopsy must be performed. Mucoepidermoid carcinomas usually present as exophytic luminal masses, which can be sessile or polypoid with a broad base connected to the bronchial wall, or pedunculated with a well-formed stalk. The cut surface is gray-white-tan with a glistening mucoid texture. Cystic degeneration can be observed in some mucoepidermoid carcinomas. The size of the tumor varies considerably within a range from several mm to 6 cm in diameter in some studies [17].

An additional chest CT scan with contrast media is necessary to visualize the size, location and involvement of the surrounding structure of the tumor. In general, lymph nodes are not involved, but they should be considered. Radiological findings include hilar or perihilar masses and associated obstructive changes (atelectasis, consolidation, bronchocele or hyperinflation) [19].

Finally, diagnosis is made histologically. As mentioned previously, mucoepidermoid carcinomas consist of three cell types that serve as one of the histologic criteria for tumor grading. The coexistence of three cell types is very characteristic for a low-grade mucoepidermoid carcinoma, but some debate remains regarding the definition of high-grade mucoepidermoid carcinoma. High-grade lesions usually demonstrate necrosis, nuclear pleomorphism, active mitosis and a solid or nested pattern of growth for the intermediate or squamous cells. In the literature, most mucoepidermoid carcinomas of the bronchus are categorized as low grade, but high-grade mucoepidermoid carcinomas arising from the bronchus have been reported in adults with a frequency as high as 50% in a few small series. Low-grade mucoepidermoid carcinoma is usually confined to the bronchus and does not involve adjacent lung parenchyma. However, in high-grade neoplasms, the tumor can infiltrate into the surrounding lung parenchyma [17, 18, 20].

Recent cytogenetic studies independently demonstrated several reciprocal chromosomal translocations frequently involving chromosome 11. Translocations of t(1;11)(p22;q13) result in overexpression of cyclin D1, and the translocations t(11;19) (q14-21;p12) and t(11; 19)(q21;p13) are capable of disrupting the Notch signaling pathway since they encode a novel fusion product, MECT1-MAML2 [17, 21].

Treatment

The regimen depends on the histological sub-type. Since low-grade tumors have a low risk of local and distal recurrences, treatment is surgical, and lung-sparing surgery is the technique of choice that can be performed as a sleeve resection, local resection, segmental resection or even lobectomy. In general, neither pneumonectomy nor endoscopic resection is recommended.

One study reported 54 patients with disease-free follow-up from 8 months up to 21 years. One patient with lymph node metastasis died, one patient developed lymph node metastasis 5 years after the initial treatment and one patient had questionable lymph node metastasis [18]. Owing to the possibility of late-onset metastatic disease, patients with mucoepidermoid carcinoma of the lung should be provided with long-term clinical follow-up. Even if the likelihood of high-grade mucoepidermoid carcinomas is extremely rare in childhood, treatment is directed by local infiltration, tumor size and lymph node metastasis. In this case, therapy is more aggressive and has to be adapted to the individual case.

5.2.4 Adenoid cystic carcinoma

The third entity of salivary gland tumors is adenoid cystic carcinoma. Typically, they arise in the lower part of the trachea or main stem bronchi, and they show extra-luminal growth [22]. These tumors are extremely rare in childhood, and only two cases have been reported [23, 24]. As for all of the other tumors described thus far, the symptoms are unspecific and include bronchial irritation or obstruction, such as cough, hemoptysis, atelectasis or pneumonitis.

The main diagnostics include a CT-scan of the chest and bronchoscopy. In contrast to bronchial carcinoids and mucoepidermoid carcinoma, adenoid cystic carcinomas are seldom observed with bronchoscopy due to the extraluminal growth.

Treatment consists of complete resection whenever feasible, adjuvant chemotherapy and radiation [5]. Neoadjuvant chemotherapy was not administered in the published reports. The surgical procedure depends on the localization and extension of the primary tumor. Resection of the trachea and reconstruction of the continuity, lobectomy, sleeve resection or even pneumonectomy are potential options.

Prognosis is poor and 8-year survival is 19.5% in adults [5]. Prognosis depends on surgery, early resection, (lung) metastasis and extra luminal extension of the tumor. Therefore, early diagnosis is mandatory for survival [5].

5.2.5 Pulmonary blastoma

Pulmonary blastomas are rare, primary lung neoplasias. The first peak incidence occurs in childhood, and 20%–25% of cases occur before 15 years of age [25]. Girls are slightly more affected (2.6:1 f:m) [26]. The etiology is still unknown, but there were some cases described in siblings with a germ-line mutation and another with proven Epstein-Barr virus infection. Finally, some pulmonary blastomas seem to arise within cystic pulmonary diseases (CPAM) [27].

These tumors are structured as fetal lung with mesenchymal and epithelial differentiation, and the primitive epithelial tissue is embedded in immature embryonic mesenchyme with areas of cartilaginous and/or striated muscle differentiation [27].

Clinical presentation

In contrast to those tumors arising in the trachea or main bronchial stem, the symptoms of pulmonary blastoma are dyspnea, fatigue, tachypnea, chest pain and recurrent pulmonary infections.

Diagnosis and imaging

This tumor appears as a solid mass, sometimes with cystic areas, on chest radiographs (Fig. 5.2.3). The space-occupying mass displaces the remaining lung and a mediastinal shift occurs [27]. Further diagnostics include a CT-scan (Fig. 5.2.4) and magnetic resonance imaging (MRI) to reveal infiltration of surrounding structures, the dimensions of the tumor, lymph node involvement and compression of the trachea and major vessels. Bronchoscopy and a biopsy complete the diagnostics [25]. Histologically, pulmonary blastoma is a biphasic tumor consisting of immature or primitive epithelial and mesenchymal components and resembles an embryonic lung. The epithelial component is composed of glands lined by columnar cells with glycogen-filled vacuoles, often resembling fetal adenocarcinomas. Squamoid morules may also be observed, and the mesenchymal component is primitive, consisting of spindle to oval cells in a myxoid stroma, sometimes including osteosarcoma, chondrosarcoma or rhabdomyosarcoma [28].

Management

Complete resection of the tumor should be targeted. However, infiltration of surrounding structures and friability of the tumor may complicate excision. In these cases,

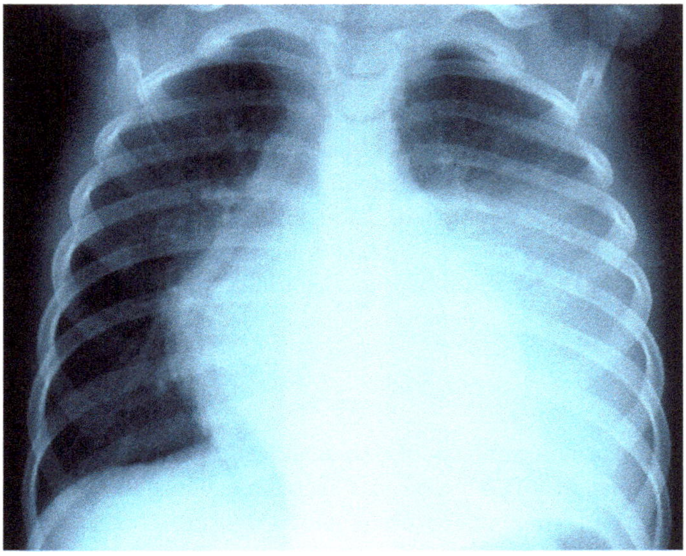

Fig. 5.2.3: Plain chest radiograph of a patient with pulmoblastoma.

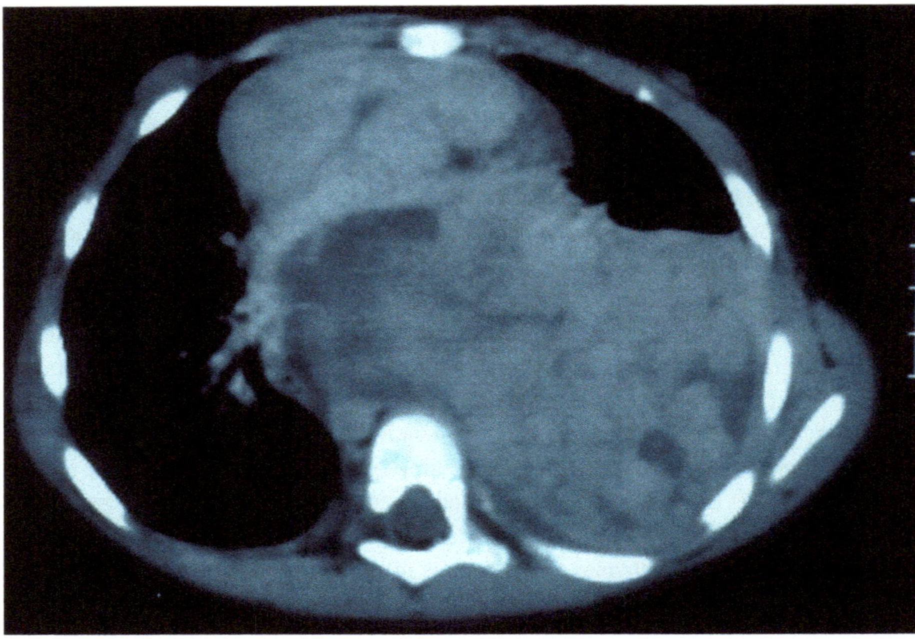

Fig. 5.2.4: Corresponding chest CT scan with large mass of pulmoblastoma.

surgery is limited to obtain tissue for histology and to reduce the tumor burden. Even in cases of macroscopically complete resections, local recurrence within a few months is quite common. Irrespective of the success of the surgery, recurrence seems to occur during the first year after diagnosis or not at all. Larsen et al. reported successful surgical excision of local recurrences in a few cases [29].

In contrast, the role of chemotherapy and radiation for the treatment of pulmonary blastoma is still unclear owing to the lack of data [29]. Sarnacki et al. reported of their experience with nine cases of pulmonary blastoma; they stated that owing to the high chemosensitivity of these tumors, pneumonectomy should be avoided for otherwise unresectable tumors and the decision to administer radiotherapy should be restricted to cases of persistent viable tumor. In order to define adjuvant chemotherapy strategies in the future, multi-institutional trials are needed.

5.2.6 Bronchioloalveolar carcinoma/adenocarcinoma in situ

Bronchioloalveolar carcinoma is a subclass of non-small-cell lung cancer and of adenocarcinomas in particular. In 2011, a revised classification renamed these tumors as adenocarcinomas in situ [30]. These tumors account for approximately 2% of malignant lung cancer in children [3]. They arise from distal bronchioles and alveoli and show a low tendency for invasive growth and metastatic spread. Rojas et al. described four cases of adenocarcinomas in situ in children [3]. None of them had metastatic disease, and the therapy of choice was complete resection with lobectomy. Radiation was not applied, and chemotherapy was administered to only one patient. Regional lymphadenectomy was performed in one patient, and none of these patients had metastases [3]. However, prognosis is excellent with a 5-year overall survival of 100% [31]. Interestingly, there are signs that adenocarcinomas in situ are associated with benign pulmonary lesions such as congenital cystic adenomatoid malformations (CPAM) or other malignant tumors [32]. Kayton et al. described in these patients with coincidental malignancies an accumulation of *KRAS* mutation or *EGRF* mutations. They proposed a lung-sparing surgery to resect the adenocarcinoma in situ.

5.2.7 Hemangiopericytoma

Hemangiopericytoma is a highly vascularized soft-tissue sarcoma (Fig. 5.2.5). These tumors are derived from fibroblastic cells and are classified as fibroblastic/ myofibroblastic tumors [33]. Most hemangiopericytomas are located at the lower extremity and the pelvis, but other regions can also be affected. Approximately 10%–20% are metastasized at the time of diagnosis, and 5%–10% of all hemangiopericytomas occur in children and adolescents. Primary lung hemangiopericytomas are extremely rare, but the lung is the primary site of metastatic disease, especially of intracranial hemangiopericytomas [34]. Interestingly, hemangiopericytomas in patients younger than 1 year show a good response to chemotherapy. Fernandez-Pineda et al. reported of good results with actinomycin D, vincristine and cyclophosphamide. The biological behavior in older children is similar to that in adults, and the response to chemotherapy is poor [33]. However, surgical resection is the most effective treatment, and complete removal of the tumor has to be sought. Results after incomplete resection are poor, and both chemotherapy and radiation are of limited value [34]. Finally, there are

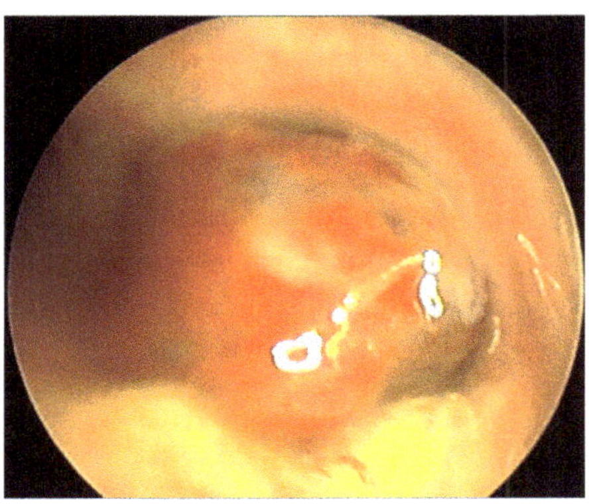

Fig. 5.2.5: Bronchoscopic view at a hemangioperizytoma.

no histological markers defining the aggressiveness of these tumors, and late recurrences are known. Therefore, a diagnostic follow-up for at least 10 years is recommended [33].

5.2.8 Inflammatory myofibroblastic tumors

Inflammatory myofibroblastic tumors are rare neoplasias that occur in children and young adults. One-third of these tumors are located in the lung, but all other sites of the body can be affected as well [35]. Inflammatory myofibroblastic tumors can arise from the lung parenchyma, bronchus and the pleura and are associated with a clinical syndrome in 15% to 30% of patients [35].

Histology

Originally, inflammatory myofibroblastic tumors were considered to be benign tumors, but there are some inflammatory myofibroblastic tumors with malignant characteristics and, occasionally, an unfavorable prognosis [36]. Additionally, identification of recurrent clonal rearrangements involving chromosome 2p in approximately 50% of cases is sufficient to characterize these tumors as true neoplasms [35].

Both the "benign" and "malignant" forms share similar morphologic features, which are not predictive of prognosis or etiology. They are characterized by fascicles of bland myofibroblasts admixed with a prominent inflammatory component [36]. Histological features include variably cellular spindle cell proliferation in a myxoid to collagenous stroma with a prominent inflammatory infiltrate composed primarily of plasma cells and lymphocytes, with occasional admixed eosinophils and neutrophils. Coffin et al. described three basic histological patterns that are often seen in combination within the same tumor: a myxoid/vascular pattern, a compact spindle cell pattern and a hypocellular fibrous (fibromatosis-like) pattern [35, 37].

Even if the etiology is still unclear, some viruses such as the Epstein-Barr virus and human herpes virus 8, have been implicated in the etiology of these tumors [36]. To date, there are no molecular markers with prognostic value.

Clinical presentation

Inflammatory myofibroblastic tumors of the lung become symptomatic with nonspecific respiratory symptoms in most cases [36]. A constitutional syndrome consisting of fever, weight loss and malaise is seen in 15%–30% of the patients [35].

Diagnosis and imaging

Laboratory tests may reveal microcytic anemia, an elevated erythrocyte sedimentation rate, thrombocytosis, and/or polyclonal hypergammaglobulinemia. In some cases, the mass may be found only after an extensive workup for a fever of unknown origin or growth failure [35]. A plain chest radiograph is useful as first-line imaging since these tumors are large enough in most cases. A chest CT scan is the next diagnostic step (Fig. 5.2.6), and the application of contrast media is advisable [38]. An additional PET-scan may be useful to screen for metastasis. However, histological examination is key to diagnosis. Biopsy can be achieved by video – assisted thoracoscopy or true-cut needle biopsy.

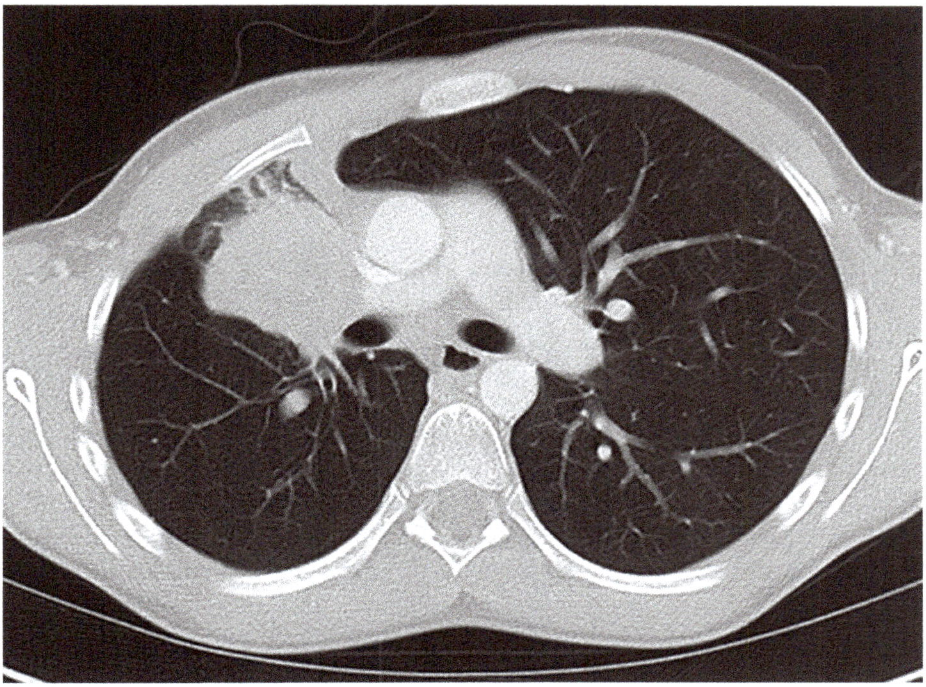

Fig. 5.2.6: CT scan with contrast of an inflammatory myofibroblastic tumor.

Treatment

After confirmation of diagnosis, complete surgical resection is the treatment option of choice. The type of resection depends on tumor localization; in any case, complete resection is mandatory, since incomplete resection is associated with high local recurrence rates [39]. In the case of giant tumors or tumors adjacent to vital structures, neoadjuvant treatment might be indicated. High-dose corticosteroids are the first-line treatment for these patients, since most inflammatory myofibroblastic tumors show a good response to treatment [39]. In the case of non-responders, rituximab is another agent with good clinical outcomes, especially in patients with orbital inflammatory disease [40]. Subsequent surgical resection can be performed

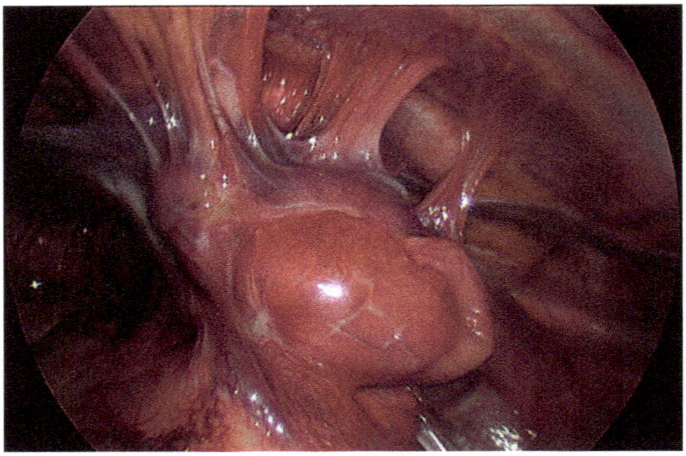

Fig. 5.2.7: Intraoperative view at the inflammatory myofibroblastic tumor.

afterwards (Fig. 5.2.7). Diagnostic follow-up should be performed for at least 10 years since cases of late, local recurrences have been described [35].

5.2.9 Pulmonary arteriovenous malformations

Pulmonary arteriovenous malformations are rare, sporadic shunts between pulmonary arteries and veins. They are characterized by a high flow, low-resistance and a right-to-left shunt. This shunt can be clinically relevant in larger malformations, resulting in hypoxia or a variety of neurologic sequelae. In most cases, these malformations are associated with the congenital, autosomal dominant, hereditary hemorrhagic telangiectasia formerly known as Osler-Weber-Rendu syndrome. Rare other causes may include trauma, cardiac surgery, malignancies and hepatopulmonary syndrome. The latter relates to the lack of the ability of the liver to metabolize vasoactive substances.

Clinical presentation

Since pulmonary arteriovenous malformations are rare diseases, it is sometimes difficult to see the link between the clinical symptoms and the underlying pathology. Therefore, pulmonary arteriovenous malformations should be considered in the evaluation of young patients who present with hypoxia/cyanosis, cerebral abscess, transient ischemic attacks (TIAs) and/or stroke [41].

Diagnosis and imaging

Seated, recumbent and post-exercise pulse oximetry may show decreased oxygen saturation on room air. An echocardiogram and electrocardiogram are mandatory to detect the ventricular load. The malformation can be seen in most cases on plain chest radiograph, but should be verified with a chest CT scan. An abdominal ultrasound is useful to exclude any other malformations. MRI of the head is mandatory in patients with neurologic disorders [41].

Treatment

Historically, pulmonary arteriovenous malformations were treated by surgical excision. To date, first-line treatment is embolization with coils by an interventional radiologist. The success rate is as high as 95%, even when including cases of recanalization [41].

Prognosis

The associated mortality of the untreated pulmonary arteriovenous malformation is estimated to range from 0% to as high as 55%, depending on the publication. Gossage et al. reviewed several studies of untreated patients and calculated a stroke incidence of 11.4%, a brain abscess incidence of 6.8% and total morbidity and mortality at 23% [42]. White et al. reported migraine headaches in 43% of patients, TIAs in 37%, stroke in 18%, brain abscess in 9% and seizures in 8% [43]. In contrast, treatment-associated complications are low and the success rate is high.

5.2.10 Hamartoma

Hamartomas of the lung are benign congenital lesions that are also called CCAM or CPAM. This entity will be described elsewhere in this book.

5.2.11 Juvenile respiratory papillomatosis

Juvenile respiratory papillomatosis is caused by infection with the human papilloma virus, serotypes 6 and 11. Multiple papillomas affect different sites of the (upper) respiratory tract, including the vocal cords, subglottic space, ventricular bands and the epiglottis. However, 5% of patients have tracheobronchial involvement, and 1% have parenchymal lung disease [44]. Hoarseness is the most common symptom of patients with papillomatosis, but every other symptom of upper airway obstruction can also be observed [45].

Diagnosis and imaging

In cases of laryngeal involvement, papillomatosis can be detected by a simple inspection of the larynx by placing a mirror into a patient's mouth. In general, a laryngotracheoscopy is needed to visualize the papillomas and perform a biopsy to test for

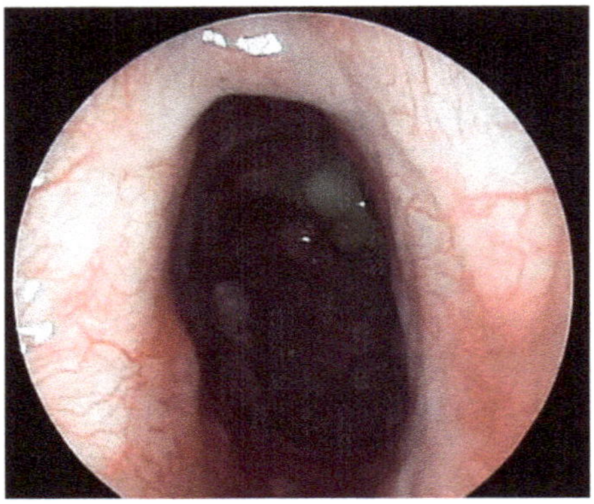

Fig. 5.2.8: Bronchoscopic view at an extensive papillomatosis.

the presence of human papilloma viruses (Fig. 5.2.8). In cases of severe papilloma burden, an additional plain chest radiograph and/or a chest CT scan might be helpful.

Treatment

The standard therapy is surgical excision with cold instruments, CO_2 laser, pulsed dye laser or microdebrider, but many surgical interventions are needed to control the disease. The mean frequency is 4.4 interventions per year. Surgical therapy can be supported by an intralesional application of cidofovir, which is an antiviral agent effective against DNA viruses [44]. Patients with severe upper airway obstruction due to tracheal papillomas require tracheostomy to secure the airways.

Prognosis

The delay between the first symptoms and initiation of therapy is prognostic for the future course of the disease. Silva et al. showed that a delayed diagnosis is negatively associated with the outcome [45]. Although juvenile respiratory papillomatosis is considered a benign disease, its potential for malignant degeneration has been described in several studies [46]. In contrast to adult-onset papillomatosis, which has a remission rate of approximately 70% [47], the juvenile form is more aggressive and more likely to spread outside the larynx [44].

5.3 Chest wall tumors in childhood and adolescence

5.3.1 General considerations

Only 20% of all thoracic tumors account for chest wall tumors. Although these tumors are rare in childhood and adolescence (1 per million children less than 15 years of age), several differential diagnoses have to be considered. There are important differences in incidence rates of different countries. While in less developed countries, tuberculosis is considered at first instance, in Europe and Northern America, malignancies are more common [48]. In contrast to adult patients in whom chondrosarcoma is the predominant malignancy, primitive neuroectodermal tumor (PNET) is the common malignancy in childhood [48].

Fortunately, technical improvements have facilitated the resection of even large tumors. New technical devices allow the resection of relevant chest areas without residual paradoxical respiration. Therefore, surgical resection of both, benign and malignant tumors, has improved over the last several decades [49].

Clinical presentation ranges from visible deformation of the thorax to respiratory distress and recurrent pulmonary infections in case of intrathoracic growth. Beyond anamnesis and physical examination, plain chest radiography is the first-line diagnostic tool. Chest radiography can detect large masses, bone erosion, pulmonary infiltration, and in some cases, mediastinal lymphadenopathy. The next step is to perform an axial thoracic computed tomography (CT) scan, which can detect the site, size, bony involvement, and infiltration into contiguous structures. CT scan is needed to screen for lung metastasis [49]. Magnetic resonance imaging (MRI) is necessary only in few cases, especially when spinal cord involvement is expected. Otherwise, CT scan is the screening method of choice. Additional positron emission tomography (PET) scan is helpful in detecting the metastatic spread of malignant tumors; however, it might also detect inflammatory processes [49]. Finally, a biopsy is needed for definitive diagnosis. Since fine-needle aspiration biopsy is insufficient to determine subtypes of malignant tumors, Tru-cut needle biopsy is the diagnostic tool of choice in most cases. Limited open biopsy is requested if larger tumor tissue samples are needed.

5.3.2 Primitive neuroectodermal tumors (PNETs)

These tumors are members of the Ewing tumor family and share the common t (11; 22) (q24; q12) translocation. They are highly malignant "small blue round cell tumors" [49]. PNETs can arise at any site of the body and a PNET of the chest wall is known as Askin tumor.

Clinical presentation

Patients with PNETs have chest wall masses and/or radicular pain. Even severe back pain can occur in case of vertebral involvement. Dyspnea and diminished breath sounds can be caused by the space occupying effect of the tumor, as well as by reactive pleural effusions.

Diagnosis and imaging

The first-line diagnostic tool is plain chest radiography where masses and bone destruction may appear. A CT and MRI scan with contrast medium would be the next step (Fig. 5.2.1), followed by PET or a whole body technetium bone scan for staging [50].

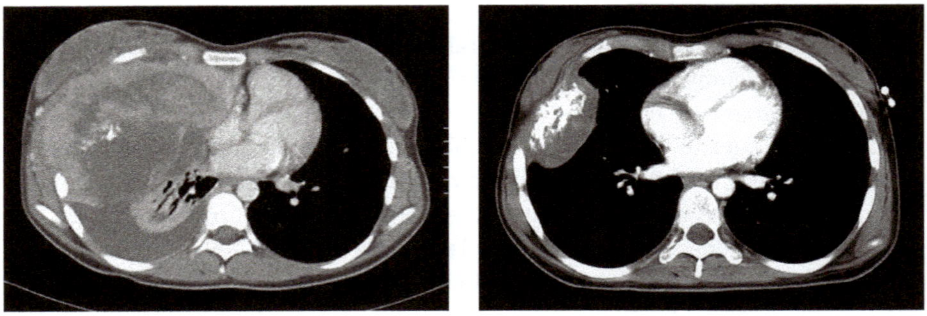

(a) (b)

Fig. 5.3.1: Initial CT scan of a Ewing sarcoma of the right chest wall (a) and same patient after neoadjuvant chemotherapy (b).

A limited biopsy would confirm the diagnosis. However, the surgeon has to determine an incisional site that would not compromise subsequent resection. Therefore, we recommend that the surgeon who would perform the resection should also perform the biopsy. Parallel to the biopsy, bone marrow aspiration should be performed [50].

Treatment and prognosis

After histologic confirmation of the diagnosis, neoadjuvant chemotherapy is administered. PNETs are treated according to the Ewing sarcoma protocol of the EURO-Ewing trial [50]. Subsequently, complete curative resection of the primary tumor is targeted (Fig. 5.3.2). Treatment continues with adjuvant chemotherapy. If feasible, resection of the metastases is performed. If residual tumor is still present, radiation therapy is an alternative for local treatment. In some cases, autologous stem-cell transplantation is required [49, 50].

Presence of metastases is the most prominent adverse prognostic factor in Ewing sarcoma. Metastases are detected at diagnosis in 15–33% of the patients, with survival rates of 9–41%, which are lower than the approximately 70% survival expectancy of patients with localized disease. Patients with primary pulmonary metastases fare better than patients with primary bone and/or bone marrow involvement do [50].

5.3.3 Rhabdomyosarcoma

Rhabdomyosarcoma arises from the primitive mesenchymal stem cells that differentiate to form the striated muscle. It can occur anywhere in the body, including the sites where striated muscle is normally not found. The incidence of rhabdomyosarcoma among children is estimated to be 4 per million in children less than 15 years of age.

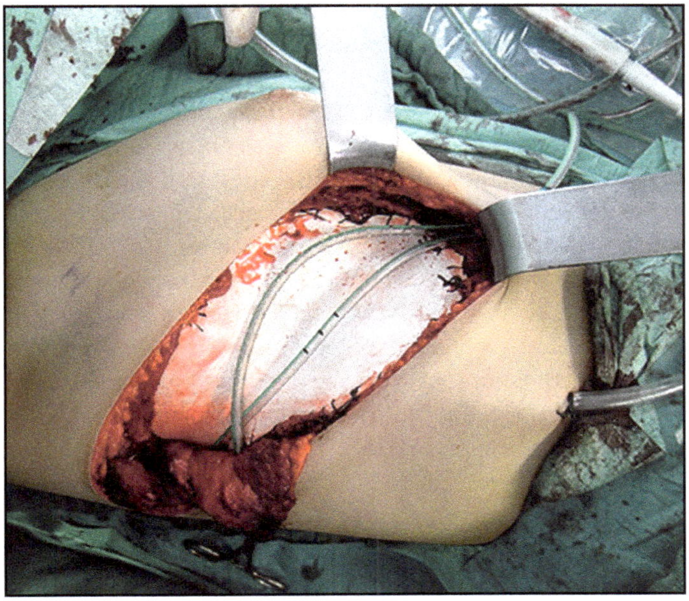

Fig. 5.3.2: Intraoperative view after complete resection of the affected ribs and the replacement by a Gore-tex® patch.

Clinical presentation

In general, symptoms are mild and not specific. In most cases, swelling and/or pain at the tumor site are the primary signs [49].

Diagnosis and imaging

As for other entities, plain chest radiography, and CT and MRI scans of the chest with contrast media, are the first-line diagnostic tools of choice. Whole-body technetium bone scan and bone marrow aspiration are needed for staging, and finally a limited biopsy is performed to confirm the diagnosis. Alternatively, an ultrasound guided Tru-cut biopsy can be performed, which would give similar results. However, the surgeon has to determine a site of incision that would not compromise subsequent resection. Therefore, we recommend that the same surgeon perform both the resection and the biopsy [48, 49].

Treatment and prognosis

Complete resection after neoadjuvant chemotherapy is the mainstay of treatment. Chemotherapy is administered according to the treatment protocols of the CWS-2007-HR Trial. Current treatment protocols recommend radiotherapy for all patients with chest wall tumors, with microscopically and macroscopically residual disease, especially because local disease control is of utmost importance. Most notably, patients with alveolar histology do benefit from radiotherapy irrespective of the postsurgical status. Therefore, radiotherapy is recommended for such patients in all cases [48].

However, prognosis depends on several factors. Alveolar rhabdomyosarcoma has worse prognosis than the embryonic type. Additionally, incomplete resection also has poor prognosis, and compared to other tumor sites, the chest wall is particularly unfavorable. Finally, lymph node involvement, tumor diameter >5 cm, and the age at diagnosis >10 years, are associated with poor prognosis [48]. Interestingly, the Intergroup Rhabdomyosarcoma Study II and III (IRS-II and II) showed that patients with microscopic residual disease had better survival than patients with microscopically complete excisions did. The latter had higher rates of local recurrence. These patients had not received any further therapy for local control, in contrast to patients with microscopically residual malignant cells. This indicates that determination of margin status might be difficult in soft-tissue tumors [48].

5.3.4 Osteosarcoma/malignant fibrohistiocytoma

These tumors are also extremely rare in childhood. The incidence is estimated to be as high as 4.8 per million in children less than 15 years of age. Only 1% are located in the chest wall and the spine. (Neo-) adjuvant chemotherapy and complete resection are crucial for treatment, because these tumors are relatively insensitive to radiotherapy. The success of resection is the main prognostic factor. Owing to multidisciplinary approaches, the overall survival increased over the last decades to 71% in children younger than 9 years of age, and to 48% in older children. Malignant fibrohistiocytomas are often mixed up with osteosarcomas. However, their incidence is approximately 10% that of the osteosarcoma incidence, and approximately 2% are located in the thoracic wall. Treatment is similar to that administered for osteosarcomas.

5.3.5 Fibrosarcoma

Two types of this rare soft-tissue sarcoma are known. Children less than 1 year of age have the infantile type of fibrosarcoma. Infantile fibrosarcoma is characterized by a t (12; 15) translocation. Infantile fibrosarcoma should be distinguished from giant cell fibroblastoma, a benign, nonmetastasizing tumor [49]. In general, infantile fibrosarcoma shows a rapid initial growth and tends to spontaneously regress. Metastatic disease is uncommon (1–13%), and the overall prognosis is good with survival rates of 80–100% [48]. Because this tumor has high chemosensitivity, neoadjuvant therapy is indicated. Chemotherapy is administered according to the CWS-2007-HR protocol. Subsequent complete resection should be targeted, followed by adjuvant chemotherapy. Radiation is only administered for local tumor control in selected cases, which are cases of incomplete resection and/or unresectable tumors [48].

Older children develop adult type fibrosarcoma with a worse prognosis. The 5-year overall survival is reported to be 51– 60%, only. Therefore complete resection should always be targeted. (Neo-) adjuvant chemotherapy is also defined in the CWS-2007-HR protocol. Radiotherapy is mandatory when clear surgical margins cannot be achieved [48].

5.3.6 Hemangiopericytoma

These soft-tissue tumors arise from mesenchymal stem cells and show pericyte differentiation. Since they commonly derive from the bronchus, they are described elsewhere in this book.

5.3.7 Langerhans cell histiocytosis (LCH)

LCH is characterized by the clonal proliferation of pathologic cells with the characteristics of Langerhans cells. Whether LCH is a malignancy is not clearly defined. It can appear in a single organ or multiple organs. Langerhans cells are bone marrow-derived dendritic cells that reside in the skin and lymph nodes. LCH is a rare disease of unknown etiology, with an estimated incidence of 8–9 cases per million in children less than 15 years of age. This disease is encountered in adult patients as well. Clinical presentation of LCH is very heterogeneous, ranging from a generally benign single-system involvement, to a multisystem life-threatening disease [51].

The role of surgery is both diagnostic and in some cases curative. Since biopsy is important for diagnosis, surgical resection is indicated in selected cases only.

In most unifocal bone lesions, a simple curettage or even a biopsy can provide diagnostic tissue and will often result in spontaneous healing. Surgical resection is usually not recommended and could potentially increase long-term deformity. Observation is restricted to LCH lesions in 'non-risk' bones in patients with a pathologic diagnosis, and to patients presenting with vertebra plana without a soft tissue mass. The risk of biopsy in these patients outweighs the benefit, and this should be carefully followed to exclude malignancies including Ewing sarcoma. Indications for treatment include cases with severe pain, restriction of mobility, lesions with a risk of imminent bone fracture, and spinal cord compression. Local therapies include steroids and irradiation. Intralesional instillation of steroids is an effective and safe treatment modality when therapy is required for a limited number of bone lesions. Low-dose radiation therapy (6–8 Gy) should be restricted to emergency situations such as spinal cord compression. Systemic therapies include indomethacin, bisphosphonates, and chemotherapy [51].

Prognosis is worse in cases of multisystem disease and depends on the involvement of the so-called risk organs, including the liver, spleen, lungs, and the hematopoietic system [48]. The role of surgery depends on diagnostic reasons. Treatment is defined in the LCH-III trial.

5.3.8 Lipoblastoma

Lipoblastoma is a slow-growing, benign tumor that presents as a chest wall mass. Pain is uncommon. Ultrasonography is of less diagnostic value, and the imaging modality of choice is MRI. These tumors give intense signals on T1-weighted MRI (Fig. 5.3.3). Local excision is the preferred treatment option. It is important to remove all of the tumor; however, mutilation has to be avoided [48].

5.3.9 Mesenchymal hamartoma

This benign tumor presents at birth or shortly after with chest deformity and respiratory distress. A calcified mass involving one or more ribs can be seen in the chest radiograph. The tumor is composed of chondroid tissue with large, endothelium-lined vascular spaces, and immature mesenchyme with large osteoclastic giant cells and osteoid. It must be differentiated from aneurysmal bone cysts, and chondromas. Although these may be large tumors, they are benign and complete resection may not be necessary, except to relieve respiratory or cardiac embarrassment [48].

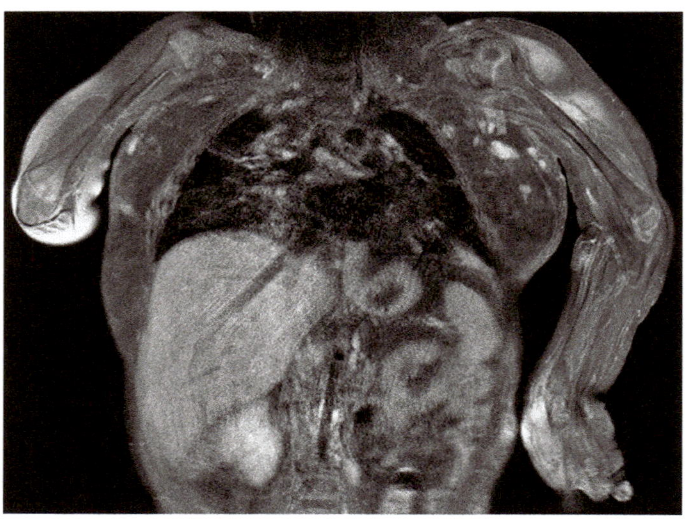

Fig. 5.3.3: CT scan of a mesenchymal hamartoma.

5.3.10 Chondroma

Chest wall chondromas are benign tumors and arise from the costochondral arches or sternum as a chest wall mass. Even histological differentiation between chondroma and chondrosarcoma can be difficult. Therefore chondromas should be excised with a wide margin. Periosteal chondromas may arise in regions of previous thoracotomy. Chondromatous hamartoma of the chest wall is a very rare lesion that arises during infancy. These usually present as large masses, and hyaline cartilage on histology, resembling that of the growth plate, spindle cells, woven bone, and hemorrhagic cysts are seen. Wide excision is recommended in such cases as well [48].

5.3.11 Desmoid tumor

Chest wall desmoid tumors are noted to be locally aggressive, but metastatic spread is uncommon. Therefore, these tumors are categorized as semi-malignant. Complete resection with negative microscopic margins is associated with the lowest rate of local recurrence. These tumors have been observed in patients with mutations of the adenomatous polyposis coli (APC) gene and in patients who previously underwent thoracotomy. Even sternal resection has been described as a treatment option [48].

5.4 Primary mediastinal tumors in childhood and adolescence

5.4.1 General considerations

Primary mediastinal tumors and cysts are relatively rare in children. In fact, the majority of mediastinal masses in children are malignant. In a recent report from seven American medical centers on cases from 1970 to date, 39% of the mediastinal masses were benign, whereas 61% were malignant. More than half of these were lymphomas. Neurogenic tumors were the most common benign lesions and the second most common malignancy. Mediastinal masses in children present in a variety of ways. Over one-half of children with mediastinal masses are symptomatic. Malignant lesions have higher chances of exhibiting symptoms than benign lesions. The most common symptoms in children are dyspnea, cough, fever, and malaise. Most mediastinal masses, regardless of whether they are malignant or benign, require surgical intervention either for diagnosis or for definitive treatment [52].

The compartmentation in anterior, middle, and posterior mediastinum is based on historical reasons. This was useful for differential diagnosis in the pre-computed tomography (pre-CT) era, since localization of tumors was assessed using lateral chest radiography. Nowadays CT scans are more precise in the diagnosis of these tumors. However, preoperative planning still orientates at this compartmentation.

Apart from chest radiography and CT scan, magnetic resonance imaging (MRI) might be another tool for diagnostic work-up. However, this examination is limited by the length of the procedure. Therefore, control of ventilation through either voluntary or mechanical ventilation is crucial. Other examinations such as myelography, barium esophagram, and/or bronchography are restricted to limited indications only. In case of neuroblastoma, an additional metaiodobenzylguanidine (MIBG) scintigraphy is demanded and in case of other suspected malignancies, a positron emission tomography (PET) should be considered [52].

Surgery is required for both diagnostic and therapeutic intervention of the mediastinal masses. Several surgical procedures are available, including fine-needle biopsy, thoracoscopy, and thoracotomy. In selected cases, mediastinoscopy might be useful [53].

Since mediastinal masses can result in airway obstruction, they can cause severe respiratory distress, with a need for immediate intubation or tracheostomy. The same is true for induction of general anesthesia for elective operations. Therefore the anesthesiologist needs to be prepared for these complications [54].

The surgeon plays a role in the diagnosis and management of mediastinal tumors. Most tumors can be accessed by sternotomy, thoracotomy, or thoracoscopy. In selected cases, access from the neck through a suprasternal approach, or from the abdomen through the diaphragm is needed [52]. Mediastinotomy is rarely used in children except for biopsy or removal of the thymus, or occasional resection of cystic hygroma of the upper mediastinum. Sternotomy is most frequently used for anterior mediastinal masses, such as thymomas, teratomas, lipomas, and vascular tumors. The biopsy of masses by a Chamberlain incision through the second intercostal space and anterior thoracotomy might be useful in case of anterior mediastinal masses as well. Occasional anterior mediastinal masses may be resected or biopsied by thoracoscopy. Posterior mediastinal masses are generally approached by posterolateral thoracotomy or thoracoscopy. Mediastinal tumors may involve adjacent structures including the nerves, vena cava, or pericardium [52]. In general, the surgeon has to keep these structures in mind while resecting the tumor in order to prevent mutilation.

5.4.2 Lymphoma

Lymphomas are the third most common childhood malignancies and the most common types of pediatric mediastinal tumors (50%). More than 60% are non-Hodgkin lymphomas, and they present with large tumor burden especially in the anterior and middle mediastinum. In general, the role of the surgeon is diagnostic. However, in almost all cases, the diagnosis can be made from cervical lymph node biopsies. In exceptional cases, the upper airway obstruction necessitates emergency intubation or tracheostomy. Otherwise, lymphomas are treated with chemotherapy.

5.4.3 Extragonadal germ cell tumors

Extragonadal germ cell tumors are typically located in the midline from the pineal gland to the coccyx. Even if 90% of the extragonadal germ cell tumors occur in adult men aged 20–35 years, there are documented pediatric cases as well as cases older than 60 years of age. The most common primary site is the anterior mediastinum followed by the retroperitoneum, with rare occurrence in the pineal gland and presacral area. There are isolated reports of extragonadal primaries in the bladder, prostate or liver. Extragonadal germ cell tumors share the gain of isochromosome 12p with gonadal germ cell tumors. Cisplatin-based chemotherapy should be administered as for the testicular germ-cell tumors (GCT). Residual disease should be considered for surgical resection in nonseminomatous extragonadal germ cell tumors.

The anterior mediastinum is the most common site of extragonadal germ cell tumors, comprising 50–70% of all extragonadal tumors. Mature benign teratoma or seminoma is most commonly observed. Malignant mediastinal germ cell tumors are divided between seminomas (40%) and nonseminomatous germ cell tumors (60%). The only known risk factor for mediastinal nonseminomatous germ cell tumors is the Klinefelter syndrome (47XXY) [55].

Treatment and prognosis

Primary mediastinal nonseminomatous germ cell tumors represent a clinically and biologically distinct subset of extragonadal germ cell tumors. Prognosis of these tumors is poor with an overall survival rate of 40–50% after platinum-based chemotherapy and surgery. The overall survival decreases to 25% if there is metastatic disease of the lung, liver, or supraclavicular lymph nodes. In contrast, mediastinal seminomas have a good prognosis with 88–90% overall survival rates [55].

Primary mediastinal nonseminomatous germ cell tumors represent the most challenging group of malignant germ cell tumors. Survival outcome depends on successful chemotherapy and surgical tumor removal. Since a testis primary is unlikely, testis ultrasound is not needed. However, the levels of tumor markers including human chorionic gonadotropin (hCG) > 1000 U/l, and/or any elevation in the α-fetoprotein (AFP) level, indicate nonseminomatous extragonadal germ cell tumors. In these cases, an additional biopsy is not needed. These extragonadal germ cell tumors can be treated using the MAKEI protocol. Patients with normal tumor markers or a mild elevation in the hCG level require a biopsy to establish a definitive diagnosis [55].

Finally, surgical tumor resection after neoadjuvant chemotherapy is required and should be performed by experienced oncosurgeons. Viable tumor is present in 30–47% of patients who undergo post-chemotherapy resection. In general, surgery for patients with testicular germ cell tumors is reserved for those with normalized markers. However, in the absence of effective salvage chemotherapy and long-term survival for patients with primary mediastinal nonseminomatous germ cell tumors, patients with local disease are likely to benefit from post-chemotherapy resection despite elevated markers before surgical resection [55].

The post-operative course depends on surgical success and histological diagnosis, and is specified in the treatment protocols such as the MAKEI protocol.

Mediastinal teratoma

Mature teratomas are large circumscribed tumors of the anterior mediastinum. These tumors are nonsecretory with normal serum hCG and AFP levels. They are only treated by surgical resection; however, in cases of secretory teratomas, chemotherapy should be considered due to the presence of malignant transformation.

The 'growing teratoma syndrome' is a special kind of presentation with a secondary cardiopulmonary deterioration due to the growing teratoma. Prompt recognition of this syndrome, discontinuation of chemotherapy, and surgical intervention can be curative [55] (Figs. 5.4.1 and 5.4.2).

Mediastinal seminoma

Mediastinal seminomas comprise 30–40% of malignant mediastinal germ cell tumors. Mediastinal seminoma has an excellent prognosis and should be treated with

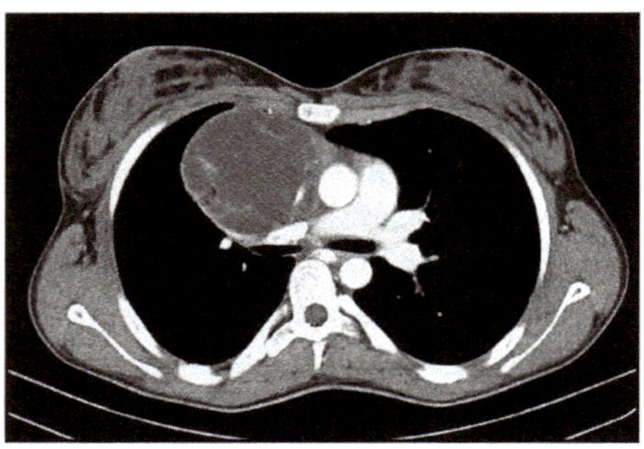

Fig. 5.4.1: CT scan of a mediastinal teratoma.

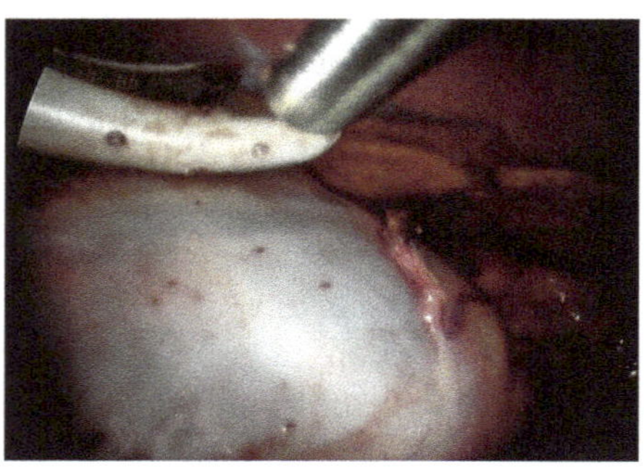

Fig. 5.4.2: Intraoperative view at the same teratoma.

a low-risk chemotherapy regimen (three cycles of bleomycin, etoposide, and platinum or four cycles of etoposide and cisplatin) with no surgical resection needed [55].

5.4.4 Thymoma and thymic carcinoma

Thymoma and thymic carcinoma are epithelial tumors arising from the anterior mediastinum. They are extremely rare in childhood and because of the role of the thymus in the immune system, these tumors are associated with autoimmune diseases in up to 40% of adult patients. Histologically, they are categorized according to the World Health Organization classification based on the presence of atypical epithelial cells, normal lymphocytes, and mimicking of the thymic architecture. Thymomas are low-grade tumors with early local invasive growth, but unlikely distal metastasis. In contrast, thymic carcinomas are highly aggressive and are characterized by early metastatic spread with a poor prognosis. They may arise from preexisting thymomas.

Clinical presentation

In some patients, local symptoms including cough, dyspnea, chest pain, respiratory distress and superior vena cava syndrome may occur; however, some of them are asymptomatic, and tumors are detected on chest radiography. Up to 15% present with paraneoplastic symptoms, such as myasthenia gravis, polymyositis, systemic lupus erythematosus, hypothyroidism, gastrointestinal disorders (chronic ulcerative colitis), collagen and autoimmune disorders (Sjögren's syndrome, scleroderma, and polymyositis), hypogammaglobulinemia, dermatologic disorders (alopecia), endocrine disorders (Cushing's syndrome), renal disease (nephrosis), and hematologic syndromes (red cell aplasia, agranulocytosis). The onset of these diseases can herald the presence of a treatable tumor [56].

Diagnosis and imaging

The first-line diagnostic tool is plain chest radiography followed by CT with contrast medium. PET may be useful as it can distinguish between hyperplasia and neoplasia. The use of semi-quantitative maximum standardized uptake value (SUVmax) may help distinguish low grade thymoma from thymic carcinoma [56]. Final diagnosis is made histologically after initial biopsy of the tumor.

Treatment and prognosis

Complete resection is crucial for treating all thymic neoplasms. However, this is difficult since most thymic neoplasms exhibit local invasive growth. Although complete resection is the best treatment option, survival after gross total resection is slightly better than after biopsy alone. Due to the rarity of these tumors, no standardized chemotherapy protocols are available. Most current protocols for patients with unresectable thymomas include cisplatin, doxorubicin, cyclophosphamide, and prednisone; however, with poor outcome. Radiotherapy might be another option in combination with chemotherapy; however, the use of radiation has to be discussed individually [56].

There are some reports of epithelial thymic tumors expressing tyrosine kinases, such as epidermal growth factor receptor (EGFR), RET, AKT1, and c-KIT. These are potential targets for EGFR or mTOR inhibitors. Octreotide, an inhibitor of the somatostatin type 2 receptor, has been efficacious in combination with prednisolone. Some authors used sunitinib and imatinib to treat thymic carcinoma. However, these are experimental approaches with lack of evidence [56].

5.4.5 Neurogenic tumors

Neurogenic tumors account for 25% of all pediatric mediastinal tumors. The majority (75%) of these tumors are benign. They arise from the peripheral nerves, sympathetic ganglia, or rarely, parasympathetic ganglia. Schwannoma, neurofibroma, and malignant nerve sheath tumor arise from the peripheral nerves. Ganglioneuroma, ganglioneuroblastoma, and neuroblastoma arise from the sympathetic ganglia. Parasympathetic ganglia tumors include nonsecretory chemodectomas and pheochromocytomas. Nerve sheath tumors are common in adult patients while sympathetic ganglia tumors predominately affect pediatric patients [57].

Schwannoma, neurofibroma, and malignant nerve-sheath tumor

Schwannomas and neurofibromas are benign, slow-growing neoplasms arising from any thoracic nerve. Schwann cells proliferating in a collagenous matrix are the origin of schwannomas. They are heterogeneous, especially when large, with areas of cystic degeneration, low cellularity, hemorrhage, myelin, and small calcifications. [57] In contrast, neurofibromas are usually homogeneous, well marginated, but nonencapsulated tumors. They result from unorganized proliferation of all nerve elements, including Schwann cells, myelinated and unmyelinated nerve fibers, and fibroblasts [57]. Despite these differences, both tumors manifest grossly as lobulated spherical masses.

A plexiform neurofibroma is a well-defined, non-encapsulated tumor that usually infiltrates along an entire nerve trunk or plexus. Multiple neurogenic tumors, or a single plexiform neurofibroma is pathognomonic of neurofibromatosis [57].

Malignant nerve sheath tumors are considered as the malignant transformation of schwannomas or neurofibromas. Especially patients suffering from neurofibromatosis are at higher risk of developing this malignancy. This pleomorphic tumor with high cellularity grows aggressively and tends to metastasize early.

Clinical presentation

Most of these tumors present with no symptoms or minor symptoms, and are incidental findings on chest radiographs due to other indications. Only few patients experience paresthesia or pain caused by the compression of adjacent structures or from intraspinal tumor extension. Some of the neurogenic tumors can expand to the spinal canal, forming the so-called 'dump-bell' or 'hourglass' tumors. In this condition, compression of the spinal cord with paraplegia may be the leading symptom. These events are emergency cases and need immediate intervention; a combined or staged neurosurgical and thoracic surgical procedure is necessary for intraspinal debulking [57].

Diagnosis and imaging

This tumor appears as a solid mass on chest radiographs. Further diagnostics include a CT scan and MRI to reveal infiltration into the surrounding structures, the spinal canal, the dimensions of the tumor, lymph node involvement, and compression of the trachea and major vessels. A biopsy completes the diagnostic procedures. Especially in patients with neurofibromatosis, a PET scan may be useful to detect transformation into malignant nerve sheath tumors [58]. In addition, the PET scan is used to detect metastatic spread of these malignant tumors.

Treatment and prognosis

Complete resection of solitary schwannomas and neurofibromas should be targeted. In case of neurofibromatosis, surgical resection is seldom reasonable, since a complete removal of the tumor might not be feasible. In our experience, neurofibromas will relapse to the initial size in a short time. Therefore, patients with neurofibromatosis need continuous follow-up, since they are at higher risk for malignant transformation. Their lifetime hazard might be as high as 10% [57].

Patients with malignant nerve sheath tumors need complete surgical resection with large margins. Otherwise, local recurrence is frequent with very poor prognosis. Adjuvant radiation therapy and chemotherapy do not seem to improve survival but may be beneficial in the treatment of metastatic disease [57].

Neuroblastoma, ganglioneuroblastoma, and ganglioneuroma

While neuroblastomas are malignant embryonic neoplasms with high maturation potential, the other two tumors represent different stages of maturation from malignant to completely differentiated tumors. Neuroblastomas arise from sympathetic ganglia such as the sympathetic trunk or the adrenal gland. They can be localized and eventually disseminate (stages 1–4). Only 20% of these tumors originate in the thorax and have better prognoses than retroperitoneal or intraabdominal neuroblastomas. The thoracic manifestations are in general as localized tumors [59]. Most of the neuroblastomas are symptomatic before 2 years of age.

Clinical presentation

Spinal cord compression, weakness, or paralyses of one upper limb, clonus, Horner's syndrome, or respiratory problems are clinical signs in approximately two thirds of the children. Another rare clinical manifestation might be the opsoclonus-myoclonus-syndrome (OMS) [60]. However, in 30% of the patients, diagnosis is incidental [57].

Diagnosis and imaging

In cases of suspected neuroblastoma or ganglioneuroblastoma, several diagnostics are needed for verification of the diagnosis and to evaluate the stage of the disease. The diagnostic imaging tools are plain chest radiography, metaiodobenzylguanidine (MIBG) scintigraphy used to estimate the stage of the disease, and CT and/or MRI scan to visualize local extension (Fig. 5.4.3). Laboratory tests include tumor markers such as lactate dehydrogenase (LDH), neuron-specific enolase (NSE), and urine catecholamines. Tumor biopsy is needed to measure molecular markers such as *MYCN* amplification and 1p deletion. These markers are needed for risk stratification. Biopsy can be performed by Tru-cut, thoracoscopic, or open biopsy. Bone marrow aspiration is also required for estimating the stage of the disease.

Treatment and prognosis

Treatment of these tumors is organized in multinational protocols, for example the protocol by the European SIOP Neuroblastoma Group (SIOPEN). These protocols

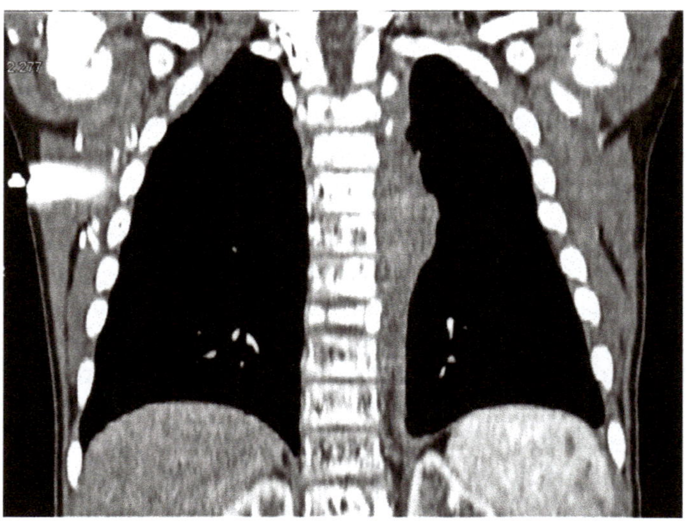

Fig. 5.4.3: MRI scan of an lipoblastoma predominately at the left hemi-thorax.

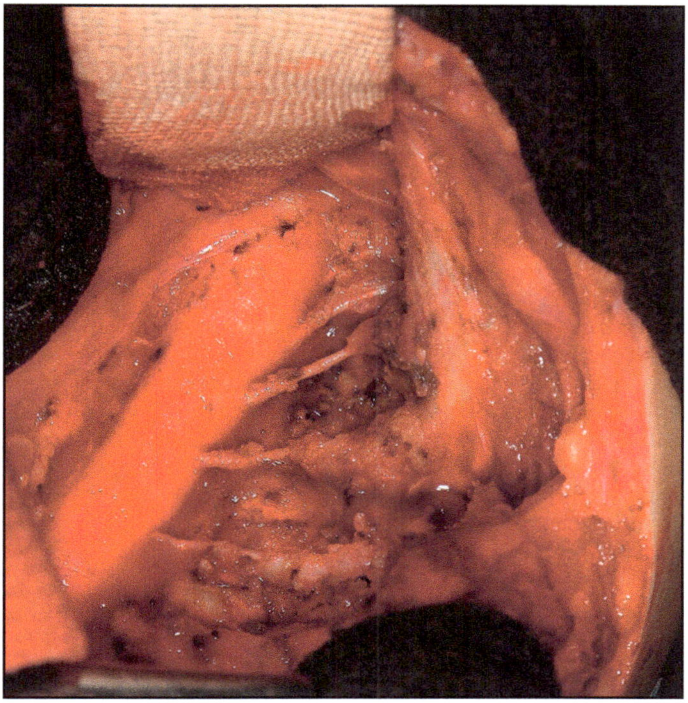

Fig. 5.4.4: Intraoperative view after resection of the neuroblastoma.

manage the use of (neo-) adjuvant chemotherapy, surgical strategies, and radiation. Because of the high grade of spontaneous maturation, the watch and wait approach has to be balanced with surgical resection. Markers indicative for resection are *MYCN* amplification, (1p deletion), clinical symptoms (i.e. OMS, spinal compression), and/or growing tumors. However, the decision for surgery is made using an interdisciplinary approach. Thoracoscopic resection is feasible in some cases. Otherwise lateral thoracotomy is the procedure of choice (Fig. 5.4.4).

5.5 Further reading

[1] Neville HL, et al. Incidence and outcomes of malignant pediatric lung neoplasms. J Surg Res 2009;156:224–230.
[2] Yu DC, et al. Primary lung tumors in children and adolescents: a 90-year experience. J Pediatr Surg 2010;45:1090–1095.
[3] Rojas Y, et al. Primary malignant pulmonary tumors in children: a review of the national cancer data base. J Pediatr Surg 2015;50:1004–1008.
[4] Al-Qahtani AR, Di Lorenzo M & Yazbeck S. Endobronchial tumors in children: Institutional experience and literature review. J Pediatr Surg 2003;38:733–736.

[5] Shadmehr MB, et al. Primary major airway tumors; management and results. Eur J Cardiothorac Surg 2011;39:749–754.
[6] Eyssartier E, et al. Characteristics of endobronchial primitive tumors in children. Pediatr Pulmonol 2014;49:E121–5.
[7] Bertino EM, Confer PD, Colonna JE, Ross P & Otterson GA. Pulmonary neuroendocrine/carcinoid tumors: a review article. Cancer 2009;115:4434–4441.
[8] Rizzardi G, Bertolaccini L & Terzi A. Bronchial carcinoid tumours in children–a review. Eur Oncol Hematol 2011.
[9] Yao JC. Neuroendocrine tumors. Molecular targeted therapy for carcinoid and islet-cell carcinoma. Best Pract Res Clin Endocrinol Metab 2007;21:163–172.
[10] Walch AK, et al. Typical and atypical carcinoid tumors of the lung are characterized by 11q deletions as detected by comparative genomic hybridization. The American Journal of Pathology 1998;153:1089–1098.
[11] Fink G, et al. Pulmonary carcinoid: presentation, diagnosis, and outcome in 142 cases in Israel and review of 640 cases from the literature. Chest 2001;119:1647–1651.
[12] Spunt SL, Pratt CB, Rao BN & Pritchard M. Childhood carcinoid tumors: The St Jude Children's Research Hospital experience. Journal of pediatric ... (2000).
[13] Lococo F, et al. PET/CT assessment of neuroendocrine tumors of the lung with special emphasis on bronchial carcinoids. Tumour Biol 2014;35:8369–8377.
[14] Rizzardi G, et al. Bronchial carcinoid tumours in children: surgical treatment and outcome in a single institution. Eur J Pediatr Surg 2009;19:228–231.
[15] Rea F, et al. Outcome and surgical strategy in bronchial carcinoid tumors: single institution experience with 252 patients. Eur J Cardiothorac Surg 2007;31:186–191.
[16] Caplin ME, et al. Pulmonary neuroendocrine (carcinoid) tumors: European Neuroendocrine Tumor Society expert consensus and recommendations for best practice for typical and atypical pulmonary carcinoids. Ann Oncol 2015;26:1604–1620.
[17] Liu X & Adams AL. Mucoepidermoid carcinoma of the bronchus: a review. Arch Pathol Lab Med 2007;131:1400–1404.
[18] Dinopoulos A, Lagona E, Stinios I, Konstadinidou A & Kattamis C. Mucoepidermoid carcinoma of the bronchus. Pediatr Hematol Oncol 2000;17:401–408.
[19] Singh D, Bhalla AS, Veedu PT & Arora A. Imaging evaluation of hemoptysis in children. World J Clin Pediatr 2013;2:54–64.
[20] Kim TS, et al. Mucoepidermoid carcinoma of the tracheobronchial tree: radiographic and CT findings in 12 patients. Radiology 1999;212:643–648.
[21] Roden AC, et al. Histopathologic immunophenotypic and cytogenetic features of pulmonary mucoepidermoid carcinoma Mod Pathol 2014;27:1479–1488.
[22] Spizarny DL, Shepard JA, McLoud TC, Grillo HC & Dedrick CG. CT of adenoid cystic carcinoma of the trachea. AJR Am J Roentgenol 1986:146:1129–1132.
[23] Roby BB, Drehner D & Sidman JD. Pediatric tracheal and endobronchial tumors: an institutional experience. Arch Otolaryngol Head Neck Surg 2011;137:925–929.
[24] Hartman GE & Shochat SJ. Primary pulmonary neoplasms of childhood: a review. The Annals of thoracic surgery 1983;36:108–119.
[25] Karnak I, Ciftci AO, Şenocak ME, Kale G & Büyükpamukçu N. Pulmonary blastoma: diagnostic and therapeutic aspects. Pediatr Surg Int 1999;15:380–382.
[26] Manivel JC, et al. Pleuropulmonary blastoma. The so-called pulmonary blastoma of childhood. Cancer 1988;62:1516–1526.
[27] Seballos RM & Klein RL. Pulmonary blastoma in children: report of two cases and review of the literature. J Pediatr Surg 1994;29:1553–1556.

[28] Cagle PT, Barrios R & Allen TC. Color Atlas and Text of Pulmonary Pathology. (Lippincott Williams & Wilkins, 2008). doi:10.1097/00024382-200507000-00018.
[29] Larsen H & Sorensen JB. Pulmonary blastoma: a review with special emphasis on prognosis and treatment. Cancer treatment reviews 1996.
[30] Travis WD, et al. International Association for the Study of Lung Cancer/American Thoracic Society/European Respiratory Society: international multidisciplinary classification of lung adenocarcinoma: executive summary. in 2011;8:381–385.
[31] Noguchi M, et al. Small adenocarcinoma of the lung. Histologic characteristics and prognosis Cancer 1995;75:2844–2852.
[32] Kayton ML, et al. Primary lung adenocarcinomas in children and adolescents treated for pediatric malignancies J Thorac Oncol 2010;5:1764–1771.
[33] Park MS & Araujo DM. New insights into the hemangiopericytoma/solitary fibrous tumor spectrum of tumors. Curr Opin Oncol 2009;21:327–331.
[34] Fernandez-Pineda I, et al. Childhood Hemangiopericytoma: Review of St Jude Children's Research Hospital. J Pediatr Hematol Oncol 2011;33:356–359.
[35] Gleason BC & Hornick JL. Inflammatory myofibroblastic tumours: where are we now? J Clin Pathol 2008;61:428–437.
[36] Alaggio R, et al. Inflammatory myofibroblastic tumors in childhood: a report from the Italian Cooperative Group studies. Cancer 2010;116:216–226.
[37] Coffin CM, Watterson J, Priest JR & Dehner LP. Extrapulmonary inflammatory myofibroblastic tumor (inflammatory pseudotumor). A clinicopathologic and immunohistochemical study of 84 cases. Am J Surg Pathol 1995;19:859–872.
[38] Kleinschmidt MC, Scherbaum CW & Müller T. Inflammatory pseudotumour of the lung as a rare differential diagnosis of a pulmonary mass - a case report and overview of the literature. Pneumologie 2010;64:246–248.
[39] Kovach SJ, et al. Inflammatory myofibroblastic tumors. J Surg Oncol 2006;94:385–391.
[40] Suhler EB, et al. Rituximab Therapy for Refractory Orbital Inflammation: Results of a Phase 1/2, Dose-Ranging, Randomized Clinical Trial. JAMA Ophthalmol 2014;132:572–578.
[41] Meek ME, Meek JC & Beheshti MV. Management of pulmonary arteriovenous malformations. Semin Intervent Radiol 2011;28:24–31.
[42] Gossage JR & Kanj G. Pulmonary arteriovenous malformations. A state of the art review. Am J Respir Crit Care Med 1998;158:643–661.
[43] White RI Jr, Lynch-Nyhan A, Terry P & Buescher PC. Pulmonary arteriovenous malformations: techniques and long-term outcome of embolotherapy. Radiology 1988; doi:10.1148/radiology.1988.169.issue-3;page:string:Article/Chapter.
[44] Ablanedo-Terrazas Y, Soda-Merhy A, Hernández-Palestina M, Ormsby CE & Reyes-Terán G. Intralesional cidofovir in severe juvenile respiratory papillomatosis. B-ENT 2012;8:197–202.
[45] Silva L, Gonçalves CP & Fernandes A. Laryngeal papillomatosis in children: The impact of late recognition over evolution. Journal of medical ... 2015; doi:10.1002/jmv.24181/epdf.
[46] Go C, Schwartz MR & Donovan DT. Molecular transformation of recurrent respiratory papillomatosis: viral typing and p53 overexpression. Ann Otol Rhinol Laryngol 2003;112:298–302.
[47] Derkay CS. Task force on recurrent respiratory papillomas. A preliminary report. Arch Otolaryngol Head Neck Surg 1995;121:1386–1391.
[48] van den Berg H, van Rijn RR & Merks JH. Management of tumors of the chest wall in childhood: a review. J Pediatr Hematol Oncol 2008;30:214–221.
[49] La Quaglia MP. Chest wall tumors in childhood and adolescence. Seminars in Pediatric Surgery 2008;17:173–180.

[50] Ladenstein R, et al. Primary disseminated multifocal Ewing sarcoma: results of the Euro-EWING 99 trial. J Clin Oncol 2010;28:3284–3291.
[51] Abla O, Egeler RM & Weitzman S. Langerhans cell histiocytosis: Current concepts and treatments. Cancer Treat Rev 2010;36:354–359.
[52] Jaggers J & Balsara K. Mediastinal masses in children. Seminars in Thoracic and Cardiovascular Surgery 2004;16:201–208.
[53] Hubertus J, Hirsch W, Burkhardt U & Korholz D. The efficacy of cervical mediastinotomy in children. Journal of Indian Association of Pediatric Surgeons 2007.
[54] Latham GJ. Anesthesia for the child with cancer. Anesthesiol Clin 2014;32:185–213.
[55] Albany C & Einhorn LH. Extragonadal germ cell tumors: clinical presentation and management. Curr Opin Oncol 2013;25:261–265.
[56] Stachowicz-Stencel T, Orbach D & Brecht I. Thymoma and thymic carcinoma in children and adolescents: A report from the European Cooperative Study Group for Pediatric Rare Tumors (EXPeRT). European Journal of Cancer 2015.
[57] Macchiarini P & Ostertag H. Uncommon primary mediastinal tumours. Lancet Oncol 2004;5:107–118.
[58] Salamon J, et al. Nerve Sheath Tumors in Neurofibromatosis Type 1: Assessment of Whole-Body Metabolic Tumor Burden Using F-18-FDG PET/CT. PLoS ONE 2015:10:e0143305.
[59] Vo K T, et al. Clinical, biologic, and prognostic differences on the basis of primary tumor site in neuroblastoma: a report from the international neuroblastoma risk group project. J Clin Oncol 2014;32:3169–3176.
[60] Hero B & Schleiermacher G. Update on pediatric opsoclonus myoclonus syndrome. Neuropediatrics 2013;44:324–329.

6 Diaphragm

6.1 Introduction

Today, a literature review of studies relating to congenital diaphragmatic hernia (CDH) reveals more than 5700 references. The sheer volume of research in this area reflects ongoing and tireless efforts to unravel the still enigmatic etiology of CDH, and to improve the pre- and postpartum treatment and surgical techniques utilized to treat this condition. The interdisciplinary group from Rotterdam, namely **Dick Tibboel, René Wijnen and Hanneke IJsselstijn** accepted the challenge of compiling an up-to-date, concise overview of contemporary research approaches and findings. The overlap between CDH and congenital diaphragmatic event ration (CDE) might be of minor relevance. However, the surgical procedure is different, and the French colleagues **Anne Schneider, Francesca Borruto and Francois Becmeur** discuss this topic in depth.

Dick Tibboel, René Wijnen, Hanneke IJsselstijn

6.2 Congenital diaphragmatic hernia (CDH)

6.2.1 Introduction

For a number of decades the overall survival rates for newborns with congenital diaphragmatic hernia (CDH) remained around 50%. A number of landmark publications have changed the landscape of the individual patient with CDH and have resulted in a higher level of agreement regarding prenatal risk factors as well as standardization of postnatal therapy [1–9]. In this respect CDH has changed from a surgical emergency for a patient in which the main focus of therapy is directed towards optimal ventilatory support and prevention of long-term pulmonary sequalae. Optimal therapy of pulmonary hypertension, which is due to the abnormal pulmonary vascular morphology, and our lack of knowledge concerning optimal medical therapy are today the main determinants of outcomes in individual patients. To this effect important international initiatives were raised such as the institution of the CDH registry in 1995 [7] as well as the establishment of the CDH EURO Consortium in 2006. More recently a Japanese working group on CDH has been established. Moreover international consensus is available now to determine the way of reporting for patients with CDH [10].

6.2.2 Epidemiology of CDH

CDH has a worldwide incidence of 1 in 2500–3000 live births. Based on international collaboration a number of candidate genes as well as environmental factors have been identified as playing a role in the occurrence of CDH in individual offspring. Most of the genes, although located at different chromosomes, are known to have strong relationships with the retinoic acid pathway [11–13]. In the most used animal model of CDH (the nitrofen rodent model) the crucial step is interference with the enzyme RALDH2 as a pivotal step in retinoic acid metabolism, at least in experimental models. CDH may occur as an isolated anomaly but the increasing use of prenatal ultrasound and MRI has revealed a significant number of fetuses with associated anomalies (cardiac, renal) while modern genetic techniques have increased the yield of genetic abnormalities (array and next-generation sequencing).

6.2.3 Pathophysiology of CDH

For a long time, the hypoplastic lungs of CDH patients have been considered as immature and resembling the lungs of preterm born infants. Although the prevalence of chronic lung disease in term-born CDH patients is around 30% and comparable with a preterm of around 1000 grams, no primary surfactant deficiency has been documented in newborns with CDH. The ongoing potential damage to the lungs by artificial ventilation may result in a secondary surfactant deficiency/inactivation. As such there is no argument to use artificial surfactant in patients with CDH and severe respiratory insufficiency. A recent trial [14] revealed that conventional artificial ventilation as initial ventilatory support is superior to high frequency oscillation. Increasingly treatment modalities are focusing on modulation of the pulmonary vascular tone as the main determinant of outcome in the majority of patients except for those who have an extreme form of pulmonary hypoplasia and the number of available alveoli is under a critical level. Our present level of knowledge of the molecular mechanisms underlying normal and abnormal pulmonary vascular development and the therapeutic targets to modulate pulmonary vascular growth and/or tone is far from complete. As a consequence our treatment of pulmonary hypertension is still trial and error as no properly designed comparative effectiveness trials have been conducted so far for CDH specifically in contrast to the body of literature on the use of inhaled NO in preterm-born infants.

6.2.4 Prenatal diagnosis

Worldwide, numerous attempts have been made to identify the optimal prenatal predictor of outcome for an individual patient with CDH. In most institutions the observed/expected (O/E) LHR (formerly LHR) which is independent of gestational age is used as a predictor of outcome of the individual patient although this use is still debated [15]. Apart from the O/E LHR, the position of the liver (liver up or down), the presence of associated anomalies (cardiac, renal, etc.) and the absence or presence of chromosomal abnormalities have all been used as predictors. It is important to understand that these values cannot be seen as independent to the standardization of postnatal care and experience of the treatment team. After years of compassionate use of fetoscopic endoluminal tracheal occlusion (FETO), to date the tracheal occlusion to accelerate lung growth (TOTAL) trial is on its way in both severe and moderate forms of prenatally diagnosed CDH guided by three European centers (Leuven, Belgium; London, UK; and Barcelona, Spain).

The results of this trial will determine the ultimate position of antenatal tracheal plugging in selected patients with prenatally diagnosed CDH. The results are expected in the next 2 years.

6.2.5 Treatment

Following the ongoing data collection within the framework of the CDH, an international debate was started about optimal ventilatory support in newborns with CDH in need of artificial ventilation. In many institutions, high frequency oscillation (HFO) was used as a rescue therapy in case of ongoing high levels of arterial PCO2 which resulted in severe selection bias and the use of this treatment modality by unexperienced hands as a last resort. To answer the question about the optimal ventilatory approach in CDH, the so-called VICI-trial was conducted in prenatally diagnosed CDH patients, which revealed the superiority of conventional ventilation [13]. Against the background of international consensus on all treatment modalities in CDH, the results of this kind of investigations are of value and should be considered as a prerequisite of treatment results.

Long-term follow-up is equally important to evaluate the result of neonatal interventions with special attention to pulmonary, gastrointestinal and neurodevelopmental outcome parameters [16]. Evaluation of the presence of an increased pulmonary vascular tone by cardiac ultrasound is one of the contemporary hallmarks of therapy. Together with the evaluation of the presence of structural cardiac anomalies, the condition of the right ventricle is an important target of medical intervention for pulmonary vascular tone. In contrast to the positive effects of inhaled NO in preterms with pulmonary hypertension, the effects of inhaled NO in CDH newborns is around 30%.

Although no properly designed trials on the use of any vasoactive drug to modulate the pulmonary vascular tone have been conducted, most institutions use a combination of enhancing the systematic blood pressure by vasoactive drugs according to local habits in combination with inhaled NO. The medical therapy should be based on translational knowledge of the different pathways of endothelial smooth muscle cell interaction [17]. As part of the standard postnatal therapy, the ultimate aim is not to reach preductal situations of 100% in the absence of any R-L shunt because this will seriously damage the lungs due to increased shear forces and oxygen toxicity to the vulnerable lungs of CDH patients. In case all treatment modalities fail, extra corporeal membrane oxygenation (ECMO) can be used for specific patients and in institutions with a proven track record and enough patients on a yearly base. Solid guidelines for early transfer and clear criteria for admission to an ECMO center are important aspects of quality of care for the use of ECMO in CDH patients. Most institutions will still use VA-ECMO but from a pathophysiological point of view there are no arguments against the use of VV-ECMO in CDH patients as this will "oxygenate" the pulmonary vasculature and eventually result in relaxation of the abnormal pulmonary vascular bed. The application of ECMO has significantly decreased in many institutions over the years and ranges from 15–25% while the overall survival is around 35% post-ECMO according to the ELSO registry (2015).

6.2.6 Surgical therapy

Timing and venue of surgery

A good outcome in pediatric surgery is not only dependent on surgical skills but even more on good collaboration between anaesthetists and surgeons. Especially for CDH this is particularly important. In the treatment of children born with CDH it was long thought that immediate closure of the defect in the diaphragm was the most important goal for both specialties. Since the 1980s, however, delayed repair of CDH became the accepted method, first allowing the infant to stabilize and obtain optimal pulmonary function prior to surgery [17]. Nevertheless, the definition of 'stable' was originally dependent on local expertise. A special sub group in this context is formed by premature babies with a CDH. Surgery within 48 hours in these infants is associated with a higher risk of intracerebral accidents. This phenomenon perhaps also holds true for instable term-born babies. The definition of early surgery in stable infants nowadays is still depending on local experiences and protocols and varies between 1 to 5 days. Until now there are no multi-center studies focussing on this issue [18].

In the 1990's ECMO was incorporated in a strategy of delayed repair of CDH and was used for preoperative stabilization in patients who were unresponsive to maximal conventional treatment. If ECMO was required for preoperative stabilization, the diaphragmatic defect was repaired while the patient was on ECMO. In early experiences with this approach, all patients suffered from bleeding complications, however, since the introduction antifibrinolitic therapy with tranexamic acid (TEA) during and immediately after CDH repair on ECMO, hemorrhagic complications are significantly reduced [19]. Also the therapeutic or prophylactic use of antithrombotic agents such as TachoSil and Tissuecol is recommended. Most of the serious cardiopulmonary instable patients in ECMO centers will be placed on ECMO within 24 hours after birth.

The timing of closure of the diaphragmatic defect in instable patients on ECMO is still being debated, however. Comparing surgery during the ECMO run with surgery after the ECMO run, further stabilization may be slightly favorable for the latter approach, at least in the CDH registry study [20]. The timing of surgery on ECMO is also being debated; either in the first 2 or 3 days on ECMO or at the expected end of the ECMO run. The advantage of early surgery is less edema but later surgery provides the opportunity to finish the ECMO run in case of bleeding.

The optimal venue for surgery is the operating room, which is a team-friendly site with enough space and availability of all facilities. However, surgery on these critically ill neonates in the intensive care unit does away with the potential risks involved in transport, such as temperature changes, metabolic de-arrangements and line or tube loss.

In addition, resuscitation procedures can be performed in an ideal environment and there will be continuity of care by the same physicians. No definitive data are available on the risk of infections.

Several papers have dealt with this issue with regard to various surgical disorders. There is only one study including CDH patients only [21]. The results of this study showed that patients operated on in the intensive care unit had a worse outcome as expressed by postoperative markers of inflammation and length of hospital stay. However, looking at the clinical characteristics, it appears that patients operated on in the intensive care unit were more severely ill than those operated on in the OR. In an attempt to exclude the impact of disease severity on the outcomes, a recent study focused on patients with a good postnatal prognosis defined as reaching stability within the first 72 hours of life [22]. In patients with high-risk CDH but a good postnatal outlook, the surgical venue does not have a significant impact on body temperature, infectious complications or respiratory outcomes.

Open surgical technique

In open surgery the most frequent incision is the subcostal one. It is essential that this incision is not too close to the ribs. Also a real transverse incision can be performed, which can give a better cosmetic result. Closing of the diaphragm depends on the size of the defect. The different phenotypes of CDH are well described by Ackerman [23]. In clinical practice and in the CDH registry the defect size is categorized into four groups: type A concerns small defects; type B are defects smaller than 50% of the diaphragm; type C defects are larger than 50% and type D concerns total agenesis [23]. Primary closure is mostly feasible for type A and small type B defects. In general this is performed with interrupted non-absorbable sutures. The larger type B, C and D defects need repair with a patch. The ideal patch material has to be strong enough to hold the sutures against abdominal pressure, pliable enough to allow natural movements and inert enough to prevent adhesions. Furthermore it would be ideal if native tissue could be incorporated to account for the rapidly expanding surface area preventing chest wall deformation. The most commonly used non-absorbable patch is made of polytetrafluorethylene (PTFE) but this does not allow incorporation of native tissue. In many small case studies absorbable patches are used, such as a-cellular porcine intestinal submucosa type 1 collagen (Surgisis), a-cellular human cadavaric dermis (AlloDerm), a-cellular porcine dermal cross-linked collagen (Permacol) or non-cross-linked collagen (Straties) [24]. In animal studies the PTFE patches show more recurrences, foreign body reactions and rib-deformation than most absorbable patches, however the long-term results in these animal models are not yet clear. Clinical data of small series with absorbable patches show recurrence rates between 14% and 40% and small bowel obstruction rates between 7% and 22%. Furthermore, these studies concern a relatively short follow-up while recurrences in the long term can also be expected due to impairment of the resulting scar tissue which is left at the place of the graft. In summary, none of the currently available patches hold all the ideal characteristics and the absorbable patches so far have not demonstrated clear advantages over the most used PTFE patch. The conventional open patch repair is with a patch the size of the defect or with an overlapping border of 1 cm circumferentially and sutured with interrupted non-absorbable material to the rim of the diaphragm. Significantly reduced recurrence rates in open repair are seen when cone-shaped PTFE patches are used [25]. The advantages of the cone-shaped patch are an increased abdominal capacity and reduction of redundant chest capacity, thereby allowing a normal physiological position of the abdominal organs, which in turn prevents gastroesophageal reflux (GER) and causes fewer recurrences because of separate fixation of the overlapping border of the cone. There are no studies comparing running and interrupted sutures; however, most centers use the latter technique. In addition to patch repair for large congenital diaphragmatic hernias a split abdominal wall muscle flap is a good alternative. A retrospective study showed a reduced risk of recurrence [26].

When closing the diaphragm, the intrathoracic abdominal organs have to be placed in the abdomen, which is sometimes too small for all these organs, in which case the abdominal cavity closing is impossible or results in abdominal compartment syndrome. In these cases, a patch is temporarily sutured in the abdominal wall. This can be performed with patches from PTFE, silicon or other materials. Normally these patches should be removed within a few weeks because of the high rate of infection. After this period, in most cases, the abdomen can be closed.

Originally thoracic drains were frequently used. It was important to have no suction on these drains, as this could move the mediastinum too much to the ipsilateral side. This can have a devastating effect on the circulatory and ventilatory stability of the patients. Today only the use of thoracic drainage is advocated in patients on ECMO.

Minimal access surgery

The traditional surgical management of CDH consists of repair by laparotomy. Since the 1990s minimal access surgery (MAS) became more popular in pediatric surgery. Therefore, laparoscopic and thoracoscopic repair techniques are being explored more in neonates with CDH. General advantages of MAS include less pain, less surgical stress, faster recovery and shorter hospitalization. Thoracoscopy for CDH can also bring a potential decrease in the occurrence of subsequent scoliosis, chest deformation, shoulder muscle girdle weakness and is associated with shorter duration of postoperative ventilation and a lesser need of narcotics. Early studies reported higher recurrence rates in the thoracoscopic repair group. This was explained by the so-called learning curve. However, more recent studies report no decrease of recurrence. Moreover, conversion of thoracoscopic surgery to open surgery is often needed (3.4% to 75.0%) because of surgical technical and ventilation problems. With respect to general complications, there is no significant difference between the approaches in the literature. In one study the mortality in the open repair group was higher due to these patients' worse condition. Those patients have more need of cardiovascular and pulmonary support and often have a larger defect with the liver protruding into the thorax. All previous studies are retrospective and non-randomized. So the two types of surgery can still not be validly compared [27].

Several articles describe selection criteria for thoracoscopic repair. The cardiovascular criteria are almost the same in these overviews, i.e. no clinical signs of persistent pulmonary hypertension, no need for inhaled nitric oxide during surgery and no need for ECMO. They all agree that the patient has to be respiratory stable, but the definition of respiratory stable differs for PIP, PEEP, FiO2 and the saturation of peripheral oxygen (SpO2). The ventilation criteria of the recommendations of the CDH consortium are a PEEP of 2 to 5 cm and in addition FiO2 < 50% with SpO2 between 85%–95%, so that both open and thoracoscopic repair are possible. These recommendations are based on non-analytic studies, case reports or expert opinions. The artificial pneumothorax needed for thoracoscopic surgery creates acidosis due to hypercapnia by CO2 insufflation. This, in combination with higher intra-abdominal pressure, is believed to be related to deficient microcirculation. Nevertheless, patients with hypercapnia showed global hyperperfusion of the cerebral blood flow.

Bishay et al. recently proved severe arterial blood gas changes during thoracoscopic repair of CDH, but this finding was based on only five patients [28]. We also showed significant differences in pH and pCO2 values before and after thoracoscopic repair. However, these differences were small and have no clinical relevance. Due to the acidosis and hypercapnia, high frequency oscillation ventilation during neonatal thoracoscopic repair has gained attention in recent years. Mortellaro et al. showed that this allowed good intraoperative exposure in correction of esophageal atresia and CDH, while allowing excellent oxygenation and elimination of carbon dioxide to prevent acidosis [29].

The long-term consequences of hypercapnia and acidosis during surgery are still unknown.

Because of the possible detrimental effect in CDH patients of thoracoscopic repair, in several centers this is only done when the patient is cardiovascular and pulmonary stable. Still, if it appears that a patch is needed the technique must be converted to open surgery. The patient who does not fulfill the above criteria will undergo open repair from the start.

Other surgeries

The most common surgeries after recovering from the diaphragmatic hernia are fundoplications and gastrostomies. A high percentage of these patients have feeding problems which frequently require an open or laparoscopic gastrostomy. Also GER is seen in a high percentage of these patients, which leads to the need of a fundoplication [30].

6.2.7 Long-term follow-up

As increasing numbers of neonates with CDH survive, attention should be directed to possibly persisting morbidity. Initially, most studies that had been published were cross-sectional and in small study populations and focusing on pulmonary or gastrointestinal morbidity. The past few years have seen a shift towards long-term multidisciplinary evaluations.

Respiratory morbidity

Despite the fact that severe respiratory failure with fulminant persistent pulmonary hypertension and the need for ECMO occurs in the neonatal period, airflow obstruction in survivors of school and adolescent age is usually mild [31, 32]. However, most studies were performed several decades ago and selection bias of the survivors may play a role as children with the most severe lung hypoplasia died. Longitudinal data in a cohort of ECMO-treated CDH patients showed that lung function seems to deteriorate over time as the children get older: mean (SE) z-score FEV1 decreased from -0.71(0.40) at 5 years to -2.73(0.61) at 12 years [33]. Airflow obstruction may occur from airway hypoplasia and fibrotic changes following lung damage caused by artificial ventilation and hyperoxia. Measured lung volumes are usually within normal limits. Most likely, the hypoplasia has been compensated for by alveolar distension and, consequently, hyperinflation. Therefore, the question arises whether measurement of lung function adequately reflects lung morphology. However, data on lung morphology are scarce and usually limited to postmortem findings. Recently, a new imaging technique has become available and the results of this technique in adult CDH survivors have been published: The use of hyperpolarized helium inhalation as contrast agent during magnetic resonance imaging (MRI) of the lungs provides the opportunity for non-invasive measurements of alveolar dimensions and evaluation of the homogeneity of ventilation (Fig. 6.2.1) [34].

Several cross-sectional studies on maximal exercise endurance at school age and adulthood are published: It is usually normal or decreased in comparison to

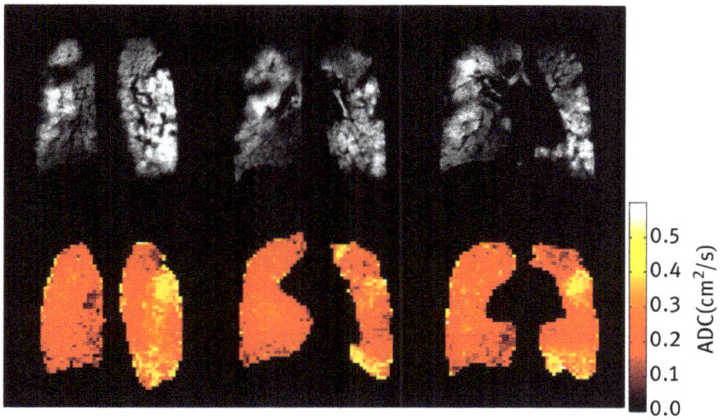

Fig. 6.2.1: Hyperpolarized 3He MR images of an 18-year-old CDH patient, treated with neonatal ECMO; (top row) ventilation-weighted images demonstrating multiple ventilation defects and (bottom row) maps of 3He apparent diffusion coefficient (ADC) showing elevated ADC in the ipsilateral lung compared to the contralateral lung consistent with enlargement of mean dimensions of the confining lung micro-structure at the alveolar level. (Images provided by Helen Marshall and Jim Wild, POLARIS, Academic Radiology, University of Sheffield, UK).

healthy peers depending on the clinical characteristics of the study population and the reference data that have been applied [32, 35–37]. In a longitudinal study in CDH-patients treated with neonatal ECMO aged 5 to 12 years, maximal exercise endurance deteriorated significantly over time, the mean (SE) z-score maximal endurance time decreased from -0.53(0.33) at 5 years to -2.23(0.52) at 12 years [38]. It is not clear why exercise capacity decreases over time. No correlation between airflow obstruction and maximal exercise endurance has been observed. However, ventilation-perfusion mismatch, which has been described in CDH patients and gets worse when the children get older, may have a role in the deterioration of exercise capacity [39]. It is unknown whether pulmonary hypertension contributes to the deterioration of exercise capacity.

Respiratory tract infections (RTI) frequently occur within the first years of life of CDH patients but may persist into adulthood [40]. Immunization to prevent respiratory syncytial viral infections within the first year, the use of prophylactic antibiotic therapy and influenza vaccinations may be important to reduce the frequency and severity of RTI. Recurrent RTI affect oral intake and physical growth and may lead to impairment of physical activity in the first years of life and beyond. This – in its turn – may reduce the opportunities to practice gross motor skills and hence lead to less physical activity.

Taking into account that more children with more severe lung hypoplasia nowadays survive long term follow-up and care even into adulthood is warranted, aiming at prevention of inhalation of toxic agents (smoking habits, exposure during practice of a profession), recurrent RTI, and physical inactivity.

Gastrointestinal morbidity and physical growth

Children with CDH are at risk for GER, feeding difficulties and growth failure. Patch repair and intrathoracic liver position have been described as predictors for GER [41]. In childhood prevalences of GER, up to 85% have been described in the literature, whereas symptoms are reported less frequently. This suggests that CDH patients have an altered perception of GER symptoms and may be at risk for development of (Barrett's) esophagitis. The question is of active screening for GER and endoscopic surveillance is warranted for this patient group. Further studies evaluating GER at older ages in CDH patients may be needed. ECMO-treated CDH patients have more severe growth failure than non-ECMO treated patients. This may be due to the more severe lung hypoplasia rather than the ECMO treatment itself. As impaired growth in CDH persists in childhood (Fig. 6.2.2) long-term follow-up – starting within the first months of life – with standardized nutritional assessment and intervention aiming at dietary management and oral intake is important.

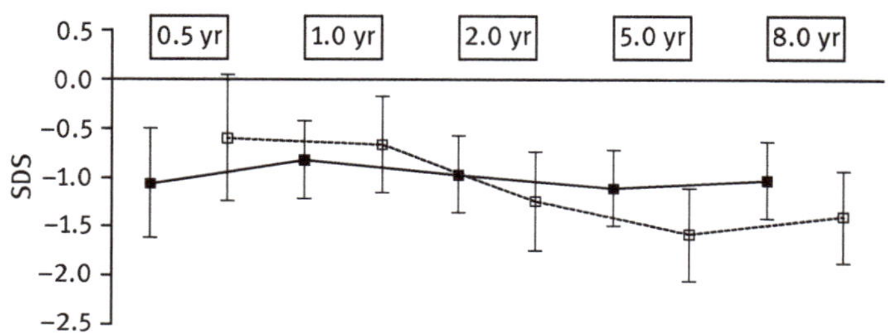

Fig. 6.2.2: Mean (95% confidence interval) SDS height corrected for parental height within first 8 years of life. Closed symbols represent CDH patients without ECMO treatment; open symbols represent ECMO-treated CDH patients.

Sensorineural hearing loss

Sensorineural hearing loss (SNHL) is another physical problem that has been reported in CDH survivors. Its prevalence varies among different studies, and risk factors seem to be related to neonatal intensive care treatment such as acidosis and use of aminoglycosides, neuromuscular blocking agents and loop diuretics rather than the underlying congenital anomaly itself [42].

Neurodevelopmental outcomes

The burden that affects quality of life and participation in society which arises from neurodevelopmental morbidity has hardly been recognized in CDH patients up till now since evaluation of neurodevelopmental outcome usually stops at school age or even earlier.

When evaluating the results of different studies on neurodevelopmental outcome we have to realize that standardized assessments cannot be performed in children with severe disabilities. Data on motor function performance in CDH patients is scarce, but problems in this domain occur in approximately 40% of children at preschool age and 20%–30% at school age. In general, ECMO-treated CDH patients show worse motor performance. Most problems are seen with gross motor function [43]. From infancy up till school age normal scores for cognition have been reported in several studies in CDH survivors. Despite an overall average cognition, however, many children (up to 50%) have problems keeping up with the regular education program and have special educational needs. The ECMO-treated CDH patients are more at risk for impaired intelligence than those who don't need ECMO [44]. The first data on neuropsychological outcomes in CDH revealed that at school age children have problems with information-processing speed and sustained attention and concentration [45]. The question arises whether these patients – and especially the most critically ill neonates who needed ECMO-treatment – are at risk for neuropsychological problems due to impaired development of executive functioning skills, which are developed in early childhood and continue development into young adulthood. These skills are needed to develop academic, behavioral and social functioning and to prepare for successful daily functioning (e.g. starting a career). Poor executive functioning skills may cause problems with functioning in a complex and demanding environment.

6.2.8 Implications and future perspectives

During the past decade survival has increased due to the introduction of standardized treatment protocols and advanced techniques in surgery and intensive care. Therefore, more children that otherwise would have died survive. The current population of adult CDH patients was treated in another era and it can be assumed that they have less severe lung hypoplasia. However, they were ventilated with less sophisticated equipment with high ventilatory pressures and high oxygen levels possibly resulting in more iatrogenic lung damage. Therefore, it is hard to predict whether microstructural morphological changes seen in the lungs of adult CDH patients will be representative of long-term respiratory morbidity in CDH survivors of today. We have to realize that standardized lung function tests provide us with indirect information on pulmonary function but not on lung structure. Future care and studies on long-term respiratory morbidity should aim at longitudinal assessments of lung function, lung imaging, exercise endurance and cardiac function. Impaired gross motor function may lead to physical inactivity and diminished exercise tolerance. An active lifestyle should be advocated with additional support to stimulate motor function if needed. Chronic malnutrition due to diminished intake or an increased energy expenditure will lead to growth failure and lethargy, which may – in its turn – also lead to physical inactivity and learning problems. At present, it is not clear which factors contribute to long-term neuropsychological morbidity but prolonged hospital stay, multiple surgeries and prolonged exposure to (toxic) sedatives and analgesic drugs may have a role. Multicenter studies in centers using similar treatment protocols and standardized follow-up programs are needed to create large enough sample sizes to study determinants of long-term morbidities in CDH.

Anne Schneider, Francesca Borruto and Francois Becmeur

6.3 Eventration

6.3.1 Introduction – definition

CDE is a serious and rare condition representing about 5% of all diaphragmatic defects [46]. It consists of a diaphragmatic outpouching allowing the displacement of the abdominal organs into the thorax due to a focal defective musculature, resulting in a partial elevation of a hemidiaphragm with lung compression. The consequences for the development of the fetal lungs are similar to CDH, but CDE presents a better prognosis. Focal lesions are more frequent, affecting the right hemidiaphragm (65%–70%), but a whole hemidiaphragm (42%) or even both sides may be involved [46–48].

6.3.2 Etiology, physiopathology

Congenital or "true diaphragmatic eventration" derives from an anomaly during the formation of the pleuroperitoneal membrane at 8–10 weeks of gestation with focal thinning and loss of normal musculature of the diaphragm, which is replaced by a tissue composed of diffuse fibroelastic changes and a paucity of muscle fibers [46–48]. The etiology of CDE is unknown, though infectious causes, such as cytomegalovirus or rubella, have been implicated, while no known familial predisposition is demonstrated [49]. Acquired CDE can derivate from birth trauma, cardiac surgery, central line placement or any injury occurring to the phrenic nerve [50]. Those patients have a normal amount of muscle fiber, but not correctly working [48].

6.3.3 Clinical presentation

Congenital

Most CDE are diagnosed in early childhood (75% within 1 year) with a peak at age 0–3 months [47]. Early clinical manifestations are not obvious and nonspecific and some children can be asymptomatic, especially if they have a focal CDE (51% in a large series of 177 pediatric cases) [47]. The main symptoms derive from the compression of the lower lobe of the lung as result of the elevated intra-abdominal organs. It involves the loss of the chest wall compliance and the mismatch of the ventilation/perfusion [48]. These factors provide recurrent respiratory infections, persistent cough or expectoration, dyspnea, vascular dysfunction and cardiac symptoms (tachycardia or arrhythmia, cyanosis). Mild gastrointestinal disorders such as nausea and vomiting or anorexia may also be associated [47]. Most rarely thorax deformity (rib deformity or pectus excavatum) may be noted.

Late presentation

Less often CDE can be detected in a late diagnosis (about 23% of patients after 1 year, and less than 5% after 3 years), which concerns mainly asymptomatic patient [46–48]. The majority present with an elevated hemidiaphragm discovered incidentally on a chest X-ray.

6.3.4 Paraclinical investigation

The thoracic prenatal MRI provides a prenatal diagnosis and detects any associated malformations. Chest X-ray (standard full-inspiration posteroanterior and lateral chest roentgenogram) shows the elevated hemidiaphragm. Pulmonary scintigraphy can highlight the entity of the hypoperfusion and the hypoventilation of the lung: the vital capacity and total lung capacity are reduced by 20% to 30% in CDE [47]. Pulmonary function tests can be used to monitor changes over time [48].

6.3.5 Treatment

Indication

Surgery is indicated only for symptomatic patients. Indications for surgery include rapid breathing without improvement under a conservative treatment, two or more recurrent ipsilateral pneumonias, one life-threatening pneumonia, inability to wean from mechanical ventilation or respiratory distress related to paradoxical motion of the diaphragm [47]. In case of asymptomatic patients and CDE incidentally detected there is still an open debate in the literature; the exuberant diaphragm may impair lung development. The current trend is that there is no indication for plication if the patient remains fully asymptomatic. But irreversible parenchyma impairment should be considered also in asymptomatic patients. Surgery allows re-expanding of the atelectatic lung, improvement in respiratory and digestive symptoms and improvement in the quality of life within 1 month if a thoracotomy or laparotomy approach is performed [47]. However ventilatory function is less impaired after a thoracoscopy than a thoracotomy so that the postoperative pulmonary function improvement is quite immediate [51].

Techniques

The principle of the operation is to manage to decrease the surface of the redundant diaphragm by plicating it to an acceptable normal level. In this way the repair improves the movement of the diaphragm during respiration and achieves physiologic pulmonary function. Care should be taken to protect the phrenic nerve.

Posterolateral thoracotomy: is the traditional approach. In a lateral decubitus position with the affected side up, using contralateral single lung ventilation. A variety of techniques have been described for the suture: U-stitches, mattress sutures, running sutures and stapling devices [48].

Laparotomy: interesting for left CDE and access to both sides of the diaphragm with a single incision [48].

Nowadays minimally invasive approaches are replacing open surgery in many areas of pediatric surgery. CDE laparoscopy and thoracoscopy avoid the morbidity associated with open procedures, such as thoracic dystrophy and scoliosis, and result in decreased pain, shorter length of stay and quicker return to normal activity [50].

Laparoscopy: provides more room for manipulation and an appropriate view of the branches of the phrenic nerve. Laparoscopy can be very useful if a thoracoscopic approach is impossible because of intrathoracic adhesions after cardiac surgery or in case of technical problems with single-lung ventilation [51].

The patient's position is supine, with the surgeon positioned between the legs. Three ports are used. The pneumoperitoneum pressure is at 8–10 mmHg [49]. The "invaginating the diaphragmatic dome" technique is performed by folding both sides of the weak areas of the diaphragm to the middle area and making interrupted nonabsorbable sutures. So the diaphragmatic dome is invaginated. The "pleating" technique consists of pleating little by little the redundant diaphragm like an accordion [49].

Thoracoscopy: can also benefit from a minithoracotomy (video-assisted thoracic surgery).

The child is placed in a lateral decubitus position with the surgeon in front of the child, and the screen behind (Fig. 6.3.1). The patient may be positioned head up to displace the intraabdominal organs downward for a better view and easy manipulation of the diaphragm. For young children, a block lying under the chest, opening the opposite intercostals spaces can be a good option. Unlike the adult surgery selective ventilation is not used: a gentle intrapleural CO_2 insufflation (4–6 mmHg) is applied to achieve the collapse of the lung. The optical port is placed just caudal to the tip of the scapula. Two operative ports are located under vision in the same intercostals space (fourth) anterior and posterior to the initial port (Fig. 6.3.2). A fourth port is sometimes necessary for pushing down the redundant diaphragm. Eventration is progressively reducted with two endoscopic graspers. The redundant diaphragm must be pulled and rolled with endoforceps and kept drawn tight when suturing it (Fig. 6.3.3). It is plicated with interrupted sutures using extracorporeal knots, or with a running suture (various nonabsorbable sutures) [51]. One of the advantages of this approach

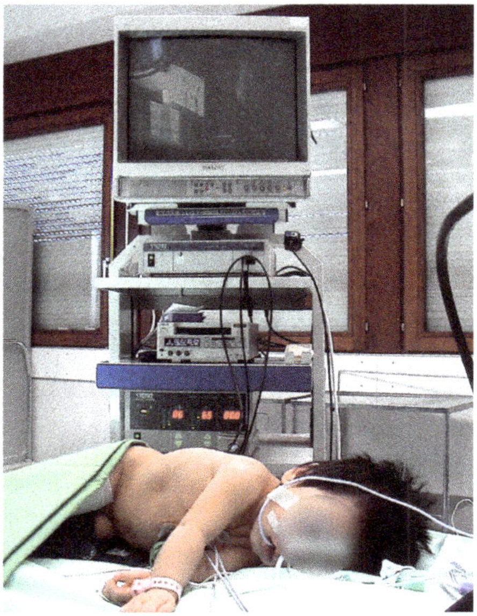

Fig. 6.3.1: Thoracoscopic approach. Patient in a lateral decubitus position, with the screen behind.

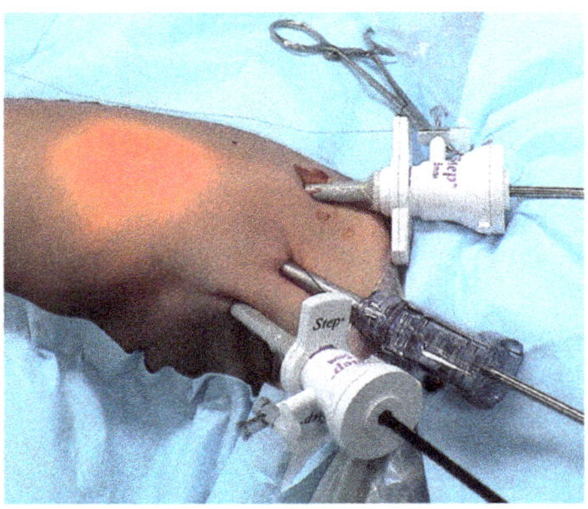

Fig. 6.3.2: Thoracoscopic approach. Port's position.

is the best view of the branches of the phrenic nerve, useful for example in case of a right eventration where the liver is an obstacle for laparoscopic plication [51].

Several plication techniques can be used and a review of the literature is presented in Tab. 6.3.1.

Tab. 6.3.1: Thoracoscopic approach for diaphragmatic eventration: review of the literature.

	Patients (n)	Median age (months)	Operating time (min)		Conversion
Becmeur, 2005 [51]	10	17.0 (6.0–41.0)	?		20%
Borruto, 2014 [52]	8	19.2 (6.0–84.0)	60.5 (40.0–85.0)		13%
Hu, 2014 [49]	8	12.7 (2.0–36.0)	“reefing the mainsail”	121.2 ± 33.6	0
	10		“invaginating the dome”	112.2 ± 25.2	
	9		“pleating”	90.6 ± 20.4	
Snyder, 2014 [50]	9	3.0 (0.2–13.2)	60.0 (50.0–84.0)		0
Kozlov, 2015 [53]	17	1.1 ± 0.6	51.8 ± 8.1		0

– Plication with interrupted sutures or a running suture: the excessive diaphragmatic remnant is left in place and not resected (Fig. 6.3.4)

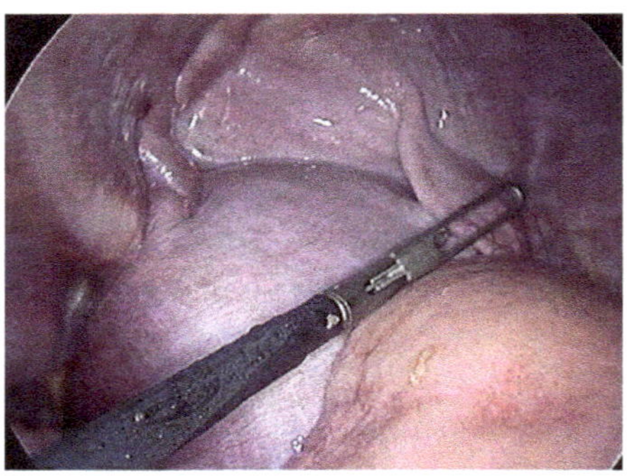

Fig. 6.3.3: Thoracoscopic approach: plication technique. Rolling the redundant diaphragm.

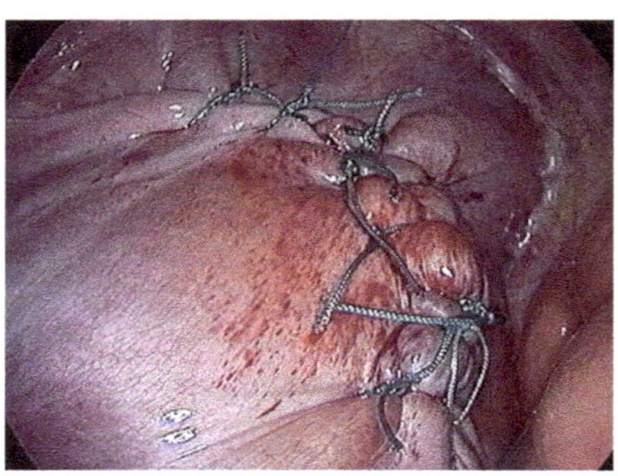

Fig. 6.3.4: Thoracoscopic approach: Port’s position. Plication with interrupted nonabsorbable sutures.

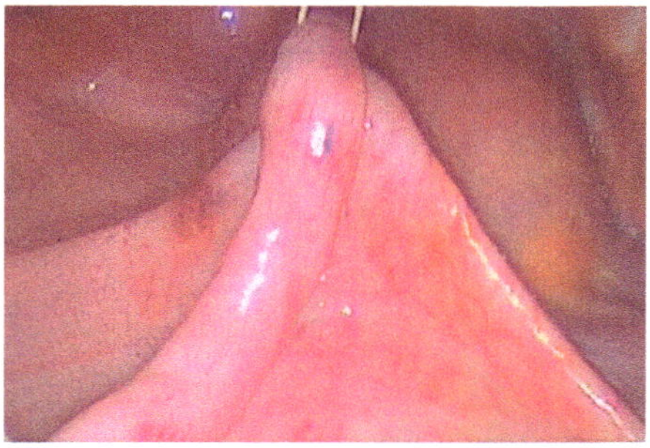

Fig. 6.3.5: Thoracoscopic approach: resection/suturing of the excessive diaphragm with the use of an endostapler. Suspension of the diaphragmatic dome.

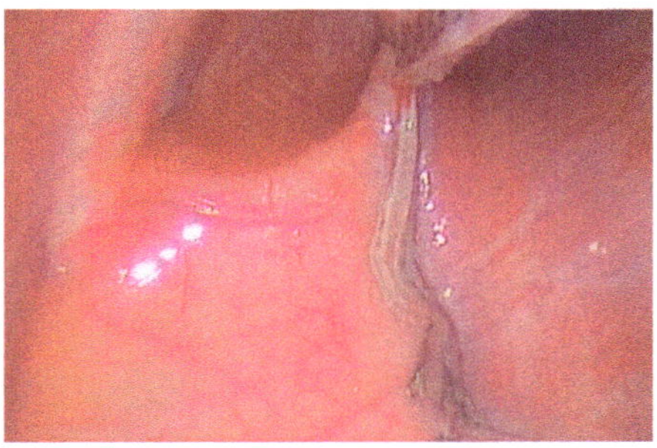

Fig. 6.3.6: Thoracoscopic approach: resection/suturing of the excessive diaphragm with the use of an endostapler. Final view of the remaining diaphragm.

- Resection/suturing of the excessive diaphragm with the use of an endostapler (Fig. 6.3.5–Fig. 6.3.7). To help exposure of the excessive diaphragmatic dome, it requires suspension to the thoracic wall by two stitches, which can avoid use of an additional port or mini-thoracotomy. It is quite easy to perform by thoracoscopy, even in small children. But resection of the diaphragm is a risky procedure and should not be generally recommended (risk of intrathoracic evisceration); this technique should be reserved for cases of excessive redundancy of the diaphragm, avoiding however the creation of excessive tensions and assuring the procedure by an additional running suture [52].
- Diaphragmatic plication using a spinal needle: an 18-gauge spinal needle is passed through the chest wall into the pleural space. The diaphragm is plicated over the needle and a non-absorbable suture is passed through the needle and tied extracorporeally. The needle is passed repeatedly until the desired degree of tension is achieved. Intracorporeal suturing, which can be technically difficult in small neonates, is avoided [49].
- "Reefing the mainsail" technique: the top of the diaphragm is folded to the opposite side and strengthened with layers of the musculus diaphragm using interrupted nonabsorbable sutures; the "invaginating the diaphragmatic dome" technique and the "pleating" technique can also be used [48].

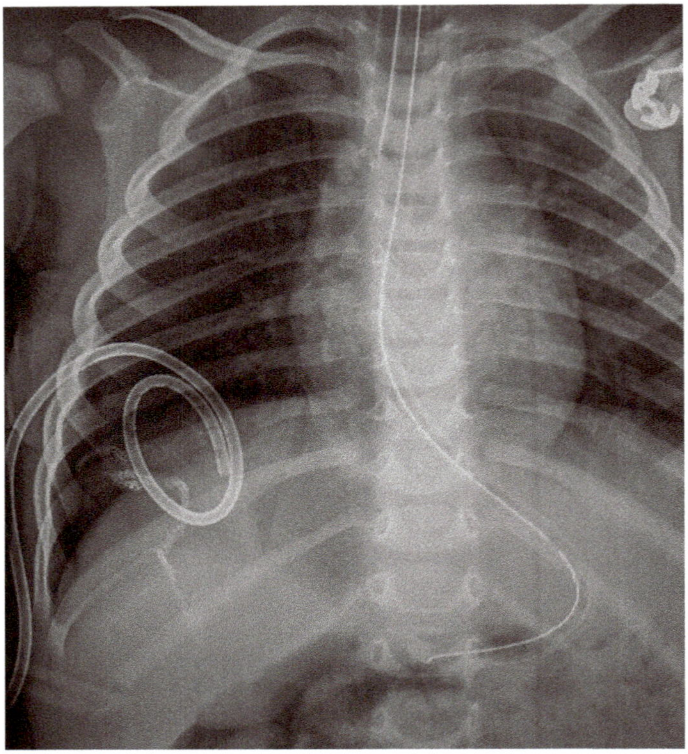

Fig. 6.3.7: Thoracoscopic approach: resection/suturing of the excessive diaphragm with the use of an endostapler. Postoperative chest X-ray showing the stapler line.

An open controversy concerns the use of a thoracic drain. Some authors assert that a gentle suction can be sufficient to re-expand the lung and remove residual air in the pleural space [51]. Surely it can reduce postoperative pain.

Complications for all approaches

In a recent study, Kozlov et al. affirmed that early postoperative complications are more frequent in the open approach (16.7% vs. 0% in the thoracoscopic group) [53]. The complications related to the surgical treatment of CDE include:

- **Recurrence:** Few data are available about recurrences in pediatric population. Only one study reported two recurrences (13%) occurring at 10 and 3 months postoperatively using the endostapler resection technique [52]. Some authors argue that interrupted sutures may better prevent recurrence than running sutures; but there is no evidence for it [49, 51]. One study compared a thoracotomy vs. thoracoscopic approach for eventration in the first 3 months of life: two recurrences (11%) occurred in the first group vs. no recurrence in the thoracoscopic group (but result not significant) [53].

- **Pneumonia** 6% [47],
- **Pleural effusions** 15% [47],
- **Pneumothorax** (0–22%) [49–50, 53],
- **Gastroesophageal reflux** (17%) [53].

Redo-procedures

A redo-procedure with a thoracoscopic approach, consisting of the resection/suture of the redundant diaphragm by an endostapler 10 months after thoracoscopic plicature, have been successful performed but there is not enough experience in the literature to confirm the technique as replicable [7].

6.3.6 Follow-up

A Chest X-ray and a clinical evaluation at 1, 6 and 12 months is recommended as follow-up [52–53].

There is little information about the long-term durability of eventration repair in children and adults: it can be hypothesized that there is some degree of recurrent diaphragmatic laxity over time [50]. In adult populations long-term follow-up data suggest that thoracoscopic diaphragmatic plication may be as effective as an open approach [48].

6.4 Further reading

[1] Wilson JM, Lund DP, Lillehei CW, Vacanti JP. Congenital diaphragmatic hernia – a tale of two cities: the Boston experience. J Pediatr Surg 1997;32:401e5.
[2] Clark RH, Hardin Jr WD, Hirschl RB, et al. Current surgical management of congenital diaphragmatic hernia: a report from the Congenital Diaphragmatic Hernia Study Group. J Pediatr Surg 1998;33:1004e9.
[3] Azarow K, Messineo A, Pearl R, Filler R, Barker G, Bohn D. Congenital diaphragmatic hernia – a tale of two cities: the Toronto experience. J Pediatr Surg 1997;32:395e400.
[4] Wung JT, Sahni R, Moffitt ST, Lipsitz E, Stolar CJ. Congenital diaphragmatic hernia: survival treated with very delayed surgery, spontaneous respiration, and no chest tube. J Pediatr Surg 995;30:406e9.
[5] UK collaborative randomised trial of neonatal extracorporeal membrane oxygenation. UK collaborative ECMO Trail Group. Lancet 1996;348(9020):75e82.
[6] Neonatal Inhaled Nitric Oxide Study Group (NINOS). Inhaled nitric oxide and hypoxic respiratory failure in infants with congenital diaphragmatic hernia. Pediatrics 1997;99:838e45.
[7] Clark RH, Kueser TJ, Walker MW, et al. Low-dose nitric oxide therapy for persistent pulmonary hypertension of the newborn. Clinical Inhaled Nitric Oxide Research Group. N Engl J Med 2000;342:469e74.
[8] Moyer V, Moya F, Tibboel R, Losty P, Nagaya M, Lally KP. Late versus early surgical correction for congenital diaphragmatic hernia in newborn infants. Cochrane Database Syst Rev 2002;(3): CD001695.
[9] Morini F, Goldman A, Pierro A. Extracorporeal membrane oxygenation in infants with congenital diaphragmatic hernia: a systematic review of the evidence. Eur J Pediatr Surg 2006;16:385e91.

[10] Lally KP, Lasky RE, Lally PA, Bagolan P, Davis CF, Frenckner BP, Hirschl RM, Langham MR, Buchmiller TL, Usui N, Tibboel D, Wilson JM. Congenital Diaphragmatic Hernia Study Group. Standardized reporting for congenital diaphragmatic hernia - an international consensus. J Pediatr Surg. 2013 Dec;48(12):2408–15.
[11] Clugston RD, Zhang W, Alvarez S, de Lera AR, Greer JJ. Understanding abnormal retinoid signaling as a causative mechanism in congenital diaphragmatic hernia. Am J Respir Cell Mol Biol 2010;42:276e85.
[12] Klaassens M, de Klein A, Tibboel D. The etiology of congenital diaphragmatic hernia: still largely unknown? Eur J Med Genet 2009;52:281e6.
[13] Clugston RD, Greer JJ. Diaphragm development and congenital diaphragmatic hernia. Semin Pediatr Surg 2007;16:94e100.
[14] Snoek KG, Capolupo I, Van Rosmalen et al. Conventional mechanical ventilation versus high-frequency ventilation for congenital diaphragmatic hernia. Annals of Surgery 2015. In press.
[15] Ba'ath ME, Jesudason EC, Losty PD. How useful is the lung-to-head ratio in predicting outcome in the fetus with congenital diaphragmatic hernia? A systematic review and meta-analysis. Ultrasound Obstet Gynecol 2007;30:897e906.
[16] Reiss I, Schaible T, van den Hout L, et al. Standardized postnatal management of infants with congenital diaphragmatic hernia in Europe: the CDH EURO Consortium consensus. Neonatology 2010;98:354e64.
[17] Humbert M, Sitbon O, Simonneau G. Treatment of pulmonary arterial hypertension. N Engl J Med 2004;351:1425e36.
[18] Harting MT, Lally KP. Surgical management of neonates with congenital diaphragmatic hernia. Semin Pediatr Surg 2007 May;16(2):109–14.
[19] van der Staak FH, de Haan AF, Geven WB, Festen C. Surgical repair of congenital diaphragmatic hernia during extracorporeal membrane oxygenation: hemorrhagic complications and the effect of tranexamic acid. J Pediatr Surg. 1997 Apr;32(4):594–9.
[20] Congenital Diaphragmatic Hernia Study Group, Bryner BS, West BT, Hirschl RB, Drongowski RA, Lally KP, Lally P, Mychaliska GB. Congenital diaphragmatic hernia requiring extracorporeal membrane oxygenation: does timing of repair matter? J. Pediatr Surg. 2009 Jun;44(6):1165–71; discussion 1171–2.
[21] Lago P, Meneghini L, Chiandetti L, Tormena F, Metrangolo S, Gamba PG. Congenital Diaphragmatic Hernia: Intensive Care Unit or Operating Room. Am. J of Perinatology 2005;22(4):189–97.
[22] Morini F, del Prete L, Capolupo I, Valfre L, Crisafull R, Dotta A, Bagolan P. Effect of surgical venue on patients with congenital diaphragmatic hernia. ICU vs OR. Presented on Biennial International CDH workshop 2015, Toronto.
[23] Ackerman KG, Pober B Congenital Diaphragmatic Hernia and Pulmonary Hypoplasia: New Insights From Developmental Biology and Genetics. Am J Med Genet C Semin Med Genet. 2007 May 15;145C(2):105–108.
[24] Romao RL, Nasr A, Chiu PP, Langer JC. What is the best prosthetic material for patch repair of congenital diaphragmatic hernia? Comparison and meta-analysis of porcine small intestinal submucosa and polytetrafluoroethylene. J Pediatr Surg. 2012 Aug;47(8):1496–500.
[25] Loff S, Wirth H, Jester I, Hosie S, Wollmann C, Schaible T, Ataman O, Waag KL. Implantation of a cone-shaped double-fixed patch increases abdominal space and prevents recurrence of large defects in congenital diaphragmatic hernia. J Pediatr Surg. 2005 Nov;40(11):1701–5.
[26] Barnhart DC, Jacques E, Scaife ER, Yoder BA, Meyers RL, Harman A, Downey EC, Rollins MD. Split abdominal wall muscle flap repair vs patch repair of large congenital diaphragmatic hernias. J Pediatr Surg. 2012 Jan;47(1):81–6.
[27] Costerus S, Zahn K, van de Ven K, Vlot J, Wessel L, Wijnen R. Thoracoscopic versus open repair of CDH in cardiovascular stable neonates. Surg Endosc. 2015 Oct 21. [Epub ahead of print]

[28] Bishay M, et al. Hypercapnia and Acidosis During Open and Thoracoscopic Repair of Congenital Diaphragmatic Hernia and Esophageal Atresia: Results of a Pilot Randomized Controlled Trial. Ann Surg. 2013 Apr 18 [Epub ahead of print].
[29] Mortellaro VE, Fike FB, Adibe OO, Juang D, Aguayo P, Ostlie DJ, Holcomb GW, St Peter SD. The use of high-frequency oscillating ventilation to facilitate stability during neonatal thoracoscopic operations. J Laparoendosc Adv Surg Tech A. 2011 Nov;21(9):877–9.
[30] Van der Hout L, Schaible T, Cohen-Overbeek TE, et al. Actual outcome in infants with congenital diaphragmatic hernia: the role of a standardized postnatal treatment protocol. Fetal Diagn Ther 2011:29;55–63.
[31] IJsselstijn H, Tibboel D, Hop WJC, Molenaar JC, Jongste de JC. Long-term pulmonary sequelae in children with congenital diaphragmatic hernia. Am J Respir Crit Care Med 1997;155:174–180.
[32] Peetsold MG, Heij HA, Nagelkerke AF, IJsselstijn H, Tibboel D, Quanjer PH, Gemke RJBJ. Pulmonary function and exercise capacity in survivors of congenital diaphragmatic hernia. Eur Respir J 2009;34:1140–1147.
[33] Spoel M, Laas R, Gischler SJ, Hop WCJ, Tibboel D, de Jongste JC, IJsselstijn H. Diagnosis-related deterioration of lung function after extracorporeal membrane oxygenation. Eur Respir J 2012;40:1531–1537.
[34] Spoel M, Marshall H, IJsselstijn H, Parra-Robles J, van der Wiel E, Swift AJ, Rajaram S, Tibboel D, Tiddens HA, Wild JM. Pulmonary ventilation and micro-structural findings in congenital diaphragmatic hernia. Pediatr Pulmonol; in press.
[35] Trachsel D, Selvadurai H, Adatia I, Bohn D, Schneiderman-Walker J, Wilkes D, Coates AL. Resting and exercise cardiorespiratory function in survivors of congenital diaphragmatic hernia. Pediatr Pulmonol 2006;41:522–9.
[36] van der Cammen-van Zijp MH, Spoel M, Laas R, Hop WC, de Jongste JC, Tibboel D, van den Berg-Emons RJ, IJsselstijn H. Exercise capacity, daily activity and severity of fatigue in term born young adults after congenital diaphragmatic hernia. Scand J Med Sci Sports 2014;24:144–151.
[37] Peetsold MG, Vonk-Noordegraaf A, Heij HH, Gemke RJ. Pulmonary function and exercise testing in adult survivors of congenital diaphragmatic hernia. Pediatr Pulmonol 2007;42:325–31.
[38] Van der Cammen-van Zijp MHM, Gischler SJ, Hop WC, de Jongste JC, Tibboel D, IJsselstijn H. Deterioration of exercise capacity after neonatal extracorporeal membrane oxygenation. Eur Respir J 2011;38:1098–1104.
[39] Hayward MJ, Kharasch V, Sheils C,et al. Predicting inadequate long-term lung development in children with congenital diaphragmatic hernia: an analysis of longitudinal changes in ventilation and perfusion. J Pediatr Surg 2007;42:112–116.
[40] Gischler SJ, van der Cammen-van Zijp MHM, Mazer P, Madern GC, Bax NMA, de Jongste JC, van Dijk M, Tibboel D, IJsselstijn H. A prospective comparative evaluation of persistent respiratory morbidity in esophageal atresia and congenital diaphragmatic hernia survivors. J Pediatr Surg 2009;44:1683–1690.
[41] Peetsold MG, Kneepkens CMF, Heij HA, IJsselstijn H, Tibboel D, Gemke RJBJ. Congenital diaphragmatic hernia: long-term risk of gastro-esophageal reflux disease. J Pediatr Gastroenterol Nutr 2010;51:448–453.
[42] Dennett KV, Fligor BJ, Tracy S, Wilson JM, Zurakowski D, Chen C. Sensorineural hearing loss in congenital diaphragmatic hernia survivors is associated with postnatal management and not defect size. J Pediatr Surg. 2014;49:895–9.
[43] Van der Cammen-van Zijp MHM, Janssen AJWM, Raets MMA, van Rosmalen J, Govaert PP, Steiner K, Gischler SJ, Tibboel D, van Heijst AFJ, IJsselstijn H. On behalf of the Dutch ECMO follow-up team. Motor performance after neonatal extracorporeal membrane oxygenation: a longitudinal evaluation. Pediatrics 2014;134:e427–435.

[44] Madderom MJ, Toussaint L, van der Cammen-van Zijp MHM, Gischler SJ, Wijnen RMH, Tibboel D, IJsselstijn H. Congenital diaphragmatic hernia with(out) ECMO: impaired development at eight years. Arch Dis Child Fetal Neonat 2013;98:F316–F322.
[45] Frisk V, Jakobson LS, Unger S, Trachsel D, O'Brien K. Long-term neurodevelopmental outcome of congenital diaphragmatic hernia survivors not treated with extracorporeal membrane oxygenation. J Pediatr Surg. 2011;46:1309–18.
[46] Alamo L, Gudinchet F, Meuli R. Imaging findings in fetal diaphragmatic abnormalities. Pediatr Radiol 2015;45:1887–900.
[47] Wu S, Zang N, Zhu J, Pan Z, Wu C. Congenital diaphragmatic eventration in children: 12 years' experience with 177 cases in a single institution. J Pediatr Surg 2015;50:1088–92.
[48] Groth SS, Andrade SR. Diaphragm plication for eventration or paralysis: a review of the literature. Ann Thorac Surg 2010;89:2146–50.
[49] Hu J, Wu Y, Wang J, Zhang C, Pan W, Zhou Y. Thoracoscopic and laparoscopic plication of the hemidiaphragm is effective in the management of diaphragmatic eventration. Pediatr Surg Int 2014;30:19–24.
[50] Snyder CW, Walford NE, Danielson PD, Chandler NM. A simple thoracoscopic plication technique for diaphragmatic eventration in neonates and infants: technical details and initial results. Pediatr Surg Int 2014;30:1013–16.
[51] Becmeur F, Talon I, Schaarschmidt K, Philippe P, Moog R, Kauffmann I, Schultz A, Grandadam S, Toledano D. Thoracoscopic diaphragmatic eventration repair in children: about 10 cases. J Pediatr Surg 2005;40:1712–5.
[52] Borruto FA, Gomes Ferreira C, Kaselas C, Schneider A, Lacreuse I, Kauffmann I, Moog R, Becmeur F. Thoracoscopic treatment of congenital diaphragmatic eventration in children: lessons learned after 15 years of experience. Eur J Pediatr Surg 2014;24:328–31.
[53] Kozlov Y, Novozhilov V. Thoracoscopic plication of the Diaphragm in Infants in the first 3 months of life. J Laparoendosc Adv Surg Tech 2015;25:342–7.

7 Thoracic wall

7.1 Introduction

Everything started in 1998 when Donald Nuss presented his 10-year experience of the minimally invasive repair of pectus excavatum. Over the years, his innovative technique rapidly gained attention and, today, it has become the standard procedure for treating patients with this condition. In this chapter, **Hans Pilegaard** describes the original procedure, its modifications and refinements, while **Hyung J. Park, Robert E. Kelly and Donald Nuss,** Dawn E. Jaroszewski and Jean-Marie Wihlm high-light several supplemental aspects of the surgery.

Horatio Abramson was the first person to transfer the principle of the Nuss procedure inversely to pectus carinatum, while **Francis Robicsek** still advocates for open repair. They comment on the chapter about pectus carinatum, contributed by **Caroline Fortmann** and **Claus Petersen**, who also describe the conservative bracing. Herein **Marcelo Martínez Ferro** offers his views on this approach. Due to the different anatomical and physical patterns of the growing skeletal system, thoracic trauma in the pediatric population differs significantly from that observed in adults, as reported by **Haiko K. Jahn** and **Sebastian van As**. Finally, the chapter concludes with **Claus Petersen** and **Frederic Lavrand's** discussion of other and rare deformities of the thoracic wall. In 2009, pediatric and thoracic surgeons founded the **Chest Wall International group (CWIG)**. For further information, please click at www.chestwall.org.

Hans Pilegaard

7.2 Pectus excavatum

Pectus excavatum (PE), funnel chest or sunken chest is the most frequent congenital anomaly of the anterior chest wall. It represents approximately 90% of these. It is more common in males compared to females with a ratio 4–6: 1. The incidence is 1 in 300–400 live-born males. It might be discovered in the first living year in around 80% but in some cases it is first seen at the beginning of puberty. A family history is present in 40%. Scoliosis is seen in about 20%. There is also a higher rate of PE in some connective tissue disorders as Marfan and Ehlers-Danlos syndromes.

Leonardo da Vinci was the first to depict it and the first description of PE was provided by Bauhinus in 1594. The first attempt to correct it was made by the German surgeon Ludwig Meyer in 1911. The modern era of correction started after 1949 where Ravitch from the US published his first paper [1]. This was an open technique with resection of ribs and cartilages. The technique was later modified with smaller incisions, preserving the perichondrium and introduction of supporting material under the sternum to retain the position. This technique was the gold standard until Nuss published his technique of minimal invasive repair in 1998 [2]. Other methods have also been used such as reversing the sternum and treatment with braces.

7.2.1 Indication

For many years it was thought that PE was only a cosmetic problem for the patients and the cosmetic complains are stated an indication in around 90% of the published papers in this field. Several papers studying the quality of life in patients with PE have shown a significantly better quality of life after correction, exhibiting higher self-esteem. More of these studies have also shown that patients after treatment feel that they have a better physical performance. More than 60% have symptoms like exercise intolerance, lack of endurance and shortness of breath [3].

It is obvious from CT-scans that the heart is moved more to the left in PE patients because of the pressure from the sternum and it is also seen in many patients that the right side of the heart is compressed. This does not influence the cardiac performance at rest but restricts the filling of the heart under physical activity. The cardiac performance is found to be reduced about 20% in adolescent age 14–17 years with a PE, but after treatment it becomes equal to normal controls [4]. In adults it has been shown that cardiac performance is significantly raised after correction by the modified Ravitch.

In most cases patients with PE have normal lung function but in the lower area. The reduced lung function has a restrictive picture. Studies have shown decreased movement of the chest in PE patients, which improves after correction.

Some surgeons use the Haller index as an indication. The Haller index is the ratio between the internal diameter of the chest at the level of the deepest point of the excavation and the distance from the backside of the sternum to the anterior part of the spine. If this is >3, 25, there might be indication for treatment. The index is dependent on the chest shape, because the same excavation seen from outside may give different indexes depending on if the chest is barrel-shaped or more flat.

There is no evidence for the optimal age for performing the procedure. In the eastern part of the world surgeons often correct patients in the age group 2–6 years. It is difficult to understand that such young children are complaining about the cosmetic and they do probably not have any symptoms. Nuss has seen that there is a trend to see more recurrences if the bar is removed before puberty, when the growth spurt starts. I would not treat a patient younger than the age of 11 years. It is important that the child understand what is going on and what one might expect in terms of postoperative pain following the correction. My optimal age is 11–13 years, but many girls are even older so they have had a demarcation of the breasts which allows placement of the incisions in the groove between the breast and the chest wall. The upper limit for doing the Nuss procedure is not defined. When the procedure was published it was said that only children and adolescents were candidates for this treatment, but with growing experience even patients older than 60 years have been corrected with good results and few complications.

7.2.2 Preoperative evaluation

Patients are seen for a clinical examination. An X-ray of the chest in the AP, and the lateral view is often sufficient. You may from this X-ray calculate a Haller index if you want, even it is not as exact as from a CT-scan. Doing only an X-ray also reduces the radiation to the patient. If there is a clinical suspicion to comorbidity in the chest it is necessary to perform a CT-scan of the chest. If Marfan syndrome is suspected, an echocardiography must also be ordered.

The patient should be informed about the expected result, which is that the excavated area will disappear. However, if flaired ribs are present, they will remain.

7.2.3 Technique

The original technique prescribed a bar extending from one mid-axillary line to the other. It is difficult to understand why the bar should be so long. The ends of the bar would only be parallel to the lateral chest wall and therefore not deliver any force from the pressure of the sternum. Placing the stabilizer(s) at the end(s) would not secure the bar against rotation.

Today more surgeons are using a shorter bar as proposed by Pilegaard [5]. A short bar is easier to place. The median length of bars is in 840 corrected patients 10". The bar may be guided in a better way through the chest and is also easier to remove. The stabilizer can be placed very close to the hinge point which gives a very stable situation, so you do not need additional sutures around the bar and the rib.

How many bars are needed in the patient is dependent on the depth of the excavation and the age of the patient. If you are in doubt of the numbers of bars needed to correct the patient it might often be better to insert two bars instead of only one to have the best correction. Two bars may in many cases be inserted through the same incisions especially in females, where the skin of the breasts is often more moveable. More bars will probably decrease the pain because they will deliver the pressure to a larger surface. In very few cases three bars may even be needed to get a good correction (Tab. 7.2.1).

One bar should normally support the deepest point. If the PE is very long, like a grand canyon type, a bar is often placed at the level of the nipples. In such a case

Tab. 7.2.1: Number of bars in 840 patients.

Number of bars	Age <18 years	18 years ≤ Age < 30 years	Age ≥ 30 years
1	75%	59%	20%
2	25%	40%	69%
3		1%	11%

a periareolar incision around the nipple on the left side makes it easier to put the stabilizer on. If the PE is very low and the deepest point is below the sternum you should use two bars where the upper one supports the sternum and the lower one is under the deepest point. The deepest point is sometimes between two levels of intercostal spaces. Here it might be a good idea to use an oblique bar (Fig. 7.2.1). If the excavation is very deep it is a good idea to place the first introducer higher than the deepest point as this will work like a crane and facilitate going under the deepest point with the next introducer. Different types of crane systems might also be used.

The procedure is done under general anesthesia. All patients should in my opinion have an epidural catheter for postoperative pain treatment. This stays for two

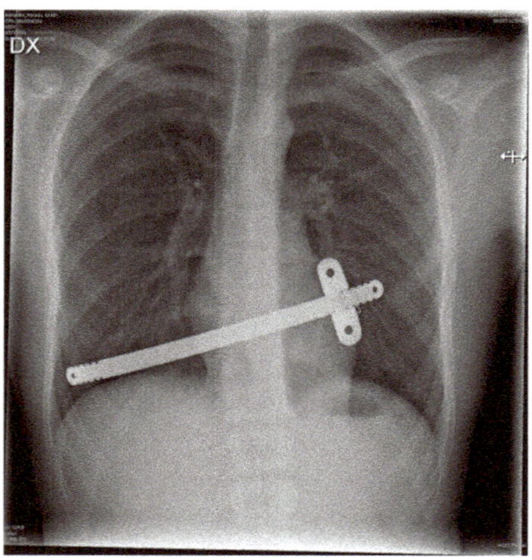

Fig. 7.2.1: The X-ray shows an oblique bar.

days. The patient is intubated with a single lumen tube, and only if you expect problems inside the chest cavity because of previous intervention or infections do you need a double lumen tube. You may use CO_2 gas to get a better view in the chest cavity, but it is often not necessary in my experience. The patient is located to the right on the table with the arm in front of the head (Fig. 7.2.2). The thoracoscope is inserted through the right lateral chest wall at the level of the nipple (Fig. 7.2.3). This gives you free movement of the scope and no problems with a very low bar.

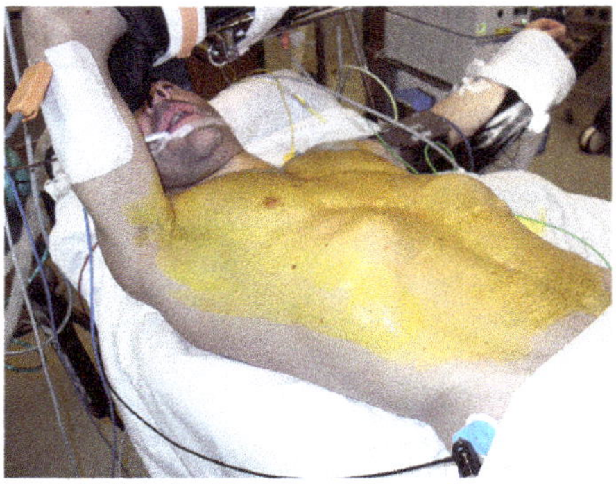

Fig. 7.2.2: The position of the patient on the table.

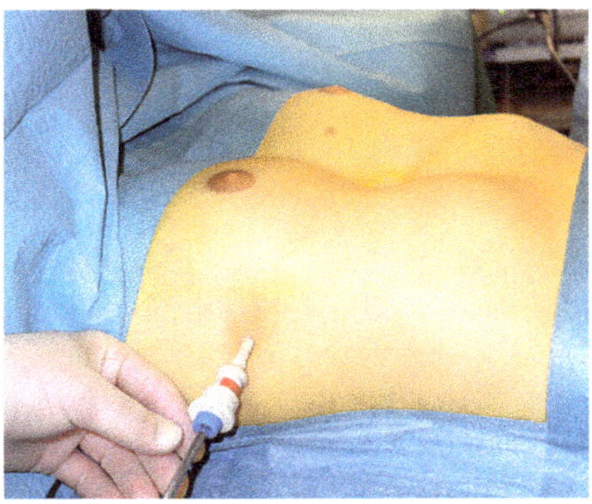

Fig. 7.2.3: The level of the insertion of the scope.

The deepest point is identified, and the intercostal spaces related to this are marked just medially to the highest point (Fig. 7.2.4). You may check this by putting a finger where you have marked and push, you can then see through the scope if it is at the correct point related to the deepest point. A template is shaped to the desired shape of the chest and even with some overcorrection (Fig. 7.2.5), because the bar will flatten in some way by the pressure from the elevated sternum (Fig. 7.2.6).

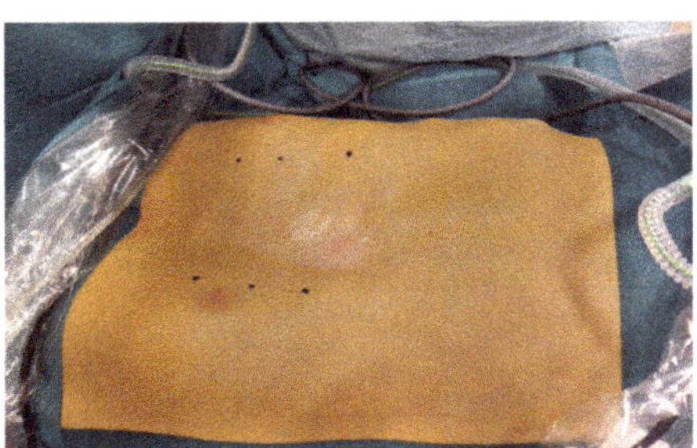

Fig. 7.2.4: Marking of the spots where the bar passes in and out of the chest.

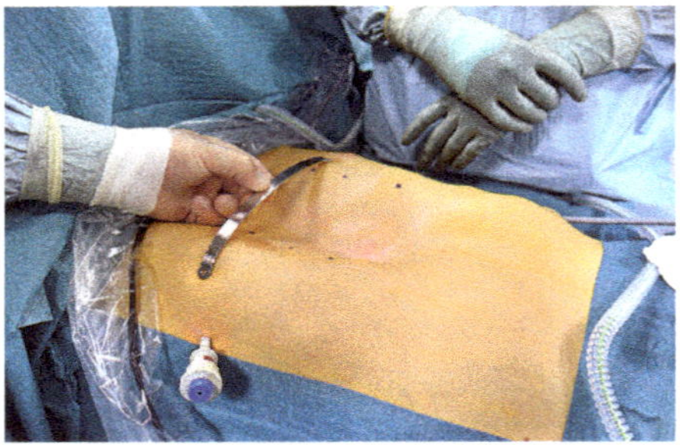

Fig. 7.2.5: Overcorrection of the bar.

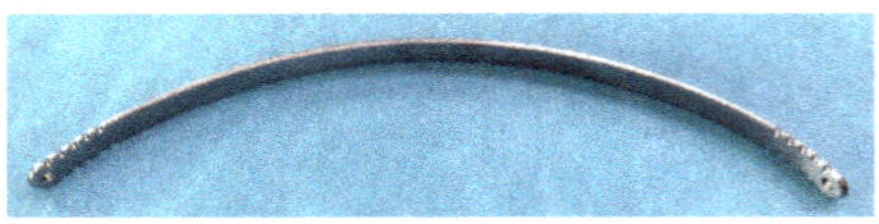

(a)

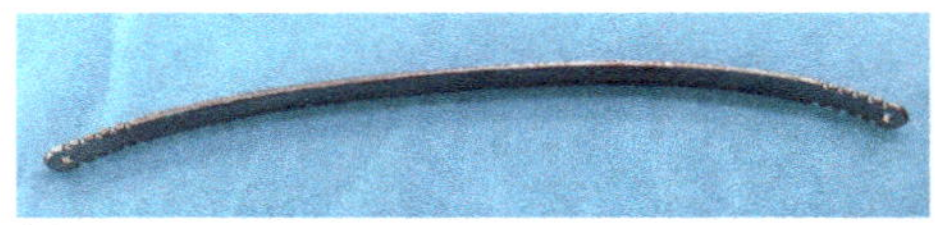

(b)

Fig. 7.2.6: Flattening of a bar after ten minutes in the body.

The bar is bent in the same way. The tunnel under the sternum is normally done by one of the introducers and the large one will in most cases be the one you should use. If there previously has been surgery inside the chest cavity and adhesions are found, they should all be cut and the tunnel created by blunt dissection using a long instrument with a peanut. If it is a long excavation and two bars are needed, it is often advantageous to place both the introducers at first and then replace one after the other with a bar (Fig. 7.2.7).

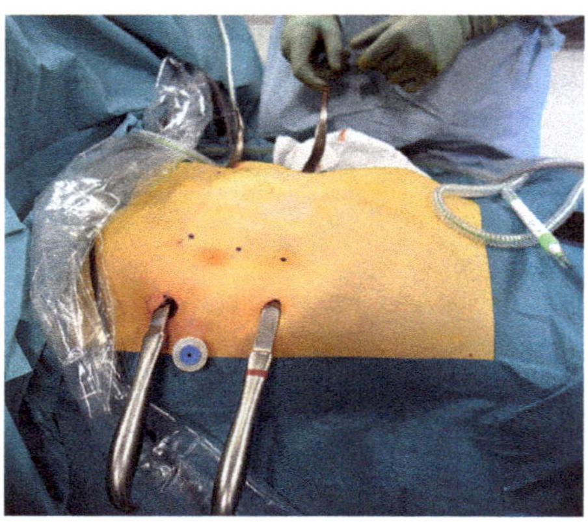

Fig. 7.2.7: Two introducers in the patient.

The bar is guided by a tape or a suture under the sternum and inserted like a U and turned 180°. Generally the stabilizer is located on the left side. The bar is placed asymmetrically on the chest, so the end with no stabilizer has a base of two ribs (Fig. 7.2.8). No additional sutures are necessary. The position of the stabilizer to the left might be a good idea to avoid compression of the heart if the end of the bar without a stabilizer should drop into the chest.

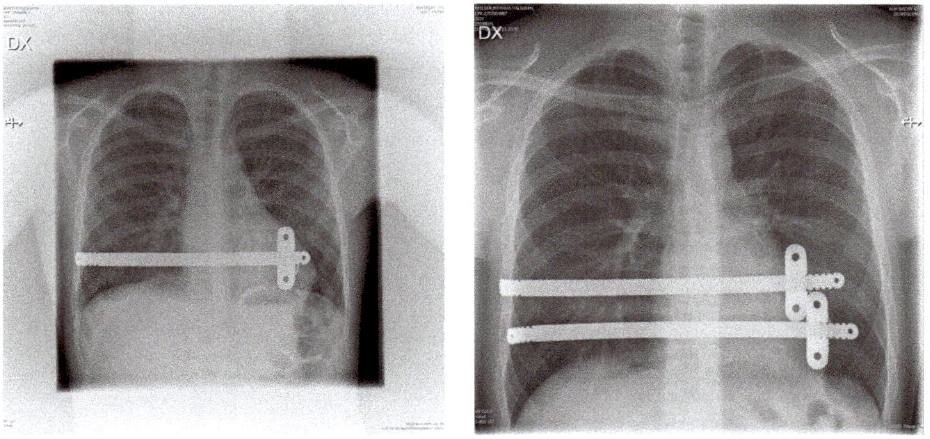

(a) (b)

Fig. 7.2.8: Asymmetric position of the bars.

The air inside the chest is exsufflated by a thin tube through the port to the scope and then the tube is removed.

The patient receives antibiotics intravenously for 3 days.

7.2.4 Postoperative care and follow up

The patient is mobilized at once after surgery and 80% can be discharged from the hospital on the second day.

In the first 6 weeks after correction there are some restrictions. The patient is not allowed to carry more than 2 kg in front of the body and 5 kg on the back. The patient is not allowed to bike or drive a car and should avoid tvisting the upper body and sleep on the back.

Pain medication is continued for 4–5 weeks and consists of morphine for 10–14 days, ibuprofene for 3–4 weeks and paracetamole for 4–5 weeks.

The patient is checked after 6 weeks with a chest X-ray and clinical control and starts then with exercises from a physiotherapist, running, swimming and biking and gradually increases the level of activity until 12 weeks postoperatively. At that time the patient should be back at the preoperative level.

As long as the bar(s) is in situ heavy contact sport should be avoided. This means ice hockey, rugby, American football and self-defense disciplines.

The bar(s) is generally removed after 3 years.

7.2.5 Complications

The complication rate should be low. The infection rate is about 1%–2%. The risk of bleeding is <1%. The rate of rotation or dislocation is approximately 1% (Tab. 7.2.2). Doing this kind of surgery you need to be able to open the chest by a sternotomy if lesions to the heart develop and there should be access to cardiac surgeons who can help if such a complication should occur. The number of procedures which is needed to keep the complication rate low and have good results are not known, but two to four cases a month might be an acceptable number.

Tab. 7.2.2: Complications in 840 patients.

	N
Bar rotation	10
Dislocation	2
Fractura sterni	1
Evolving of PC	3
Deep infection	1
Pneumonia	2
Removal of stabilizer – pain	5
Sternotomi	1
One more bar	3
Removal before time – pain	3
Pneumothorax	1
Additional drain	2

Even you exsufflate the air after surgery you will see that about 50% have a small pneumothorax. It is generally not necessary to treat this because it will be absorbed in few days. Even if the pneumothorax is larger, observation might be sufficient if the patient has no symptoms.

7.2.6 Removal of the bar(s)

This is done 3 years after insertion as an outpatient surgery procedure in most cases. The patient comes to the hospital in the morning prepared for general anesthesia. The bar is removed and the patient may be discharged later in the day without further control [6].

The recurrence rate is low, around 1%.

Hyung J. Park

Comment

The surgical treatment for pectus deformity utilizing the pectus bar continues to evolve since its first introduction by Donald Nuss in 1997. During the past 15 years, we have made tremendous strides in surgical techniques and devices for morphological diversity and different age groups. No matter the technique, it is mandatory to have a good remodeling of the entire chest wall, preserve its integrity, as well as patients' safety.

There have been four major issues to improve pectus repair. First, how to correct the asymmetric deformity to a symmetric one. Second, how to prevent pectus bar displacement. Third, how to make the repair procedure easy and solid for heavy adult chests. And last, how to guarantee the safety of the patients, due to its proximity to the heart.

My principles for symmetric repair for asymmetrical types are the morphological classification, and the morphology tailored repair technique (Terrain Contour Matching, TERCOM): asymmetric bar technique, crest compression technique, and the press-molding (the sandwich) technique for pectus carinatum [7, 8].

Pectus bar displacement has been overcome mainly by two different approaches: the one is the shorter bar technique by Dr. Pilegaard as described in the text, and the other is my approach with inventions of new devices to make the bar un-rotatable.

Dr. Pilegaard's superb technique using the shorter bar overcomes the issues of bar displacement nicely. The principle of the technique is placing the chest wall entry points (the hinge points) more medially, at the anterior aspect of the chest wall. The stabilizers on the anterior wall make it prop against the wall and thus, prevents the bar rotation [9].

His shorter bar technique has a very low bar displacement rate, but not without drawbacks. First, the short bar only covers a smaller area of the chest wall to remodel, whereas the regular bar can lift the whole anterior chest wall. Second, the shorter bar requires the skin incisions at the anterior chest. Third, this technique may not be efficient for eccentric asymmetry repair. Fourth, the bar may sink into the chest cavity when the hinge points are not supportive.

However, I have tried to resolve this crucial issue without hurting the quality of repair and ended up inventing new devices, which was different from the conventional stabilizer. My devices are devised to fix the bar to the ribs, the strongest structure in the chest wall. The claw fixator (Fig. 7.2.9), the hinge plate and the bridge connection in the parallel bars and the crossed bars (Fig. 7.2.10) covers all different mechanisms of bar dislocations. Consequently, these devices have made the bar displacement rate of "zero," "Pectus repair without bar dislocations!" The crane system and pectoscope have ushered the Pectus surgery into a new era; making the pectus repair procedure exceptionally safe and easy [10, 11].

In conclusion, Dr. Pilegaard's technique has shown a high achievement in pectus bar security and in setting adult pectus repair on the track. My techniques and devices may also contribute to a better outcome for the patients: "Zero" bar dislocations; no devastating complications; more surgeon friendly; and the only technique to repair all different asymmetric pectus excavatum and pectus carinatum.

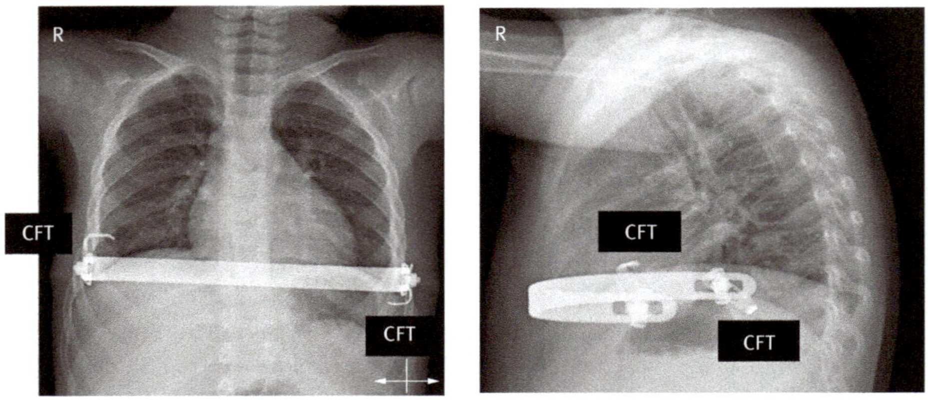

Fig. 7.2.9: The claw fixators to fix the bar to the ribs. CFT: Claw Fixator.

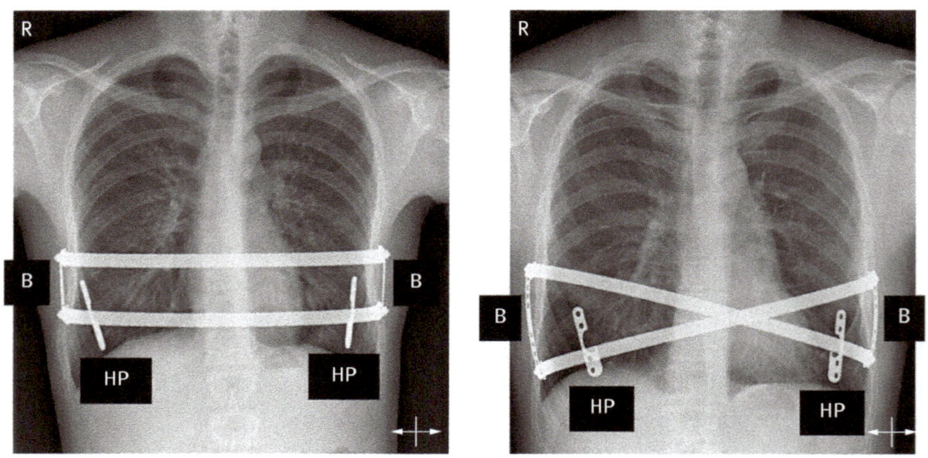

(a) (b)

Fig. 7.2.10: The hinge plates to prevent intercostal muscle stripping at the hinge points. The bridge connection of the two bars in the parallel bar technique (a), and in the crossed bar technique (b). B: Bridge; HP: Hinge Plate.

Robert E. Kelly, Donald Nuss

Comment

Prof. Pilegaard has presented his excellent experience with pectus excavatum. In our experience 8% of the patients presented before 5 years, 13% before 10 years, 47% between 11 and 15 years and 32% thereafter. We also favor doing the repair during the pubertal growth spurt but will do the repair earlier if indicated. We only operate on patients who are symptomatic and have a severe degree of deformity with evidence of cardiac and/or pulmonary compression on CT or ECHO. All surgical candidates are tested for metal allergy.

The mild and moderate degrees of pectus deformity patients are treated with a breathing and exercise protocol and if indicated the Klobe vacuum bell.

Since publication of the minimally invasive technique there has been a huge increase in the number of patients requesting repair – we only did 45 cases in the ten years from 1987 to 1996 and over a 1000 cases in the next decade. This dramatic increase in numbers has allowed numerous centers to study the cardiopulmonary effects of pectus excavatum and the outcome of the repair. These studies have confirmed what the patients have been telling us for seventy years, namely that there is right heart compression with decreased filling and increased resistance, which is corrected immediately after repair, and that that there is a restrictive pulmonary effect which is significantly improved after the bar is removed. We have reported on static (resting) pulmonary function in a multi-institutional study which showed a decrease of 10%–15% or about one standard deviation [12], and is related to depth of the depression [13]. There was significant improvement after surgical correction [14]. The mechanism appears to be poor movement of the sternum: instead of the normal motion with inspiration the lower sternum is fixed. This poor bellows action is reversed with surgical correction, and chest wall motion after the Nuss procedure is indistinguishable from controls [15]. Exercise and ECHO studies by Pilegaard from Denmark, by Sigalet from Canada, Coln and Jaroszewki from the US have confirmed the cardiopulmonary effects mentioned above with significant increase in stroke volume, cardiac output, cardiac index, oxygen pulse and VO2 max after repair. In our series 14% of patients had mitral valve prolapse pre-operative and in half of those it was resolved postoperatively, which is consistent with findings by Schamberger and Coln.

Body image concern is one of major reasons patients seek treatment. Patients frequently avoid activities which require taking their shirts off in public to swim or exercise which leads to social withdrawal. After repair, patients' body image concerns are dramatically improved [13, 16].

Technical points include proper bar length [17]; we continue to have good results with a bar 2.5 cm shorter than the distance between mid-axillary lines, which is slightly longer than Pilegaards bar but it is symmetric and we have had no problems with bar migration. Thoracoscopy is essential. We strongly endorse sternal elevation with crane, vacuum bell or subxiphoid bone hook to improve visualization and minimize any chance of cardiac injury during sub-sternal dissection. Two bars should be used if they will better distribute the force of the chest wall than a single bar. The bar must be prevented from rotating, with a stabilizer on the left side and PDS wraps of the bar/rib crossings. We do not use thoracic epidural anesthesia.

We generally hospitalize until the fourth post-operative day. Pain medications are stopped by 4 weeks post-op. Return to activity is similar. Bar removal is 2 to 3 years later. Bar removal includes opening both incisions, removing any bony overgrowth until the bar moves easily in its fibrous tunnel, flattening the bar at both ends, not twisting the bar, and applying gentle traction. Recurrence is less than 1%.

Dawn E. Jaroszewski

Comment

Treatment of pectus excavatum (PE) has evolved over the past century with minimally invasive repair techniques being recommended for the majority of symptomatic, severe patients. Symptoms such as exertional dyspnea, chest pain, palpitations and exercise intolerance have been shown to result from the cardiopulmonary restriction of the defect and are mostly resolved with surgical repair [20]. With surgical repair, right heart compression is relieved and increased right-sided cardiac output can be expected for most patients [18].

There are a number of technique modifications from the original procedure as published by Nuss [21]. These modifications have been useful for the extension of the minimally invasive repair technique into the repair of older patients and include placement of multiple support bars [22] and assisted sternal elevation [19]. The use of thoracoscopy and forced elevation prior to passing the introducer and bars improves visualization and may also decrease procedure risks (Fig. 7.2.11a–c). In agreement with Dr. Pilegaard, our own experience has led to the use of multiple bars in older patients with more than 40% of our adult patient receiving three support bars.

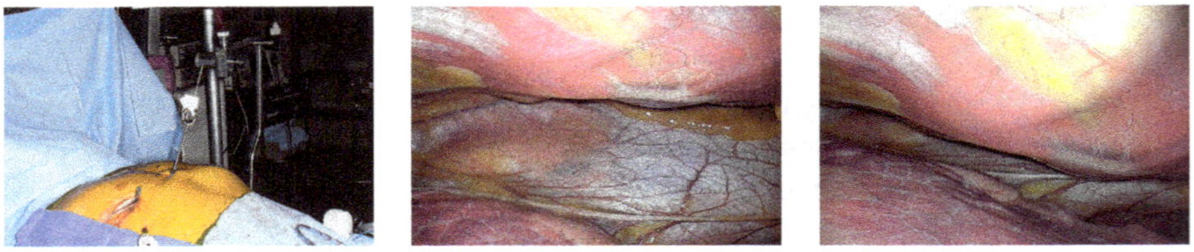

(a) (b) (c)

Fig. 7.2.11: (a) perforating bone clamp is placed on the sternum and attached to the bedside RulTract retractor forced sternal elevation. (b) and (c) thoracoscopic view of excavatum defect and cardiac compression before (left) and after (right) forced elevation with RulTract.

Good postoperative pain control is essential in this patient population. Epidurals, intravenous patient controlled anesthesia and subcutaneous pain catheters have all been reported with excellent results. In our adult patient experience, the use of a tunneled On-Q catheter with oral analgesics (ibuprofen, gabapentin and oxycodone) has been successful with few complications. At completion of the procedure, 7.5-inch soaker catheters (PM050-A, On-Q, Halyard Health, Inc, Irvine, CA) are placed anterior along the ribs using a disposable, 17-gauge, 10-inch tunneling system (Model T17X10, On-Q, Halyard Health, Inc) (Fig. 7.2.12a). The On-Q catheters are primed and attached to a 750-mL reservoir (Fig. 7.2.12b). Variable rate controllers (Select-A-Flow, Halyard Health, Inc) are locked at a rate of 7 mL/h, infusing ropivacaine, 0.2%. The reservoir is refilled at 48 hours and patients are discharged home with catheters in place. Removal is planned on day 4–5.

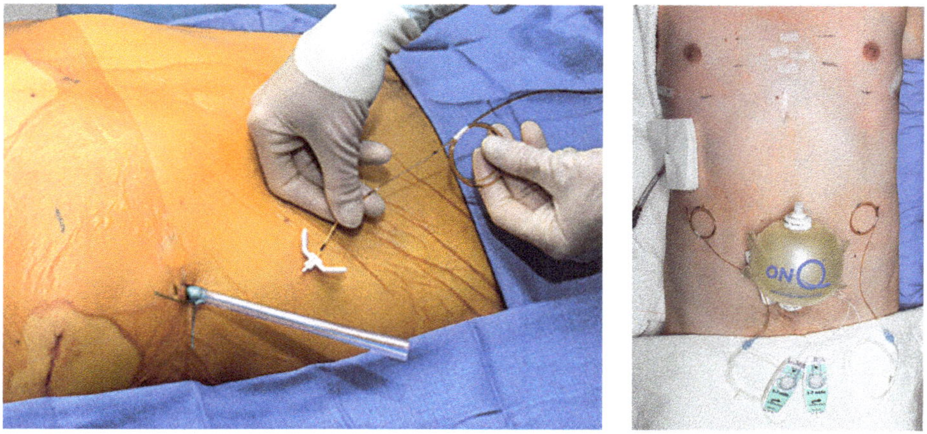

Fig. 7.2.12: 7.5-inch soaker catheters placed anterior along the ribs (a) and On-Q catheters attached to a 750-mL reservoir (b).

Patient satisfaction and quality of life are improved with repair of severe, symptomatic PE. An increasing amount of data is being published documenting the cardiopulmonary benefits and psychosocial benefits of repair. Even advanced aged patients can be candidates for minimally invasive repair and should be considered.

Jean-Marie Wihlm

Comment

Based on an important personal experience, H. Pilegaard gives an overview of the Nuss technique, also named Minimally Invasive Repair of Pectus Excavatum (MIRPE) that is likely to become the new gold standard for the next 20 years.

However, some points regarding indications are still debated: many surgeons consider this technique for mild to moderate deformities only with moderate asymmetry and sternal rotation less than 15–20°. The most controversial point is the presence of inferior costal flaring, as can be seen on Fig. 7.2.2 in an adult patient. Such an important component may only be completely treated by open surgery including inferior costo-chondroplasty during a Ravitch-type correction of PE [23] (Fig. 7.2.13).

The optimal age for MIRPE is increasing in a worldwide trend in recent publications and I personally favor the age of 15 years, considering that the age for bar removal will then be 18 years, corresponding to both the end of growth and a definitive reduced risk of recurrence.

But the most important parameter of a good indication, regardless of age, is the general flexibility of the chest and especially the anterior plastron, not considered here. This clinical evaluation is easy and simply consists of an "auto-correction" test: the patient is asked to do a strong Valsalva manoeuvre which acts like a "pneumatic

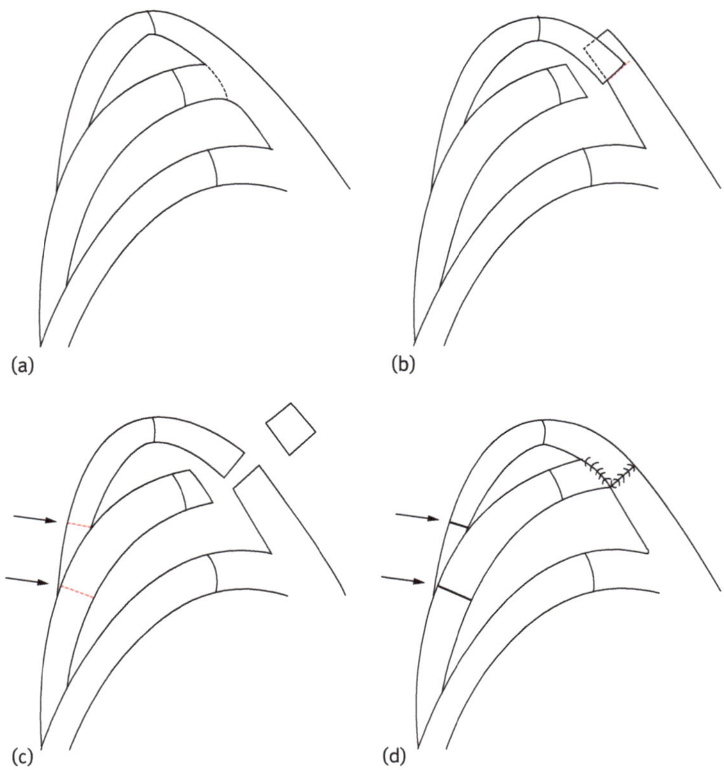

Fig. 7.2.13: Costo-chondroplasty for inferior costal flaring.

Nuss" and shows the potential of reduction of the deformity Fig. 7.2.14. This test is best made in front of a mirror, to show the patient (and the parents) an instant level of correction of 60%–70% of action of the definitive bar(s) (Fig. 7.2.14 and Video 7.1 Cavum excavatum).

Video showing a man with a cavum excavatum
https://www.degruyter.com/view/supplement/9783110419825_Cavum_excavatum.mp4

Preoperative evaluation must also include a routine CT scan (using new protocols with low doses) that allows surgeons to better assess cardiac compression, asymmetry, a

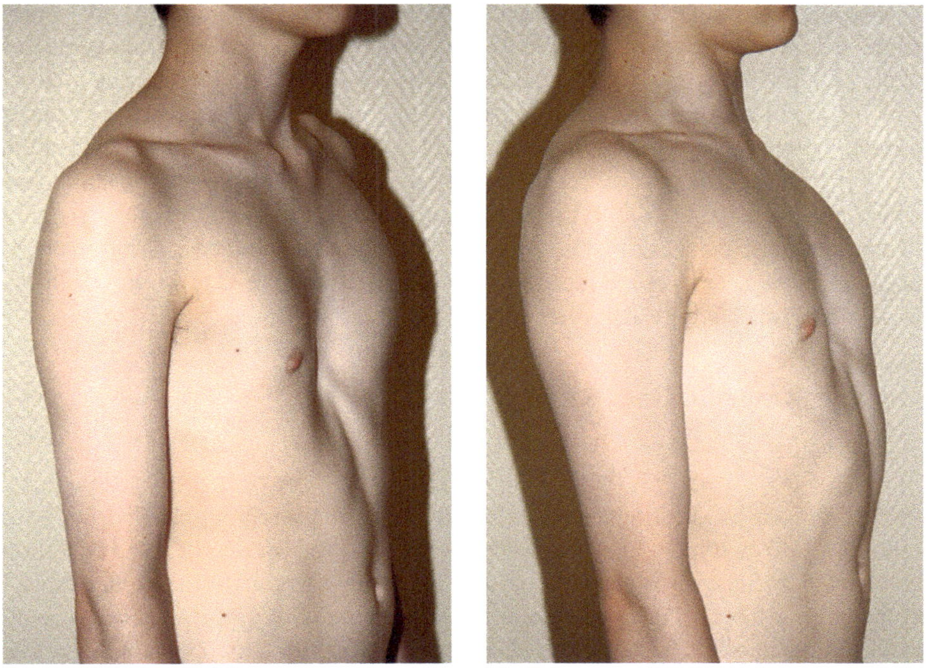

(a) (b)

Fig. 7.2.14: Auto-correction test.

prospective sternal rotation (not seen on chest X-rays only) and inferior costal flaring in 3D reconstruction [24]. CT scan data may not only change the indication for MIRPE, but may also help to better plan placement and shaping of the bars.

A routine echocardiography is mandatory as well, especially in case of clinical heart murmur, to disclose the known association of PE with mitral valve abnormalities (prolapse or insufficiency) or others, including aortic root enlargement in Marfan patients [25].

There is no mention about a possible allergy to the alloy of the stainless steel bar containing chrome and nickel, which can be tested by a 48-hour skin-test using a small bar sample.

In the Nuss procedure technique, the reason for the original bar length was obviously to have the support of at least two or three (with the stabilizers) levels of ribs bilaterally to counteract the pressure of the corrected plastron and sternum and distribute the forces on several ribs on each side and in a balanced way. Such a placement may be observed in Fig. 7.2.8 but only on the right side for both cases, instead of an equal distribution bilaterally with a classical length. On Fig. 7.2.1, the right bar support is only a single rib and there is a risk of droping in the chest in case of sliding, being more likely with short bars.

Having the end of the bars paralell to the lateral chest wall was actually not recommended to avoid an "hour glass" effect, especially in still growing teenagers. For many authors, the proper length is today one or two inches shorter than the original with a support zone on both anterior axillary line, but not as short as Dr. Pilegaard's concept however [26]. The oblique contact of both ends allows lateral growing of the rib cage during the 3 years and some manufacturers developped sliding stabilizers which may be placed closer to the hinge points but still keeping the initial security of medium size bars against lateral sliding [27]. Another advantage is a slight antero-posterior movement possible during respiratory cycle compared to wired stabilizers as seen on Figs. 7.2.1 and 7.2.8, thereby reducing pain.

Caroline Fortmann, Claus Petersen

7.3 Pectus carinatum

In 1987 Donald Nuss introduced a minimally invasive procedure, entitled the Nuss procedure, which transformed the treatment of pectus excavatum (PE). The operation involved inserting a stainless steel bar to correct any deformity of the anterior wall of the chest. After further research and trials spanning 7 years, the procedures involved in PE were effectively transferred to pectus carinatum (PC). This approach was based on the assumption that both pectus excavatum and carinatum share common characteristics and require similar therapeutic strategies. However, is that true? As we know, both deformities of the anterior chest wall are frequent, and boys are more often affected than girls. It is also a known fact that both entities can concomitantly occur together with scoliosis, whereas it is unclear whether one or the other deformity induces or interferes with the other, or if they are distinct phenomena. Similarly to PE, a genetic predisposition of PC is likely, although the onset of the latter corresponds more frequently to the beginning of puberty. Research in the associated symptoms, such as dyspnea, palpitations, etc. are inconsistent in PC, while both deformities are concomitant features in patients with Marfan and Noonan Syndrome [28]. For the sake of completeness, it should be noted that many chest wall deformities, including PC, can also occur as a result of a surgical procedure to correct a congenital disease, e.g. diaphragmatic hernia, or following sternotomy, which is mostly performed in cardiosurgical procedures.

In terms of the developmental process, a similar pathomechanism is suggested for both kinds of sternal dislocation. Researchers agree that the inappropriate growth of the costosternal cartilage can result in sternal shifting. However, it remains unclear as to which factor determines whether the sternum moves to a position above or below the ideal line, and why these osteochondral deformities occur either symmetrically or asymmetrically. It is also enigmatic whether additional pathologic angulations of the sternum are due to the abovementioned mechanism, or if another factor solely targets the osseous malformation. Another unanswered question concerns the onset of chest wall deformities, because PE, more often than PC, occurs in early infancy and remains stable over years before a rapid dislodgment of the sternum progresses as puberty starts [28].

Therapeutic concepts for the surgical repair of PC date from the early 1950s, when Ravitch published his technique for the correction of both pectus excavatum and carinatum [29]. However, this topic received very little attention from researchers and scientists and, over the course of 50 years following the introduction of Ravitch's technique, just three papers per year on average were published that examined PE and PC. The majority of those studies that were published described an individual's experience with surgery in PC, but the operative concept remained largely rare.

This situation did not change until 2005, at which point Abramson demonstrated the inverse use of the Nuss pectus bar [30]. His concept spurred the community as a whole to pay more attention to the use of surgical concepts to correct PC, and research into the modification of instruments and implants commenced. Stimulated by this discussion, promoters of the open repair of PC reappeared in the field, advocating for the open approach and refining their technique and implants. From that point onwards, the frequency of PC-related publications increased to up to 17 papers on average per year. However, in contrast to the treatment of pectus excavatum, for which the Nuss procedure had already become state of the art, the diverging concepts on how to best treat PC remained open to debate. In the meantime, the conservative approach to treating PC, which was first proposed in the mid-1970s, experienced a renaissance. Pediatric surgeons from Argentina [31] and Canada [32] introduced their newly developed devices, protocols and study results. They demonstrated that bracing PC patients during puberty had a high success rate. However, treatment strategies for PC remain under debate to this day. Table 7.3.1 focuses on the pros and cons of the three diverging approaches, while Table 7.3.2 (supplementary material online: http://www.degruyter.com/books/9783110425291) compares the results and outcomes of existing studies in this area.

The crucial and most diverging point about the treatment of chest wall deformities is to define the right indication, particularly for major procedures, including the risks and side effects of radiation, anesthesia and surgery. Despite the fact that recent studies demonstrate a slight improvement in cardiopulmonary function following PE repair, it is still the patients with PC and PE who indicate the time and mode of the procedure. In other words, we are experiencing a paradigm shift through which the affected young people do not visit cosmetic surgeons but requiring surgery that is predominantly not medically indicated from thoracic and pediatric surgeons. All the more, it remains the surgeon's responsibility to decide whether or not to follow the patient's desire. However, those adolescents who suffer from conspicuous thoracic deformities, or who suffer greatly from an impairment of self-image, should be considered candidates for surgery, even when the indication is primarily not medical. In consequence, the outcome measures also have to be newly defined. Meeting the patients' expectations is the main goal to be achieved, and success rates of either procedure have to be measured against the satisfaction of the patient and the improvement of his or her self-esteem.

Taking into account the fact that patients with PC do not suffer from physical limitations, further medical investigation depends on the therapeutic concept. Planning a surgical procedure requires appropriate diagnostic work, while scanning the thoracic surface without radiation and photographic documentation are sufficient for bracing therapy. Unnecessary exposure to radiation has to be avoided whenever possible.

Most open procedures for PC repair follow the principle of Ravitch's technique [29]. The key steps in this approach involve the dissection of the pectoralis muscles, resection of the costosternal cartilages, osteotomy of the sternum, if necessary, and intermediate fixation of the corrected sternum with variable devices and material. Several authors have published methods that incorporate slight modifications to the technique, the majority of which involve shortening the skin incision, minimizing the surgical trauma and avoiding secondary interventions for the removal of implants. The overall results of open surgery for PC are good according to the abovementioned parameters.

The inverse use of the pectus bars for PC was introduced by Abramson [31]. He showed how the protruding sternum could be pressed down into a normal position and fixed by use of an individually bent bar, which was subcutaneously introduced. The principle of this procedure was adopted by other authors, whereby they developed different solutions as to how to fix the bars to the ribs. However, the flexibility of the sternum is a crucial precondition for the use of this approach.

The flexibility of the thorax is also essential for the conservative approach to PC. Herein, thoracic plasticity can be tested by slow, but forced, manual pressure on the prominent sternum. When the sternum can be replaced into a normal position, bracing is a promising option (Fig. 7.3.1). Several studies have already shown that the effect of this treatment can be observed within a few weeks, and complete reposition is a question of months [32]. The most striking argument for this orthopedic approach is that no side effects are threatening, except for skin irritation and general discomfort when using the device. On the other hand, no evidence is given when diverging concepts are recommended concerning the design of the brace, minimal and maximal pressure rates and the appropriate time of use. Another advantage is that, in case of a relapse, the same treatment can be started once again with a reasonable chance of success.

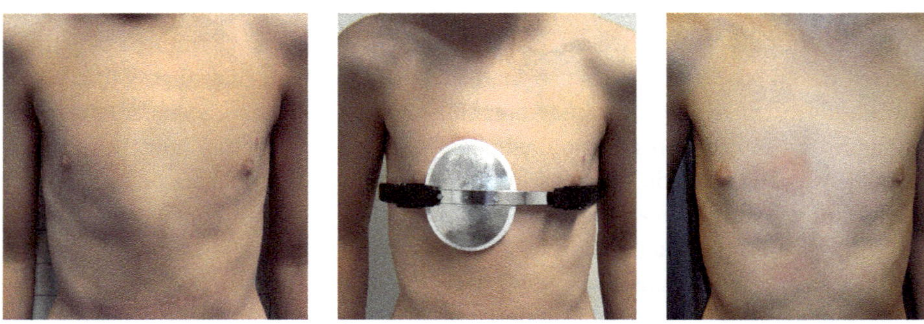

(a) (b) (c)

Fig. 7.3.1: Patient with PC before treatment (a), under treatment with a brace (b) and after treatment (c).

In contrast to PE patients, where surgical correction should preferably be scheduled for late adolescence, the orthopedic approach to PC has to be started as soon as the deformity becomes evident. This alleged contradiction has to be passed to the pediatricians, orthopedics and surgeons who see those patients first. Pros and cons of three different approaches are listed in Tab. 7.3.1. The challenge for the upcoming years will be to optimize the treatment modality of the non-operative approach to PC and to elucidate the complexity of thoracic and concomitant spinal deformities.

Tab. 7.3.1: Treatment of pectus carinatum: pros and cons of three diverging approaches.

	Open surgery	Minimally invasive surgery	Compression therapy
First described	1952	2005	1979
by	Ravitch	Abramson	Haje & Raymundo
Key steps	Resection of deformed costal cartilages + sternal osteotomy	Subcutaneous metal bar compresses protrusion	Greatest external forces by custom-fitted brace
Advancement	Various modifications of the technique (including use of metal bars for stabilization)	Combined with orthotic bracing prior to surgery in rigid chest (Various bars and stabilization systems)	1) Dynamic compressor system (DMS) + pressure measuring device (PMD) by Martinez-Ferro and Fraire, 2008 2) Calgary protocol: self-adjustable device + protocol for bracing, 2006
Pros	Possible even in rigid deformities (including chondromanubrial forms) and severe asymmetry	Small incisions, extrathoracic surgery, shorter operation time, faster recovery	No surgical risks, low-cost (various self-designed bars), no hospital stay
Cons	Major surgical procedure with variety of complications, recurrence	Wire breakage, seroma, infection, allergic reaction, recurrence	Erythema, discomfort, recurrence
Results	Mixed (worsening cosmetic results, decreased chest wall compliance), improving in last decades: excellent – very good	Excellent – good	Excellent – good
Comment	In case of bar implantation second operation needed for removal	Second operationen needed for bar removal	Compliance needed

Horatio Abramson

Comment

The establishment of appropriate techniques to correct asymmetric malformations of the thorax is challenging. The fixing plate's location, the length and shape of the compressing bar and the horizontal or oblique position of the bar are the key to achieve a successful result Fig. 7.3.2. In those patients presenting PC with contra-lateral PE, it is important to consider the extent to which the use of one bar to compress the protruded region will cause an elevation of the PE. In patients with predominant PE with contra-lateral PC, it is important to predict if the use of the retro-sternal bar alone will be sufficient. Patients that exhibit asymmetric PE or PC with the contralateral side of a standard shape can be treated with only pre-sternal or retro-sternal implants.

Other therapeutic alternatives are a) insertion of one retro-sternal bar and another pre-sternal either simultaneously or in sequence; b) insertion of a pre-sternal bar then, in a deferred action, removing it and inserting another in a lower position; c) implanting a bar with intra-thoracic journey in the depressed hemithorax and pre-sternal position in the protruded hemithorax; d) resection of costal fragments favoring compression.

In order to effectively deal with asymmetric malformations the surgeon and his team need to have extensive experience in choosing and recommending the best approach to the patient.

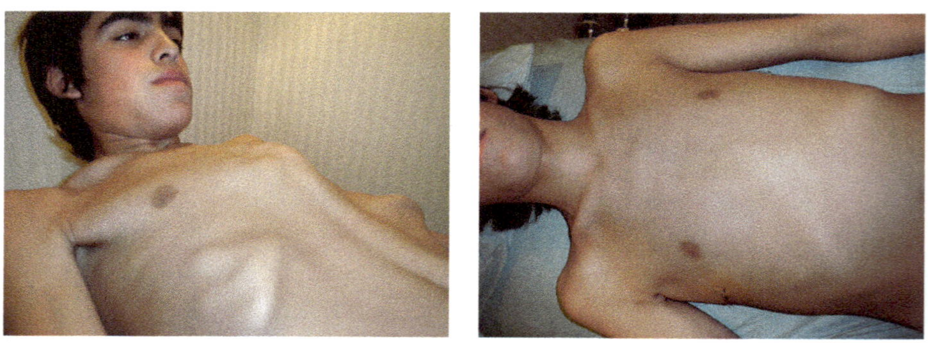

(a) (b)

Fig. 7.3.2: Pectus carinatum before (a) and after (b) minimally invasive surgical repair correction.

Marcelo Martínez Ferro

Comment

By the year 1999, with the exception of the pioneer papers of Haje and coworkers, no other authors advocated a non-operative approach. At that time, it was commonly believed that measuring the pressure exerted to the protrusion would be crucial for understanding and treating patients with PC.

Consequently, two different pressure measurements were established: pressure of correction (PC) and pressure of treatment (PT). When analyzing the recorded pressure data, it was concluded that PC indirectly measures the thoracic elasticity, increases with age and can be used to predict the treatment duration. We observed that patients with lower pressures ended the treatment faster and that PC could also help to predict the final cosmetic outcome, albeit with less precision. However, PT measurement enabled the additional observation that applying pressures greater than 2.5 PSI diminished tolerance, mostly because of skin irritation and ulceration. Accordingly, in the last 251 patients treated with the device, PT was set up with equal or less than 2.5 PSI and, as a result, the FMF® Dynamic Compressor System resulted in satisfactory treatment tolerance and compliance (see also supplementary material Figs. 7.3.3 and 7.3.4, http://www.degruyter.com/books/9783110425291).

Francis Robicsek

Comment

In treatises written on the treatment of pectus deformities, we have to cease using the long time defunct "Ravitch procedure" as a "straw man". However, contrary to those who recommend that PC should be treated conservatively or using temporarily in-dwelling rods, we believe that PC, just like it's "sister deformity" PE, should be treated by up to date, minimally invasive, open technique in line with the following principles [33].

- The treatment should be one-stage, it should be simple and swift.
- Should not leave rigid foreign material in the body. (in case of carinatum, no foreign material at all).
- Should not create a potential for complications. Serious morbidity, especially iatrogenic injuries and mortality, are unacceptable.
- Should provide uniformly excellent cosmetic and functional results.
- Should not necessitate extended follow-up.
- Should not require re-intervention.

In PC, a condition that fits best with the term of "keel chest", the sternum broadly arches forward. It has two common varieties:

Type A pectus carinatum is characterized by protrusion of the lower portion of the sternum and formation of 90 degree backward open angle with the xiphoid process Fig 7.3.3.

Type B pectus carinatum, the lower portion of the sternum is protruding but the longitudinal axis of the xiphoid process remains "in line" with it.

In the Type A deformity, the lower sternum is exposed through a 4–5 cm long, anterior transverse skin incision. The full-thickness flap is made mobile enough to be moved around to provide access to the entire operative field. The pectoralis major muscles are detached from the sternum bilaterally. A transverse sternal wedge-osteotomy is made at the upper limit of the deformity. The corresponding cartilages are subperichondrally resected. The xyphoid process is detached. In Type A, a short 4–6 cm portion is resected from the lower tip of the sternum, and then the sternum is forcefully bent backward to achieve a normal straight axis. The xiphoid process is re-attached to the resected stump of the sternum with a

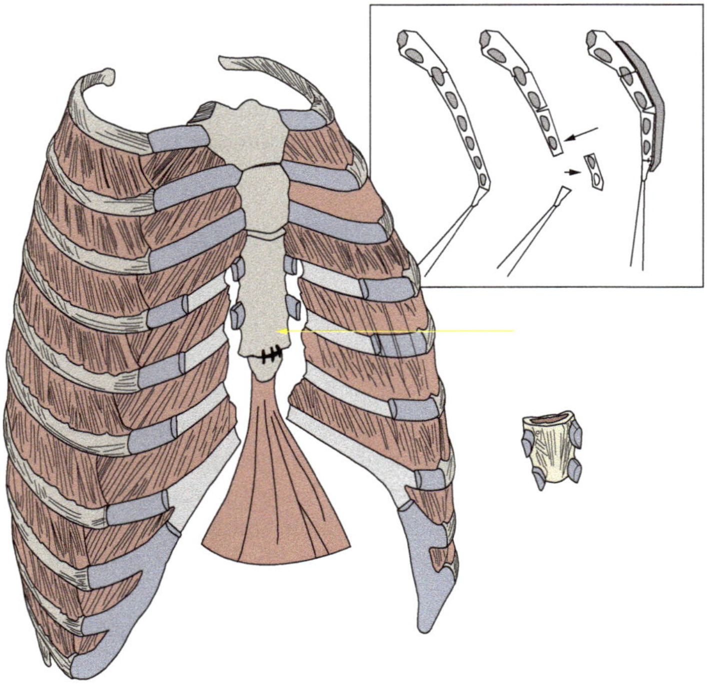

Fig. 7.3.3: In Type A pectus carinatum, the lower position of the sternum forms a 90 degree angle with the xiphoid process. After performing a transverse sternotomy, bilateral chondral resection and correction of the sternal axis, a short portion is resected from the lower sternum and the xiphoid process is reattached to the sternal stump. In the Type B anomaly, the sternal resection may be omitted. Presternal closure of the pectoral major muscles assures the corrected position of the sternum and a smooth anterior chest wall.

pair of stainless steel wire sutures. This way the pulling effect of the rectus abdominis muscles will preserve the sternum in its corrected position, which is further secured by closing the previously detached pectoralis muscles pre-sternally. In *Type B*, where the xiphoid process is "in line" with the sternal axis, sternum shortening and detachment of the xiphoid process is usually deemed unnecessary. The wound is drained with a small caliber suction device, closed and a moderately compressive dressing applied. The procedure usually requires an overnight stay and very limited follow-up [34–38].

Claus Petersen

7.4 Miscellaneous

7.4.1 Poland syndrome

In the mid-19th century, A. Poland was the first to describe the single-sided absence of pectoralis and serratus anterior muscles. Over 100 years later, his observation was recovered and more features were observed, resulting in the development of a definition of a complex anatomical defect. The nature and severity of Poland syndrome ranges from hypo- or aplasia of the nipple in combination with muscular defects, through to deformities of the thoracic cage, including ipsilateral hypo- and dysplasia of the ribs and sternum, potentially associated with anomalies of the upper limb. Disagreement still exists with regards to the etiology (e.g. intrauterine ischemia of the subclavian artery supplied structures) and classification of this complex entity. Depending on the severity of the defects, surgical reconstruction is indicated for cosmetic and/or functional improvement. In terms of minor defects, soft tissue reconstruction is required, which involves transferring the latissimus dorsi flaps, and the use of lipofilling and silicone implants alone or in combination. In females, complete reconstruction or correction of hypoplastic or absent mammae is mandatory and, if necessary, is accompanied by nipple reconstruction and tattooing.

The most complex, but rare, deformity results from bony hypoplasia and defects of the thoracic cage. Very few reports are available that address how missing ribs can partially or totally be replaced in order to close the defect and provide a supporting surface for the transferred muscles. Herein, the crucial point is that osteosynthetic devices were originally developed to compensate for bony instability while they are not intended for use with moving structures like ribs. For this reason, reconstructive surgery of defects of the thoracic cage continues to represent a challenge for innovative teams. In conclusion, patients that suffer from Poland syndrome exhibit a wide range of visible and functional defects that require individually customized treatment algorithms to meet each patient's distinct needs with minimal complication and requirement for revision.

7.4.2 Jeune syndrome

The most common feature of Jeune syndrome, which was first described in 1956, is an asphyxiating thoracic dystrophy. In this rare autosomal recessive disorder, the intrathoracic organs are squeezed into a small restrictive chest cage that doesn't grow adequately. Respiratory failure and recurrent brochopulmonary infections, together with increasing right ventricular load, can have potentially life-threatening consequences, and untreated patients often die within their first years of life. Very few reports on early surgical inventions that can successfully bridge patients from infancy to childhood are available. Of the surgery that is described, two principal procedures are employed: distraction of the sternum after longitudinal splitting with or without interposition of autologous rib grafts and other material; and the use of posterior osteotomies that are fixated with expandable implants, e.g. vertically expandable prosthetic titanium rib (VEPTR) to enlarge the thoracic cavity. However, surgical interventions that successfully treat Jeune syndrome are not yet well established and stagnate on the level of experimental procedures.

7.4.3 Sternal defects

Total or incomplete fusion of the sternum is the underlying pathomechanism of sternal clefts, ranging from isolated superior V-shaped clefts to ectopia cordis and Cantrell's pentalogy, when the abdominal wall and diaphragmatic defects are associated. Surgical repair of minor defects is recommended during the neonatal period when the sternum edges are still movable and can be easily approximated. The survival rate of babies that suffer from the extremely rare true ectopia cordis is low, due to compromised blood flow in the great vessels on the attempt to replace the heart into the mediastinum. In patients with thoracoabdominal defects, coverage of the heart, liver and intestine is the priority, followed by repair of the diaphragm and cardio surgical procedures. Despite the severity of this malformation, the outcome is much better than that associated with isolated ectopia cordis.

7.4.4 Defects of the thoracic wall

Bony defects of the thoracic cage before adulthood mostly result from small to large tumor resections. The crucial problem is that defects and the fusion of ribs frequently result in the development of scoliosis. It is nearly impossible to tackle this problem in the growing organism, because no self-expending stabilizing devices are available. After puberty, persisting defects are often required to be closed for medical and cosmetic purposes. At this time, reconstruction of the bony structures should be considered in order to prevent the underlying organs from sustaining mechanical injury and to provide a stable substructure for muscular shaping and reconstruction of the breast in females. For this indication, new implants for stabilizing or replacing ribs are available. However, in the meantime, and awaiting the development of more effective techniques, the coverage of the defect with biological or synthetic material as well as muscle flaps and soft tissue is currently common practice and is forecast to remain as such for the foreseeable future.

Frédéric Lavrand

Comment

The correction of chest wall defects requires both the ability to perform control imaging and to limit spinal or chest wall deformities in adulthood [116–124].

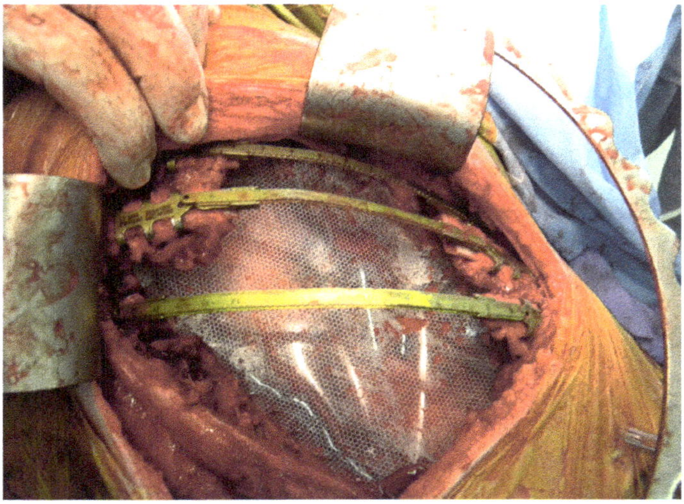

Fig. 7.4.1: The STRATOS® system.

In this sense we have used the STRATOS® system (MedXpert GmbH) for five patients since 2008 the titanium connecting bar and rib clip allow a horizontal semi rigid correction rib by rib, or more often by two, enabling the MRI control and ensuring stability of the thorax. In addition this type of correction allows a subnormal thoracic mechanism of respiration and shape of the thorax (Fig. 7.4.1).

The goal is to restore in a single step the maximum thoracic volume.

For a child the problem is growing, so it is possible to unlock one side of the connecting bar to allow the latter to slide in the titanium clip to compensate for

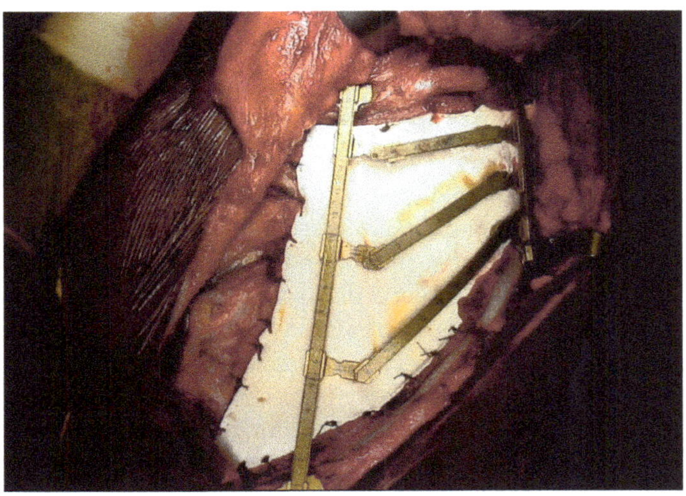

Fig. 7.4.2: Horizontal and vertical reconstruction in the same time with the MTS®.

horizontal growing of the intercostal spaces located below and above. At this time, no device failure is implicated. Protection of lung and pericardium is provided by an oversized PTFE or Silastic plate.

Unsightly muscle defects can be either treated by muscle transfer (Latimus dorsi flap) or protheses after the end of growth.

Now it is possible to perform a horizontal and vertical reconstruction at the same time with the use of MTS® (Multidirectional Thoracic Wall Stabilization) the latest evolution of the STRATOS® (Fig. 7.4.2). Its articulated staples allow reconstruction in the absence of a costal stump necessary to the previous version, close to the sternum or in the posterior chest wall close to the spine. Moreover, mobility of this device and possibility to perform bi dimensional reconstruction allows to the "respiratory pump" continue to function closely normal allowing all thoracic reconstructions.

Haiko K. Jahn, Sebastian van As

7.5 Trauma

7.5.1 Introduction

Globally, trauma remains the leading cause of death, hospitalization and long-term disabilities in the first four decades of life [39]. According to global surveys 10% of trauma-related hospital admissions are due to thoracic injuries. Thoracic injuries account for 25% of trauma related deaths [39, 40]. Isolated thoracic trauma in children accounts for 5% mortality. This increases dramatically up to 40% with associated injuries, especially with head and abdominal injuries [41].

Thoracic trauma may be classified by mechanism, anatomical site and severity (immediately or potentially life threatening). The vast majority are the result of blunt trauma. Children are usually injured as pedestrians hit by motor vehicles rather than as motor vehicles passengers [44–46]. Other mechanisms include bikes, falls and non-accidental injury (NAI) [46]. In children under three years of age rib fractures in the absence of any underlying medical problem or motor vehicle accident are highly suggestive of non-accidental injury (NAI) [69].

Less than 5% of thoracic trauma is attributable to penetrating injuries, which is largely a single-system injury and carries a high risk of requiring surgical intervention [47]. This becomes more significant in adolescences and is often the result of stab and gunshot wounds. These include BB or pellets fired from recreational air guns that can produce life-threatening injuries. In penetrating trauma almost all of the deaths are attributed to the thoracic injury. Other unusual causes of penetrating trauma seen in children 12 years old or younger include impalement onto shards of broken glass or metal rods [46].

7.5.2 Biomechanics and anatomy

The majority of pediatric data with regards to biomechanics is derived from work done by the motor industry [49, 50]. In children, the chest wall is thinner and is extremely compliant because of greater cartilage content and incomplete ossification of the ribs. This makes rib fractures rare [50, 57]. Their thoracic volume is smaller and the arrangement of vital structures is more compact than in adults [57]. This results in unusual injuries such as traumatic asphyxia and commotio cordis [53]. Rib fractures and mediastinal injuries are therefore uncommon in children. Their presence indicates the transfer of massive amounts of energy to the thoracic and abdominal organs raising the possibility of multiple serious organ injuries [42, 49].

The mediastinum in children is more flexible and mobile, lowering the incidence of major vessel trauma, but allowing a visceral shift which can result in the displacement of the heart and trachea, with pneumothorax, hemothorax and diaphragmatic rupture [50, 51, 53–55]. Displacement of the heart kinks the mediastinum compromising preload and leading to decreased cardiac output and profound hypotension [57]. Angulation of the trachea and compression of the lung by the mediastinum may produce respiratory compromise [53, 54].

Children rely on the diaphragm for ventilation because of their more compliant ribs and weak intercostal muscles. In the setting of trauma (even without abdominal injury) the majority of children hyperventilate and swallow air (arerophagia) leading to gastric distension resulting in elevation and splinting of the diaphragm and respiratory distress. Therefore gastric decompression with a nasogastric or orogastric tube in the presence of head trauma is key to ensure adequate ventilation [46, 58, 59].

7.5.3 General evaluation and initial management of the child with chest injuries

Chest injuries include damage to the chest wall, diaphragm, lungs and mediastinal structures. The guiding principles as outlined by the Advanced Trauma Life Support (ATLS) course should be followed [60]. The severity of chest trauma in children ranges from minor to rapidly fatal. The presence of chest injury often portends involvement of other organs, reflecting the transmission of substantial force to the child's compact body [46]. Therefore it is important to have a high index of suspicion for these injuries, as physical examination is highly unreliable [44–46] (Figs. 7.5.2 & 7.5.3). Theses injuries can be classified into six lethal injuries that need excluding in the primary survey and six hidden injuries that must be considered in the secondary survey and non-life threatening injuries [44, 53, 61–63] (Tab. 7.5.1).

Children with multi-trauma and chest injury are more unstable, with significantly worse Revised Trauma Scores (RTS), Injury Severity Scores (ISS) and Glasgow Coma

Scale scores (GCS) compared to those without chest trauma [44–46, 54]. Approximately two-thirds of deaths from thoracic trauma occur after the patient reaches the hospital. Therefore pediatric trauma scores may help to identify these high risk patients and ensure timely diagnosis and treatment [61].

In multi-trauma chest injury: lung or pleural space involvement was associated with a mortality of 20%, diaphragm involvement with a mortality of nearly 30%, heart involvement with a mortality of nearly 40% and blood vessel involvement with a more than 50% mortality [66]. With regards to extra-thoracic injury, mortality increased to 20% in conjunction with abdominal injury, to 35% with head injury and to 39% with all three [41].

Intra-thoracic injuries such as pulmonary contusions, great vessel injuries, esophageal perforation, thoracic duct rupture leading to chylothorax and diaphragmatic ruptures may not present with immediate symptoms making prompt diagnosis difficult. The underlying thoracic injuries are often disproportionately severe compared with the visible surface injuries (Figs. 7.5.2 & 7.5.3). At the same time concomitant extra-thoracic injuries may obscure the presence of serious chest injuries [39–46].

Signs and symptoms associated with blunt chest injuries include chest crepitation, subcutaneous emphysema, nasal flaring, chest retractions, diminished or absent breath sounds, tachypnea, dyspnea and low oxygen saturation [44–46].

Children with physical findings suggestive of chest injury or that have sustained a high-energy deceleration mechanism of trauma require chest imaging. Standard

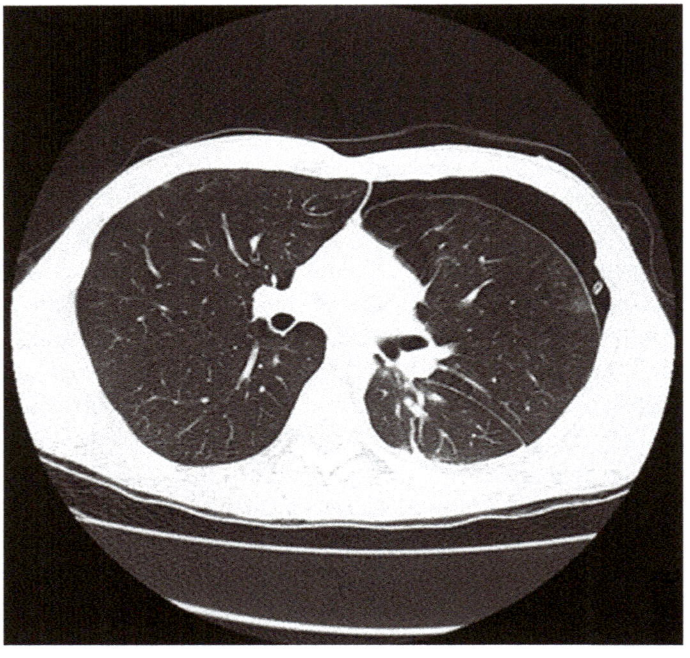

Fig. 7.5.1: CT scan of the chest demonstrating an anterior pneumothorax that cannot be diagnosed with an AP chest radiograph.

anterior-posterior (AP) chest radiographs provide a low-cost screening tool and will be abnormal in 60%–90% of children with significant injuries [44, 45, 64, 65].

However, not all thoracic injuries can be detected on plain radiography, and CT scanning of the chest may be indicated. (Fig. 7.5.1)

Children with abnormal mediastinal silhouettes should undergo helical chest computed tomography (CT). Helical CT scans can define whether an abnormal mediastinal contour on a chest radiograph represents a thymic silhouette, a mediastinal hematoma or an aortic injury. Helical chest CT scans can also demonstrate pulmonary contusions and rib fractures, and may identify additional unsuspected injuries in 15% of children with normal routine radiographs [64, 65].

Despite this, most pediatric chest trauma can be managed with a tube thoracostomy and supportive measures [44–46, 61].

Tab. 7.5.1: Classification of thoracic injuries according to their risk to life [46, 47, 61–63, 66].

Life-threatening	Potentially life-threatening	Non life-threatening
Airway obstruction	Pulmonary contusion	Rib fractures
Tension pneumothorax	Diaphragmatic rupture	Simple pneumothorax
Open pneumothorax	Myocardial contusion	Simple hemothorax
Massive hemothorax	Esophageal rupture	Chest wall contusion
Flail chest	Tracheo-bronchial injuries	
Cardiac tamponade	Great vessel injuries	

7.5.4 Airway obstruction

Children's airways are small. They have narrow nasal passages, large tongues and enlarged adenoids. Therefore small changes in diameter can lead to rapid respiratory compromise. Due to their higher metabolic rate they have a higher oxygen demand per kilogram of body weight. Management of airway obstruction follows standard resuscitation guidelines for obtaining and securing a patent airway [59].

7.5.5 Traumatic asphyxia

Traumatic asphyxia usually occurs as a result of crushing injuries to the thorax and abdomen. The exact pathophysiology is not clearly understood, but the proposed mechanism is a closed glottis and tensed abdominal muscles, causing the force of the injury to displace blood from the right atrium and through the valveless jugular and innominate veins to the head and neck, with subsequent rupture of the superficial blood vessels. Usually, the child presents tachypnoeic with petechiae over the face, neck, and chest. The face might also be blue and swollen, and fundoscopy might reveal retinal hemorrhages [46].

Children suffering from traumatic asphyxia should be very carefully examined for underlying injuries of the vital organs. One third of children with traumatic asphyxia will have associated pulmonary contusions, hypoxia or hemoptysis.

Treatment should be supportive and since these children are likely to develop respiratory insufficiency and they should be managed in a pediatric intensive care unit (PICU). In isolated traumatic asphyxia, long-term follow up has shown a general good prognosis [44–46].

7.5.6 Chest wall injuries

The elasticity and flexibility of a child's chest cage often protect the child from a serious injury. Rib fractures are rare in children occurring in only 1% to 2% of trauma victims. Flail chest occurs in only 1% to 2% of those children with rib injuries [39–46, 68]. The increased compliance of children's ribs allows the ribs to bend without fracturing. Rib fractures are usually a sign of a major energy transfer to the child's chest. In children under 3 years of age it is estimated that 39% to 82% of rib fractures are the result of non-accidental injury. In the same age group the positive predictive value of rib fractures for non-accidental injury is 95%, and rises to 100% when other causes such as motor vehicle causes or predisposing medical conditions can be excluded [69].

Anatomical position of rib fractures can predict potential underlying injuries. The commonest sites of rib fractures are posterolaterally from the 4th to the 10th rib. Greater force is required to fracture the upper four ribs as they are protected by the bony shoulder girdle, which the potential to injure the trachea, main stem bronchi, and great vessels. Equally a greater force is needed to fracture the lowest three ribs as they are not attached to the sternum and may injury the underlying organs (liver, spleen or kidneys) [44–46].

In the setting of chest trauma fractures of the clavicle, the first rib and the scapula raise the possibility of major intrathoracic and vascular injuries due the greater transmitted force and their anatomical relation to the great vessels [44–46].

Therapy is guided by patient's vital signs and physical examination along with the radiographic findings.

A portable anteroposterior (AP) chest radiograph remains the most common first radiograph obtained in most trauma patients, although STATSCAN (Lodox Systems, Sandton, South Africa), a low-radiation dose, fan-beam digital radiography unit, is an alternative in the assessment of polytrauma [46] (Figs. 7.5.2 & 7.5.3). Computed tomography (CT) scans are more reliable in diagnosing and localizing the rib fractures, but are only indicated if associated injuries are suspected [44–46, 64, 65].

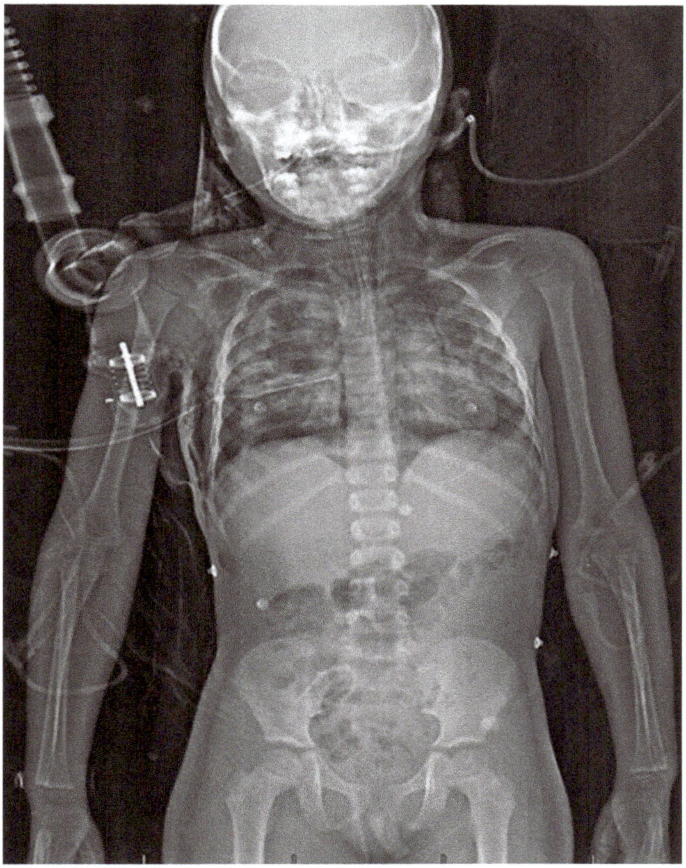

Fig. 7.5.2: A total body (Lodox©) scan of the chest demonstrating discrepancies between visible bony injuries and underlying chest injury. This patient sustained bilateral pulmonary contusions, lacerations and hemopneumothoraces, cardiac contusion, left first rib and right scapula fracture, right bronchial rupture extensive surgical emphysema, liver laceration and splenic laceration.

Inefficient ventilation is much more serious with rib fractures of the lateral and posterior chest wall since they interfere more significantly with diaphragmatic movement, an essential part in pediatric respiration [61].

Rib fractures are extremely painful. Immobilization is practically impossible. It is important to pay attention to the underlying lung contusion that can easily be overlooked in the early stages of chest imaging [44–46].

Most rib fractures are managed with adequate and appropriate analgesics that include paracetamol, nonsteroidal anti-inflammatory drugs and opiates

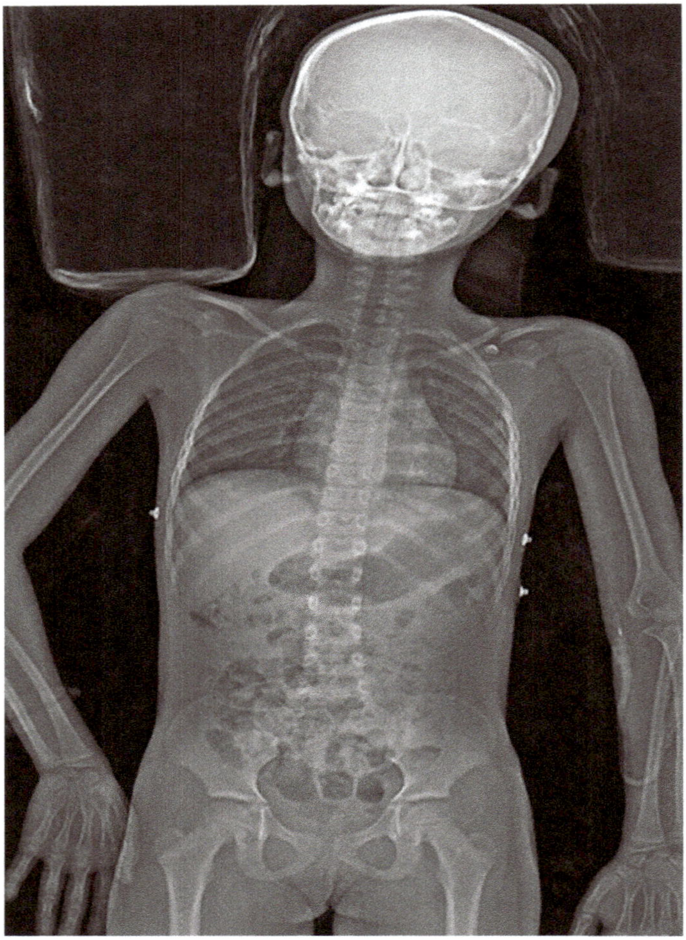

Fig. 7.5.3: A total body (Lodox©) scan of the chest demonstrating discrepancies between visible bony injuries and underlying chest injury. The image demonstrates a left clavicle fracture, posterior rib fractures 1–9 left, left lung contusion. The patient developed a left-sided chylothorax on day 5, however never required any ventilator support.

when needed. Intercostal nerve blocks may be used when the pain interferes with breathing. This ensures adequate breathing and prevents complications such as atelectasis and pneumonia, secondary to the inability to cough. Therefore respiratory exercises are an essential part of proper management. In the case of multiple rib fractures admission to a specialized trauma unit with availability of continuous chest physiotherapy is preferred [39–46, 63]. As a significant force is required to produce a flail chest segment, it is a marker of trauma severity and should raise the suspicion for other potential injuries [70]. Initial treatment involves direct pressure over the flail segment. Extensive rib fractures including a flail segment might require mechanical ventilation to improve gaseous exchange, physiotherapy and pulmonary toilet including suction, postural drainage and bronchoscopy [39–45].

7.5.7 Pulmonary injuries

Blunt pulmonary parenchymal injuries include pulmonary contusions, traumatic pneumatoceles and pulmonary lacerations and are generally the result of motor vehicle crashes, pedestrian accidents and falls [44–46].

The pliable thorax in children allows the transmission of energy through the chest wall to the underlying parenchyma. Nearly one half of children with pulmonary injury have no evidence of external chest wall trauma [39–46, 71, 72].

Lung contusions

Lung contusions occur in approximately two-thirds of all cases of chest trauma and are the most common chest injury in children. They are produced by a combination of shearing and bursting effects on the lung parenchyma that result in alveolar disruption, alveolar hemorrhage and interstitial edema. The mechanism is usually a rapid acceleration/deceleration type injury. Lung contusions occur within minutes after the injury and are mostly localized to a (lower) segment or lobe of the lung. Progressive inflammation and edema of the lung parenchyma occurs within the first 24 to 48 hours after injury. This can result in ventilation/perfusion mismatch, intrapulmonary shunting, increased lung water, decreased lung compliance, atelectasis and pulmonary consolidation [39–46, 71, 72].

Initial chest radiographs are abnormal in 67% to 90% of children with pulmonary contusions, but a normal radiograph does not exclude this injury. Radiographic changes may take 4 to 6 hours after injury to develop and include opacification and obscuration of the lung parenchyma. Aspiration may produce similar changes [44, 45, 71, 72].

Lung contusions not evident on chest radiograph can be demonstrated by helical chest CT. Ventilator support for lung contusions can be predicted if they involve more than 28% of the lung. In patients with less than 18% of lung volume involved, mechanical ventilation is rarely required [73].

Serious complications associated with lung contusion include pneumonia (20%), acute respiratory distress syndrome (ARDS, 5% to 20%) and death (15% to 20%) similar in all age groups. The risk of acute respiratory distress syndrome is highest in the first 24 hours and low after 72 hours [44, 45, 71, 72].

Management of lung contusions is supportive, consisting of adequate analgesia, supplemental oxygen, chest physical therapy and good pulmonary toilet. Mechanical ventilation is required in about a third of children with pulmonary contusions in the initial phase to prevent respiratory collapse and to achieve adequate oxygenation. Judicious fluid resuscitation and strict attention to fluid management may limit alveolar edema. Most pulmonary contusions have a good prognosis and resolve in 7 to 10 days [46].

Pulmonary hematoma is rare. It is usually caused by an injury to a major blood vessel within the lung, creating a so-called coin-lesion in the lung tissue. Management is non-operative, except in massive bleeds.

Traumatic pneumatoceles are thought to be the result of parenchymal cavitation from blunt trauma and appear as air or fluid cysts on chest imaging. They may increase in size over the first 1–2 weeks before gradually resolving and rarely cause any complications requiring surgical intervention [74–76]. Posttraumatic pseudocysts are rare and generally run a benign course resolving within 2 to 3 months. However close follow-up is recommended because of rare but serious complications such as hemothorax, pneumothorax or infection of the cyst [74].

Pulmonary lacerations are rare in children but carry a 43% mortality [41]. Clinically they may present as a hemopneumothorax with respiratory distress and may cause persitant bleeding. A chest thoracostomy tube should be placed to drain blood and air. Once drained most small pulmonary lacerations generally seal spontaneously. Large lacerations may continue to bleed requiring expeditious surgical repair [44–46].

Bronchoscopy may be required to exclude an associated tracheobronchial injury when a persistent air leak from a parenchymal laceration occurs [44, 45].

In blunt thoracic trauma surgical intervention is rarely needed, however up to one-third of patients who do require thoracotomy undergo pulmonary resection. Both formal lobectomy and pneumonectomy in acute trauma carry mortalities rates as high as 55% and 100%, respectively [79, 80].

Pneumothorax

Pneumothorax is a common occurrence in childhood chest injury. The collapse of the lung might be caused by a penetrating injury, rupture of lung parenchyma or a tear in the esophagus or tracheobronchial tree.

Air accumulates in the pleural space, leading to loss of the negative intrapleural pressure and partial or complete collapse of the lung. It can be classified as open or closed and with or without tension and is often categorized as a hemopneumothorax in in conjunction with a hemothorax. Their incidence varies between 12% to 38% and is associated with 15% mortality. The presence of pneumothorax and hemothorax increases length of hospital stay whilst pulmonary contusions and rib fractures do not. They are also associated with significantly higher Injury Severity Score (ISS) and more associated injuries. The majority of pneumothoraces are not clinically significant unless ventilator support is needed; they have the potential to develop in to a life-threatening tension pneumothorax if undiagnosed and not drained they are associated with 15% mortality [39–46].

Simple pneumothorax

Signs and symptoms in a simple (closed) pneumothorax can range from asymptomatic to respiratory distress and tachycardia with visible/palpable unequal chest movement, decreased or absent breath sounds and a hyper resonant note to percussion over the affected side.

Treatment consists of a tube thoracostomy in the fourth intercostal space, in the anterior axillary line, under adequate analgesia. Care should be taken not to cause injury tov the lung parenchyma or diaphragm during the insertion of the tube. An underwater seal should immediately be connected to the bottle. If the child is asymptomatic and can be closely monitored, aspiration or even observation of a simple pneumothorax may be appropriate. The resources to rapidly insert a chest tube should be available in the event of any deterioration [44–46]. Chest radiograph and chest CT are sensitive in demonstrating these intrapleural injuries. Small pneumothoraces noted on chest or abdominal CT scans are of questionable clinical significance and rarely require intervention. Treatment usually consists of tube thoracostomy [45–46].

Tension pneumothorax

A tension pneumothorax is the result of progressive accumulation of air under pressure in the pleural space and usually due to a valve-effect tear in the lung parenchyma. This may be more common in young children who have a more mobile mediastinum than adults [78]. It may lead to ipsilateral collapse of the lung and mediastinal shift, thereby compressing the (only properly ventilating) contralateral lung. This may result in severe impairment of ventilation as well as compromise of the venous return to the heart, and is often a lethal condition if not acted upon rapidly. (Fig. 7.5.4)

Diagnosis should be made clinically. Decreased breathing sounds, a hyperinflated ipsilateral hemithorax, tracheal deviation to the contralateral side, and a severely distressed patient all indicate that a fast needle-puncture (Thoraco-centesis) of the anterior chest (2nd intercostal space, midclavicular line) will be life-saving. The needle has to be replaced by a proper tube thoracostomy as soon as possible because blockage occurs frequently, and the excursions of an inflated lung will damage its visceral pleural surface against the sharp tip of the needle.

The following three iatrogenic pitfalls can mimic a tension pneumothorax [44, 45, 78]:

1. Children have a relatively short trachea, making it easy to intubate the right main bronchus, collapsing the left lung.
2. Luminal obstruction can have a “ball valve” effect causing progressive accumulation of pressure in the lung, and leading to reduced venous return and respiratory distress.
3. If no nasogastric tube is inserted, gastric distension can displace the left hemi-diaphragm into the chest, reducing ventilation.

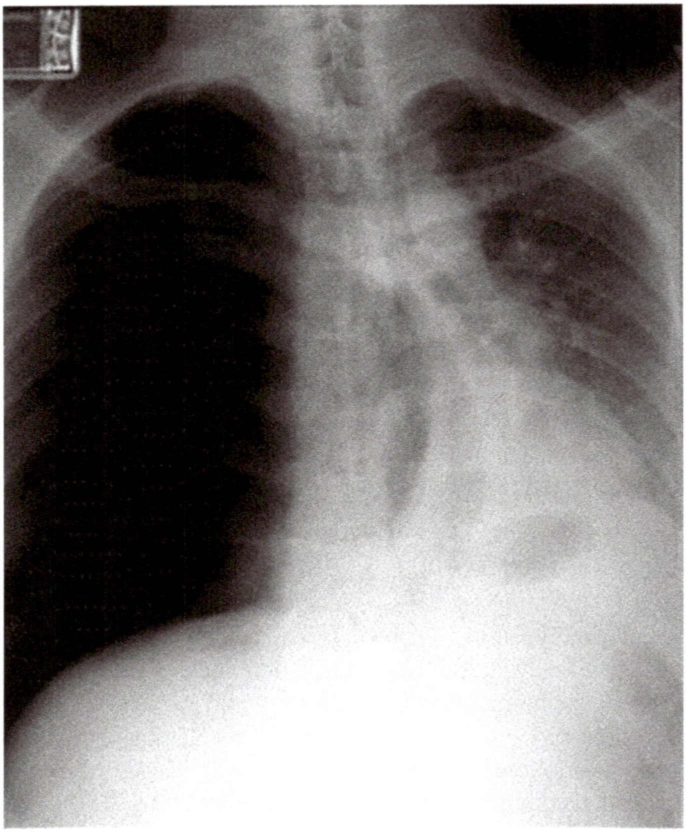

Fig. 7.5.4: Example of a radiograph with a right-side tension pneumothorax.

Open pneumothorax

Open pneumothorax is a result of a penetrating injury putting the pleural space in direct communication with the outside environment. This causes the intrathoracic and the atmospheric pressure to equilibrate, collapsing the underlying lung, If the chest wound is two-thirds the diameter of the trachea or greater, then on inspiration air will be sucked from atmosphere through the defect into the pleural space, collapsing the lung and causing mediastinal shift and subsequent cardiovascular and respiratory compromise. Therefore symptoms and signs are proportional to the wound size.

Patients present with respiratory distress and tachycardia, a visible chest wound, reduced breath sounds, and a hyper resonant percussion note over the affected side and blood-stained air bubbling. Subcutaneous emphysema may be seen or palpated at the penetration site.

Management involves preventing air from entering via the wound site with an occlusive dressing applied over the wound, taped down over three sides, creating a

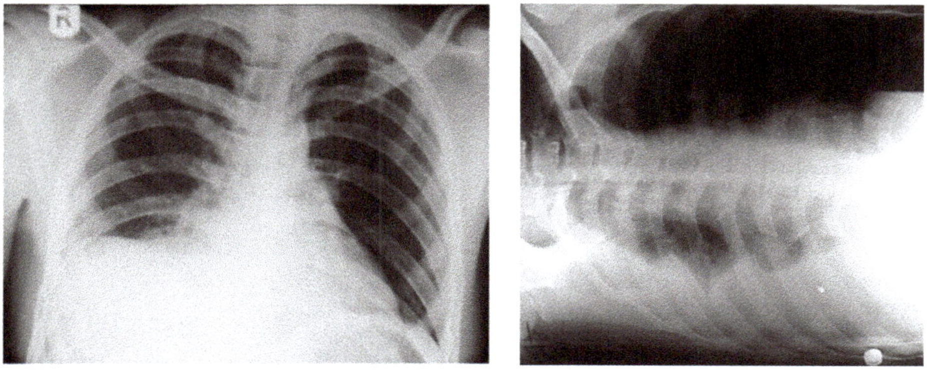

(a) (b)

Fig. 7.5.5: Chest radiograph demonstrating a *subpulmonic* hemothorax, difficult to diagnose on the AP view (a) but becoming apparent on the right side down decubitus view (b).

one-way valve. The remaining air is drained via a thoracostomy tube. The wound may need surgical debridement and closure [58, 61].

Hemothorax

Hemothorax is the accumulation of blood in the pleural space. It occurs in up to a third of cases of chest trauma, often in conjunction with a pneumothorax and is associated with a mortality of up to 53% [41, 44–46]. The most common sources for significant intrapleural blood are lacerated intercostal vessels or pulmonary parenchymal lacerations. It may also be a sign of great vessel injury. Up to 40% of the circulating blood volume can easily be lost in one pleural cavity leading to profound circulatory failure [44]. In the case of a large volume hemothorax. Volume restoration takes precedence over drainage. Intravenous access with two wide bore lines must be obtained prior to drainage, as decompression may result in further bleeding as the tamponade effect is lost [58]. The diagnosis is made clinically and confirmed with an erect chest radiograph. Blood in the lower part of the pleural cavity often causes referred pain in the upper abdomen. Once the hemothorax is drained, these abdominal symptoms disappear.

Subpulmonic hemothorax, in which blood only accumulates under the base of the lung, represents a challenge for diagnosis, particular on the right side, but a lateral decubitus radiograph will prove the condition. (Fig. 7.5.5)

On rare occasions, a massive hemothorax may lead to a tension hemothorax with respiratory and cardiovascular compromise resulting in deviation of the heart and mediastinum to the opposite side. However compared to a tension pneumothorax the neck veins are flat with hypovolemia, and there is a dull percussion note over the affected side.

Treatment consists of wide bore tube thoracostomy to drain the hemothorax (Tab. 7.5.2); only rarely a thoracotomy is indicated. When diagnosed blood

Tab. 7.5.2: Chest drain tube size by age-based guidelines [58].

Age	Chest drain size (French gauge)
0–12 months	12–16
1–5 years	16–20
5–10 years	20–24
10–15 years	24–28

should be promptly evacuated from the pleural space with tube thoracostomy, since

1. blood left in the pleural space can produce fibrous scar tissue, causing restrictive lung disease;
2. blood acts as a perfect culture media promoting sepsis and pneumonia (empyema);
3. drainage allows accurate measurements of the blood loss for replacement, determining further treatment [44–46, 77].

Intrathoracic blood should be evacuated within 1 week of injury by either thoracotomy or thoracoscopy [44–46]. The main indications for thoracotomy are ongoing active bleed while an intercostal drain is in place especially if initial blood loss >15 mL/kg, continues drainage of blood >3 mL/kg/hr for more than 4 hours or an infected hemothorax usually 5–7 days after injury [77].

Pneumomediastinum

In blunt chest injury in children pneumomediastinum is a sign of potential injury to the tracheobronchial tree, esophagus or vascular injury. It gives a streaky appearance on the radiograph, and it often extends beyond the pleural space into the neck or the abdomen. Pneumomediastinum in the absence of radiographic or clinical evidence of other thoracic injuries does not routinely require further investigations and resolves with no intervention [71, 72].

7.5.8 Tracheobronchial injuries

Tracheobronchial ruptures are rare occurrences in pediatric chest injuries that carry a 30% mortality with half of the deaths occurring within 1 hour of injury [86–88]. Generally they are a result of anterior-posterior compression of the flexible chest wall. The sternum is forced against the spine, displacing the lungs laterally and disrupting the tracheobronchial tree at the carina [86, 88]. Other mechanisms include direct tracheal injury or the “tracheal blast” effect when intratracheal pressure rises rapidly against a closed glottis from chest compression [85, 89]. Usually there is complete rupture of the trachea or bronchi with associated vascular and esophageal injuries mostly within 2.5 cm from the carina [86, 88].

Symptoms range from minimal to hemothorax, pneumomediastinum, hemoptysis and subcutaneous emphysema. This type of injury should also be suspected when a pneumothorax fails to resolve after tube thoracostomy, a continuous air leak develops or a persistent pneumomediastinum is present [81, 85, 86]. Rib fractures are present in a quarter of children [81, 86]. Whilst chest radiographs and CT scans may show a pneumothorax, they rarely demonstrate a clear disruption of the trachea or bronchus [82, 86]. Bronchoscopy aids the diagnosis and localization of the injury and may permit passage of an endotracheal tube beyond the injury for ventilation [81, 85].

Management depends on the size of the injury and the ability to adequately ventilate the child. Injuries involving less than one-third of the diameter of the bronchus may be treated non-operatively depending on the respiratory status of the child [81, 85].

More significant injuries require thoracotomy and repair using interrupted absorbable sutures applied with minimal tension while knots should be tied outside the lumen. The repair can be reinforced with a vascularized tissue buttress. In a tracheoesophageal injury a muscular (Sternocleidomastoid) or pleura flap between the injuries can be utilized to prevent a fistula formation. Complications include bronchopleural fistulas, bronchial stenosis and persistent pulmonary sepsis [57, 81, 85, 91].

7.5.9 Esophageal injuries

The esophagus is well protected, as it lies deep within the mediastinum, making esophageal injuries rare in chest trauma. There is often a delay in diagnosis and other associated injuries. Esphageal perforations are most rapidly fatal injuries of the gastrointestinal tract [89]. Blunt trauma is a rare etiology as the esophagus can decompress into the stomach, is flexible and compliant [78].

The three proposed mechanisms of injury in blunt trauma are rapid rise in intraluminal pressure against a closed glottis from a severe blow to the upper abdomen; deceleration injury, causing disruption of the blood supply, leading to ischemia and subsequent perforation; and “blast effect” injury from concomitant tracheal injury. Most cases are due to impact from steering wheels [57].

Transmitted pressure from the stomach may cause either Mallory-Weiss bleeding (if the lower esophageal sphincter is closed) or the more sinister Boerhaave syndrome, characterized by perforation of the lower esophagus into the left chest cavity (if the upper esophageal sphincter is closed). The espophagus has no serosal cover, therefore any perforation leads directly into mediastinum or pleural space [46].

Also negative intrathoracic pressure pulls the esophageal contents (bacteria and enzymes) and air into the mediastinum or pleural space leading to pneumomediastinum, pneumothorax and subcutaneous emphysema. This then results in rapidly progressing mediastinitis, abscesses and sepsis leading to multi-organ failure and death [44–46].

Penetrating injuries may also cause esophageal injuries if they are transthoracic [46]. Injury at the level of the neck usually presents with local pain, swelling and dysphagia [70]. In the mediastinum it may present with chest pain, fever, sub-cutaneous emphysema, dysponea and vomiting, circulatory failure and pneumothorax. Chest radiographs may demonstrate a pneumothorax, pneumomediastinum, pleural effusion and subcutaneous emphysema, but can also be normal in 12%–33% of cases [62, 70, 83].

The signs and symptoms are non-specific in the child with multiple injuries and one has to be vigilant for the rare possible esphageal injury to avoid diagnostic delay [46].

Investigations include water-soluble contrast study and/or endoscopy. Most injuries should be detected by oesophagram, however if there are any on going concerns endoscopy should be performed. Both have high false negative rates [57]. Salivary amylase in the chest drain would be highly suggestive of an esophageal perforation [70].

The treatment depends on the nature and the location of the injury. It includes non-operative management, esophageal exclusion and diversion or primary repair. The preferred management is primary esophageal repair within 24 hours of the injury. This has been performed safely even in delayed diagnosis [89]. Children with mediastinitis should have exclusion of the esophagus with concomitant wide mediastinal drainage [89]. Contained esophageal perforations without evidence of mediastinitis may be managed non-operatively.

7.5.10 Diaphragmatic injuries

Traumatic disruption of the diaphragm, occuring in 1% to 2% of children, is generally the result of blunt trauma. The diagnosis remains challenging and delays in diagnosis occur in 15% to 77% of patients [84]. The majority is left-sided, however the right side may sustain more unrecognized injuries. They generally result from high velocity injury, such as from motor vehicle collisions and falls from a height and require a considerable amount of force. Associated intra-thoracic, intra-abdominal as well as extra-truncal injuries are common [45, 46].

The clinical presentation varies according to the associated injuries and may be difficult to separate from concomitant chest and abdominal injuries. Signs include respiratory distress, chest pain, absent breath sounds on the affected side and bowel sounds in the chest. An isolated diaphragmatic rupture can be easily misdiagnosed, as children may have no external evidence of trauma with only minimal findings on physical examination. In children diaphragmatic rupture more commonly occurs along the periphery of the diaphragm, most likely due to the increased pliability of the thorax in young children Herniation of abdominal viscera into the thorax is common and may lead to strangulation.

Diagnosis is made on an erect chest radiograph (Fig. 7.5.6), which typically shows the nasogastric tube in the stomach above the diaphragm. However the appearance of the stomach below the diaphragm does not exclude a diaphragmatic rupture. Other radiological findings suggestive of a diaphragmatic injury include an elevated diaphragm, gastric or bowel gas patterns in the chest or an indistinct diaphragmatic contour. Other imaging modalities include contrast studies to demonstrate the stomach or bowel traversing the diaphragmatic defect. Fluoroscopy and ultrasound may be used to assess diaphragmatic movement with paradoxical or impaired motion being suggestive of diaphragmatic injury. When imaging is non-diagnostic for a diaphragmatic hernia, but there is a high clinical suspicion, laparotomy, laparoscopy or thoracoscopy should be considered [45, 46].

The diaphragm can also be injured in penetrating injuries to the lower half of the chest or the upper abdomen. Whilst this rarely leads to herniation in the acute phase, an undiagnosed hole can result in long-term complications. This should be repaired via a laparotomy given the high frequency of associated liver, spleen or bowel injuries. In delayed diagnoses the repair is generally performed through the chest [84, 92–98].

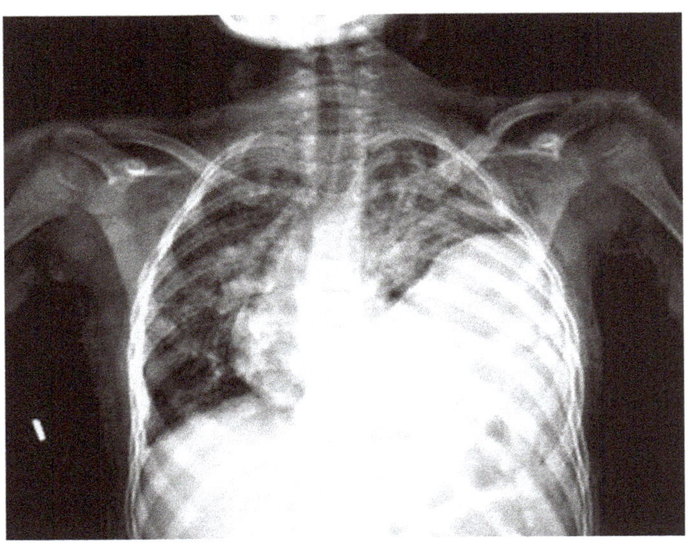

Fig. 7.5.6: Example of a radiograph of a left-sided diaphragmatic rupture with mediastinal shift to the right.

7.5.11 Great vessel injuries

Blunt injuries to the thoracic aorta and great vessels are rare in children but are lethal if missed. The majority of blunt aortic injuries die at the scene of the injury or during transport. About a third of those who reach hospital die within 6 hours making expedient evaluation mandatory [99–102].

The most common causes are motor vehicle accidents and falls from height. The abdominal aorta rather than the thoracic aorta is more commonly involved in restrained as compared to unrestrained children [57, 99–104]. The typical location of the injury is at the aortic isthmus distal to the left subclavian artery at the ligamentum arteriosum. Clinical findings suggestive of aortic injury include first rib and sternal fractures, paraplegia, upper extremity hypertension or lower extremity pulse deficits. On chest radiograph a widened mediastinum, loss of the normal aortic contour, deviation of the course of the nasogastric tube and first rib fractures would suggest aortic injury and further imaging should be performed with either a helical chest CT, transesophageal echocardiography (TEE), intravascular ultrasound (IVUS) or aortic arch arteriography [46, 57, 99–104].

Operative repair remains the standard therapy with aggressive preoperative blood pressure control with beta-blockers to reduce shear on the aortic wall to decrease the risk of free rupture [100, 102, 103]. In cases where concomitant injuries preclude thoracotomy, delayed aortic repair, endovascular stent grafting or expectant management can be considered [100, 102, 103]. If the aortic repair is delayed because of concomitant injuries aggressive blood pressure control and serial CT scans are required to monitor changes in the aortic hematoma [105, 106].

In children with minimal aortic injuries (small intimal flaps) or in situations in which the child has a limited life expectancy due to other injuries non-operative management has been used [106–107].

Other great vessel injuries (pulmonary vessels, superior and inferior vena cavae, proximal carotid, subclavian, innominate arteries) are extremely rare [46, 57].

7.5.12 Heart and pericardium

In children cardiac injury is a rare occurrence with blunt trauma. Penetrating trauma can involve the heart and/or the great vessels resulting in severe hemorrhage and cardiac tamponade with a large and rapidly lethal hemothorax.

Cardiac injuries include concussions, contusions and frank rupture of the myocardium, a valve, a septum and rarely a coronary artery [44–46]. Pericardial tears leading to herniation of the heart often present with a diminished cardiac function and a low output state. Occult structural cardiac injuries (i.e. atrial or ventricular septal defects, valvular insufficiency and ventricular aneurysm formation) can also occur and present without physiologic signs of injury. Often, these injuries are identified only after a new murmur or a change in the electrocardiogram (ECG) is noted. Echocardiography can assist to confirm the diagnosis.

Another rare condition is commotio cordis, most commonly seen in teenagers (mean age, 12 to 13 years) as a result of non-penetrating chest wall impact in the absence of any identifiable injury to the heart or chest wall. It is commonly associated with sports such as baseball, hockey, football and lacrosse. Defibrillation may be life-saving [53].

Myocardial contusion

Myocardial contusions are the most common type of cardiac injury in children with blunt chest trauma. They produce focal damage to the heart that can be seen histologically, unlike myocardial concussions, and often have an associated chest wall injury [46, 107].

Cardiac contusions have a full spectrum of presentation and outcomes, ranging from simple electrocardiogram (ECG) or cardiac enzyme abnormalities to fatal arrhythmias, myocardial pump failure with hypotension and cardiac rupture. They may not be apparent for the first 6–12 hrs, but the majority will present within the first 24 hrs, as the injured muscle becomes ischaemic by 18–24 hrs secondary to stagnant blood. Therefore most life-threatening cardiac contusions present either initially or within 48 hrs. The necrotic muscle is then replaced with fibrous vascularized scar tissue over a period of weeks making the heart susceptible to dysfunction, arrhythmia, aneurysm formation, rupture and thrombus formation.

Many diagnostic tools for cardiac contusions have been proposed including serial blood pressure, echocardiography, electrocardiography, cardiac isoenzymes (CPKMB, troponin I) and nuclear imaging, but there is no definitive diagnostic test. A 12-lead ECG is the simplest test and may be normal or show T-wave inversion, ST ischemic changes, varying degrees of heart block and supraventricular and ventricular arrhythmias. However it is difficult to predict clinical outcome based on these changes. Tropinin I has been found to be more sensitive than CPK-MB for diagnosing cardiac contusions [110, 111].

Echocardiography is useful in symptomatic cardiac contusions to demonstrate reduced ejection fraction, localized systolic wall motion abnormalities and areas of increased end-diastolic wall thickness and echogenicity [44–46, 107, 108].

Antiarrhythmic agents may be needed for persistent arrhythmias and inotropic drugs may be needed to restore blood pressure and perfusion [44–46].

A hemodynamically stable child in normal sinus rhythm with suspected blunt cardiac injury is unlikely to develop a serious arrhythmia or pump failure [107, 108].

The management of myocardial contusions is supportive, treating any hypotension or disrythmia as required. Patiens should be managed with cardiac monitoring, serial electrocardiogram and cardiac enzymes and echocardiogram in case of any arrhythmia or unexpected hypotension.

Complications are rare, however, and include mitral or tricuspid insufficiency or ventral septal defect mandating follow up for these patients [44–46, 107, 108].

Myocardial rupture and valve injury

The majority of cases of myocardial rupture result in rapid death and are due to high-energy impacts such as motor vehicle collisions or falls from great height. The right ventricle is the most common site of rupture. The child will present *in extremis* with pericardial tamponade. Early diagnosis and repair is key for survival from these lethal injuries [44–46]. Traumatic atrial or ventricular septal defects may present with a new murmur only. Valvular injuries may also occur but are rare. The atrioventricular valves are most commonly affected with damage to the valve apparatus (i.e. annulus, ruptured chorda tendinae or papillary muscle). Elective repair is an option in clinically stable patients [46, 107].

Pericardial tamponade

Cardiac tamponade is the result of blood entering the pericardial sac resulting in limited diastolic filling and reduced cardiac output, either as a result of blunt or penetrating trauma. As the pericardium is fibrous and non-pliable a small amount of blood can have a dramatic effect.

In children this may present with a range of clinical signs including tachycardia; peripheral vasoconstriction. Beck's triad of jugular venous distention, persistent hypotension unresponsive to aggressive fluid resuscitation and muffled heart sounds may be difficult to appreciate. Children have short fat necks making jugular veins difficult to see and much thinner chest walls allowing more transmission of cardiac sounds [45, 46].

This diagnosis should be considered in any child with persistent hypotension despite fluid resuscitation and adequate ventilation. Investigations include FAST scan, echocardiography and chest radiograph which may show an enlarged globular heart shadow.

7.5.13 Resuscitative thoracotomy

Immediate resuscitative thoracotomy can be a dramatic and potentially life-saving procedure, when performed in children with penetrating trauma who arrive pulseless, but with myocardial electrical activity. However it has little utility in children with cardiac arrest following blunt trauma with a reported survival rate of 2.3% from the four largest case series. Therefore in children with cardiac arrest after blunt trauma resuscitative thoracotomy should be limited to those who arrive in the hospital with vitals signs and have a witnessed arrest [111–115].

7.5.14 Pitfalls in pediatric thoracic trauma

There are a number of pitfalls in pediatric chest trauma.

- The extent of the chest injury is commonly underestimated at the initial survey because of little external evidence of injury and equally on the supine chest radiograph.
- Excessive fluid resuscitation can aggravate pulmonary contusion and edema.
- Adequate analgesia and chest physiotherapy are key to preventing the retention of secretions, which can lead to pulmonary infection.
- Iatrogenic damage can occur as part of emergency (and faulty) procedures such as endotracheal intubation, chest drain insertion and central line insertion.

7.5.15 Conclusion

Thoracic trauma is the second most common course of trauma mortality in children. It generally occurs as part of multisystem trauma in the pediatric population with increasing frequency owing to high-speed travel and violence. In multisystem trauma, chest trauma usually is a marker of increased injury severity and resulting in increased mortality. Most of the chest trauma can be managed conservatively or by tube thoracotomy. Early diagnosis and management is key to improving outcome.

A primary survey should address the life-threatening injuries adhering to basic ATLS principles. Often there are few if any external markers of injury with non-specific clinical signs and investigations can easily miss or underestimate the severity of injuries. Therefore it is important to have a high index of suspicion for potential intra-thoracic injuries based on the mechanism of injury and the understanding of a child's response to trauma.

Active exclusion of the six lethal injuries on primary survey and the six potential life-threatening injuries on secondary survey can guide the thorough assessment and management of the child with thoracic trauma.

Any rib fractures in a child under the age of 3 years without an adequate mechanism of injury should be considered as a potential, non-accidental injuries.

The top three causes of child mortality from unintentional injury are road traffic collisions (32%), drowning (17%), and burns (9%), which are all preventable.

To achieve this will require the concerted efforts of government, civil society and advocacy of the medical profession. Prevention of road traffic collisions in particular will decrease pediatric trauma in general and therefore will also lead to a reduction of thoracic injuries in children.

7.6 Further reading

[1] Ravitch MM. The Operative Treatment of Pectus Excavatum. Ann Surg 1949;129:429–44.

[2] Nuss D, Kelly RE, Jr., Croitoru DP, Katz ME. A 10-year review of a minimally invasive technique for the correction of pectus excavatum. J Pediatr Surg 1998;33:545–52.

[3] Kelly RE, Jr. Pectus excavatum: historical background, clinical picture, preoperative evaluation and criteria for operation. Semin Pediatr Surg 2008;17:181–93.

[4] Maagaard M, Tang M, Ringgaard S, Nielsen HH, Frokiaer J, Haubuf M, Pilegaard HK, Hjortdal VE. Normalized cardiopulmonary exercise function in patients with pectus excavatum three years after operation. Ann Thorac Surg 2013;96:272–78.

[5] Pilegaard HK, Licht PB. Can absorbable stabilizers be used routinely in the Nuss procedure? Eur J Cardiothorac Surg 2009;35:561–64.

[6] Nyboe C, Knudsen MR, Pilegaard HK. Elective pectus bar removal following Nuss procedure for pectus excavatum: a single-institution experience. Eur J Cardiothorac Surg 2011;39:1040–42.

[7] Park HJ, Lee SY, Lee CS, Youm W, Lee KR. The Nuss Procedure For Pectus Excavatum: An Evolution Of Techniques And Results On 322 Patients. Ann Thorac Surg 2004;77:289–95.

[8] Park HJ, Jeong JY, Jo WM, Shin JS, Lee IS, Kim KT, Choi YH. Minimally Invasive Repair of Pectus Excavatum: A Novel Morphology-Tailored Patient-Specific Approach. J Thorac Cardiovasc Surg 2010;139:379–86.

[9] Pilegaard HK, Licht PB. Can absorbable stabilizers be used routinely in the Nuss procedure? Eur J Cardiothorac Surg 2009;35:561–64.

[10] Park HJ, Kim KS, Lee S, Jeon HW. A Next-Generation Pectus Excavatum Repair Technique: New Devices Make a Difference. Ann Thorac Surg 2015;99:455–61.

[11] Park HJ, Kim KS, Moon YK, Lee SS. The Bridge Technique for Pectus Bar Fixation: A Method to Make the Bar Un-Rotatable. J Pediatr Surg 2015;50:1320–22.

[12] Kelly RE, Shamberger RC, Mellins RB, et al. Prospective multicenter study of surgical correction of Pectus excavatum: Design, perioperative complications, pain, and baseline pulmonary function facilitated by internet-based data collection. J Am Coll Surg 2007;205:205–16.

[13] Lawson ML, Mellins RB, Paulson JF, et al. Increasing severity of Pectus excavatum is associated with reduced pulmonary function. J Pediatr 2011;159:256–61.

[14] Kelly RE, Mellins RB, Shamberger RC, et al. Multicenter study of Pectus excavatum, final report: complications, static/exercise pulmonary function, and anatomic outcomes. J Am Coll Surg 2013; 217:1080–9.

[15] Redlinger R, Wooten A, Kelly RE, et al. Optoelectronic plethysmography demonstrates abrogation of normal chest wall motion dysfunction in patients with Pectus excavatum after Nuss repair. J Pediatr Surg 2012;47:160–4.

[16] Kelly RE, Goretsky MJ, Obermeyer R, et al. Twenty-one years of experience with Minimally invasive repair of Pectus excavatum by the Nuss procedure in 1215 patients. Ann Surg 2010;252:1072–81.6.

[17] Nuss D, Kelly RE Jr. The minimally invasive repair of Pectus excavatum. Operative Techniques in Thorac Cardiovasc Surg 2014;19:324–27.

[18] Chao CJ, Jaroszewski DE, Kumar PN, et al. Surgical repair of pectus excavatum relieves right heart chamber compression and improves cardiac output in adult patients-an intraoperative transesophageal echocardiographic study. Am J Surg 2015;210:1118–25.

[19] Jaroszewski DE, Johnson K, McMahon L, Notrica D. Sternal elevation before passing bars: A technique for improving visualization and facilitating minimally invasive pectus excavatum repair in adult patients. J Thorac and Cardiovasc Surg 2013;147(3): 1093–5.

[20] Kragten HA, Siebenga J, Hoppener PF, Verburg R, Visker N. Symptomatic pectus excavatum in seniors (SPES): a cardiovascular problem? Neth Heart J 2011;19:73–8.
[21] Nuss D, Kelly RE, Jr., Croitoru DP, Katz ME. A 10-year review of a minimally invasive technique for the correction of pectus excavatum. J Pediatr Surg 1998;33:545–52.
[22] Pilegaard HK. Extending the use of Nuss procedure in patients older than 30 years. Euro J Cardiothorac Surg 2011;40(2):334–7.
[23] Wihlm JM. «Open repair of Pectus Excavatum and Pectus Carinatum». In ESTS Textbook of Thoracic Surgery, ed Jaroslaw Kuzdzal. Cracow: Medycyna Praktyczna; 2015: Vol. 2: 67–85.
[24] Calloway EH, Chhotani AN, Lee YZ, Phillips JD. Three-dimensional computed tomography for evaluation and management of children with complex chest wall anomalies: useful information or just pretty pictures? J Pediatr Surg. 2011;46(4):640–7.
[25] Brochhausen Ch, Turial S, Müller F, Schmitt V, Coerdt W, Wihlm JM, Schier F, Kirkpatrick J. Pectus excavatum: history, hypotheses and treatment options. Interact Cardiovasc Thorac Surg; 2012;14(6):801–6.
[26] Kadlec J, Wihlm JM, Coonar A. «Surgery for pectus and other congenital chest wall disorders». In Core Topics in Thoracic Surgery. Eds. Marco Scarci, Aman Coonar, Tom Routledge and Francis Wells. Cambridge: Cambridge University Press, 2016.
[27] Milanez de Campos JR, Das Neves Pereira JC, Lopes KM, Jatene FB. Technical modifications in stabilisers and in bar removal in the Nuss procedure. Eur J Cardio-thoracic Surg. 2009;36:410–12.
[28] Cobben JM, Oostra RJ, van Dijk FS. Pectus excavatum and carinatum. Eur J Med Genet 2014;57:414–17.
[29] Desmarais TJ, Keller MS. Pectus carinatum. Curr Opin Pediatr 2013;25:375–81.
[30] Abramson H, D'Agostino J, Wuscovi S. A 5-year experience with a minimally invasive technique for pectus carinatum repair. J Pediatr Surg 2009;44:118–23.
[31] Martinez-Ferro M, Fraire C, Bernard S. Dynamic compression system for the correction of pectus carinatum. Semin Pediatr Surg 2008;17:194–200.
[32] Lee RT, Moorman S, Schneider M, Sigalet DL. Bracing is an effective therapy for pectus carinatum: interim results. J Pediatr Surg 2013;48:184–90.
[33] Robicsek F. Editorial Comment: The Nuss procedure: not so fast! Eur J Cardiothorac Surg February 2011;39(2):159. Krasopoulos G, Goldstraw P. Minimally invasive repair of pectus excavatum deformity. Eur J Cardiothorac Surg 2011;39:149–58.
[34] Robicsek F. Sanger PW, Taylor FH, et al. The surgical treatment of chondrosternal prominence (pectus carinatum). J Thorac Cardiovasc Surg 1963;45:691–701.
[35] Robicsek F. Surgical Treatment of Pectus Carinatum. Robicsek F, Faber LP, eds. Chest Surgery Clinics of North America. Vol.2. Philadelphia: W. B. Saunders Company; 2000:357–76.
[36] Robicsek F, Fokin AA. Pectus carinatum, Poland's syndrome, cleft sternum and acquired restrictive thoracic dystrophy. In: Encyclopedia of Respiratory Medicine. #523. Laurent GJ, Shapiro SD, Editors, Oxford, UK. Elsevier, (ISBN: 0124383602) Academic Press 2006, p. 159–67.
[37] Robicsek F. Surgical repair of pectus excavatum and carinatum. Semin Thorac Cardiovasc Surg Apr 2009:64–75.
[38] Robicsek F, Watts LT. Pectus Carinatum. Guest Editor Gaetano Rocco, Thorac Surg Clin November 2010, Vol. 20;4:563–74.
[39] Buntain WL (ed). Management of pediatric trauma. Saunders, 1995.
[40] Eichelberger MR (ed). Pediatric trauma: prevention, acute care, rehabilitation. Mosby, 1993.
[41] Peclet M, Newman K, Eichelberger M, Gotschall C, Garcia V, Bowman L. Thoracic trauma in children: an indicator of increased mortality. Journal of Pediatric Surgery 1990;25:961–66.

[42] Allen G, Cox C, Moore F, Duke J, Andrassy R. Pulmonary contusions in children: are children different? Journal of American College of Surgeons 1997;185:239–43.
[43] Ruddy R. Trauma and the pediatric lung. Paediatric Respiratory Review 2005;6:61–67.
[44] Kerr M & Maconochie I. Paediatric chest trauma (part 1) – Initial Lethal Injuries. Trauma 2008;10:183–94.
[45] Kerr M & Maconochie I. Paediatric chest trauma (part 2) – Hidden Injuries. Trauma 2008;10:195–210.
[46] Ameh E, et al. Paediatric Surgery: A Comprehensive Text for Africa Global HELP, Seattle, WA, US, 2011.
[47] Reinhorn M, Kaufman H, Hirsch E, Millham F. Penetrating thoracic trauma in a pediatric population. Annals of Thoracic Surgery 1996;61:1501–05.
[48] Sturtz G. Biomechanical data of children. In: 24th Stapp Car Crash Conference, 1980, pp. 511–559.
[49] Huelke D. An overview of anatomical considerations of infants and children in the adult world of automobile safety design. In: 42nd Annual Proceedings Association for the Advancement o Automotive Medicine, October 1998;5–7:93–113.
[50] Nakayama DK, Ramenofsky ML, Row MI. Chest injuries in childhood. Ann Surg 1989;210:770–775.
[51] Roux P, Fisher RM. Chest injuries in children: An analysis of 100 cases of blunt chest trauma from motor vehicle accidents. J Pediatr Surg 1992;27:551–55.
[52] Riley JP, Brandt ML, Mattox KL, et al. Thoracic trauma in children. J Trauma 1993;34:329–33.
[53] Maron BJ, Gohman TE, Kyle SB, et al. Clinical profile and spectrum of commotion cordis. JAMA 2002;287:1142–11416.
[54] Black TL, Synder CL, Miller JP, et al. Significance of chest trauma in children. South Med J 1996;89:494–96.
[55] Sarihan H, Abbes M, Akyazici R, et al. Blunt thoracic trauma in children. J Cardiovasc Surg 1996;37:525–28.
[56] Kisson N, Dreyer J, Walai N. Pediatric trauma: Differences in pathophysiology, injury patterns and treatment compared with adult trauma. Can Med Assoc J 1990;142:27–34.
[57] Sartorelli K, Vane D. The diagnosis and management of children with blunt injury of the chest. Seminars in Pediatric Surgery 2004;13:98–105.
[58] Greaves I, Porter K, Ryan J. Trauma care manual Hodder Headline Group: London 2001.
[59] European Resuscitation Council. European paediatric life support, 2nd ed. Resuscitation Council UK: London 2006.
[60] American College of Surgeons Committee on Trauma. Advanced Trauma Life Support for Doctors, 8th edition. 2008.
[61] Beaver B, Laschinger J. Pediatric thoracic trauma. Seminars in Thoracic and Cardiovascular Surgery 1992;4:255–62.
[62] Yamamoto L, Schroeder C, Beliveau C. Thoracic trauma. The deadly dozen. Critical Care Nursing Quarterly 2005;28:22–40.
[63] Tovar J. The lung and pediatric trauma. Seminars in Pediatric Surgery 2008;17:53–59.
[64] Sivit C. Pediatric thoracic trauma: imaging considerations. Emergency Radiology 2002;9:21–25.
[65] Hall A, Johnson K. The imaging of pediatric thoracic trauma. Pediatric Respiratory Reviews 2002;3:241–47.
[66] Cooper A, Barlow B, DiScala C, String D. Mortality and truncal injury: the pediatric perspective. Journal of Pediatric Surgery 1994;29:33–38.
[67] Tovar J & Vazquez J. Management of Chest Trauma in Children, Paediatric Respiratory Reviews 2013;14(2013): 86–91.
[68] Garcia VF, Gotschall CS, Eichelberger MR, et al. Rib fractures in children: A marker of severe injury. J Trauma 1990;30:695–700.

[69] Barsness KA, Cha E, Bensard DD, et al. The positive predictive value of rib fractures as an indicator of nonaccidental trauma in children. J Trauma 2003;54:1107–10.
[70] Dickenson D. Thoracic trauma in children. Critical Care Nursing Clinics of North America 1991;3:423–32.
[71] Allen GS, Cox CS, Moore FA, et al. Pulmonary contusion: Are children different? J Am Coll Surg 1997;185:229–33.
[72] Allen GS, Cox CS. Pulmonary contusion in children: Diagnosis and management. South Med J 1998;91:1099–06.
[73] Wagner RB, Jamieson PM. Pulmonary contusion: evaluation and classification by computed tomography. Surg Clin North Am.
[74] Stathopoulos G, Chrysikoppulou E, Kalogeromitros A, et al. Bilateral traumatic pulmonary psuedocysts: Case report and literature review. J Trauma 2002;53:993–96.
[75] Schimpl G, Schneider U. Traumatic pneumatoceles in an infant: Case report and review of the literature. Eur J Pediatr Surg 1996;6:104–6.
[76] Galea MH, Williams N, Nayell MJ. Traumatic pneumatocele. J Pediatr Surg 1992;27:1523–24.
[77] Cullen M. Pulmonary and respiratory complications of pediatric trauma. Respiratory care clinics of North America 2001;7(1):59–77.
[78] Bliss D, Silen M. Pediatric thoracic trauma. Critical Care Medicine 2002;30:409–15.
[79] Karmy-Jones R, Jurkovich GJ, Shatz DV, et al. Management of traumatic lung injury: A Western Trauma Association multicenter review. J Trauma 2001;51:1049–53.
[80] Stewart KC, Urschel JD, Nakai SS, et al. Pulmonary resection for lung trauma. Ann Thorac Surg 1997;63:1587–88.
[81] Ait Ali Alimane A, Becmeur D, Aubert F, et al. Tracheobronchial ruptures from blunt thoracic trauma in children. J Pediatr Surg 1999;34:1847–50.
[82] Grant WJ, Meyers RL, Jaffe RL, et al. Tracheobronchial injuries after blunt trauma in children-hidden pathology. J Pediatr Surg 1998;33:1707–11.
[83] Demirbag S, Tiryaki T, Atabek C, Surer I, Ozturk H, Cetinkursun S. Conservative approach to the mediastinits in childhood secondary to esophageal perforation. Clinical Pediatrics 2005:131–34.
[84] Brandt ML, Luks FI, Nitsana A, et al. Diaphragmatic injury in children. J Trauma 1992;32:298–301.
[85] van As S, et al. 2013 Treatment of Thoracic Trauma in Children: Literature Review, Red Cross War Memorial Children's Hospital Data Analysis, and Guidelines for Management. Eur J Pediatr Surg 2013;23:434–43.
[86] Hancock BJ, Weisman NE. Tracheobronchial injuries in children. J Pediatr Surg 1991;26:1316–19.
[87] Mordehai J, Kurzbart E, Kapuller V, et al. Tracheal rupture after blunt chest trauma in a child. J Pediatr Surg 1997;32:104–5.
[88] Swan KG Jr, Swan BC, Swan KG. Deceleration thoracic injury. J Trauma 2001;51:970–74.
[89] Sartorelli KH, McBride WJ, Vane DW. Perforation of the intrabdominal esophagus from blunt trauma in a child: case report and review of the literature. J Pediatr Surg 1999;34:495–97.
[90] Ozdulger A, Cetin G, Erkemen Gulhan S, et al. A review of 24 patients with bronchial ruptures: Is delay in diagnosis more common in children? Eur J Cardiothorac Surg 2003;23:379–83.
[91] Wright CD, Graham BB, Grillo HC, et al. Pediatric tracheal surgery. Ann Thorac Surg 2002;74:308–14.
[92] Karnak I, Senocak ME, Tanyel FC, et al. Diaphragmatic injuries in childhood. Surg Today 2001;31:5–11.
[93] Sharma AK, Kothari SK, Gupta C, et al. Rupture of the right hemidiaphragm due to blunt trauma in children: A diagnostic dilemma. Pediatr Surg Int 2002;18:173–74.
[94] Mihos P, Konstantinos P, Gakidis J, et al. Traumatic rupture of the diaphragm: experience with 65 patients. Injury 2003;34:169–72.
[95] Shah R, Sabanathan S, Mearns AJ, et al. Traumatic rupture of the diaphragm. Ann Thorac Surg 1995;60:1440–49.
[96] McQuay N, Britt LD. Laparoscopy in the evaluation of thoracoabdominal penetrating trauma. Am Surg 2003;69:788–91.

[97] Martinez M, Briz JE, Carillo EH. Video thoracoscopy expedites the diagnosis and treatment of penetrating diaphragmatic injuries. Surg Endosc 2001;15:28–32.
[98] Pitcher G. Fiber-endoscopic thoracoscopy for diaphragmatic injury in children. Semin Pediatr Surg 2001;10:17–19.
[99] Hormuth D, Cefali D, Rouse T, et al. Traumatic disruption of the thoracic aorta in children. Arch Surg 1999;134:759–63.
[100] Karmy-Jones R, Hoffer E, Meissner M, et al. Management of traumatic rupture of the thoracic aorta in pediatric patients. Ann Thorac Surg 2003;75:1513–17.
[101] Trachiotis GD, Sell JE, Pearson GD. Traumatic thoracic aortic rupture in children. Ann Thorac Surg 1996;62:724–32.
[102] Lowe LH, Bulas DJ, Eichelberger MD, et al. Traumatic aortic injuries in children: Radiological evaluation. Am J Roentgenol 1998;170:39–42.
[103] Parmley LF, Mattingly TW, Manion WC, et al. Nonpenetrating traumatic injury of the thoracic aorta. Circulation 1958;17:1086–1101.
[104] Hunt JP, Baker CC, Lentz CW, et al. Thoracic aorta injuries: Management and outcome of 144 patients. J Trauma 1996;40:547–54.
[105] Fabian TC, Richardson JD, Croce MR, et al. Prospective study of blunt aortic-injury: Multicenter trial of the American Association for the Surgery of Trauma. J Trauma 1997;42:374–83.
[106] Fabian TC, Davis KA, Gavant ML, et al. Prospective study of blunt aortic injury: helical CT is diagnostic and antihypertensive therapy reduces rupture. Ann Surg 1998;227:666–76.
[107] Dowd DM, Krug MD, et al. Pediatric blunt cardiac injury: Epidemiology, clinical features, and diagnosis. J Trauma 1996;40:61–67.
[108] Scorpio RJ, Wesson DE, Smith CR, et al. Blunt cardiac injuries in children: A post mortem study. J Trauma 1996;41:306–09.
[109] Salim A, Velmahos GC, Jindal A, et al. Clinically significant blunt cardiac trauma: Role of serum troponin levels combined with electrocardiographic findings. J Trauma 2001;50:237–43.
[110] Hirsch R, Landt Y, Porter S, et al. Cardiac troponin I in pediatrics: Normal values and use in the assessment of cardiac injury. J Pediatr 1997;130:872–77.
[111] Beaver B, Colambani P, Buck J, et al. Efficacy of emergency room thoracotomy in pediatric trauma. J Pediatr Surg 1987;22:9–23.
[112] Powell R, Gill E, Jurkovich G, et al. Resuscitative thoracotomy in children and adolescents. Am Surg 1988;54:188–191.
[113] Rothenberg SS, Moore EE, Moore FA, et al. Emergency department thoracotomy in children-a critical analysis. J Trauma 1989;29:1322–25.
[114] Sheikh A, Culbertson C. Emergency department thoracotomy in children: Rational for selective application. J Trauma 1993;34:323–28.
[115] Abdessalam SF, Keller A, Groner JI, Kable K, Krishnaswami S, Nwomeh BC. An analysis of children receiving cardiopulmonary resuscitation (CPR) following cardiac arrest with blunt trauma. J Am Coll Surg 2004;199(3S):S53.
[116] Anderson CJ, Spruiell MD, Wylie EF, Mc Gowan CM, Deleyiannis FW, Donaldson NJ, Heare TC. A technique for pediatric chest wall reconstruction using custom-designed titanium implants: description and report of two cases. J Child Orthop 2016 Jan 18.
[117] Azoury SC, Grimm JC, Tuffaha SH, Broyles JM, Fischer AC, Yang SC, Tufaro AP. Chest Wall Reconstruction: Evolution over a decade and experience with a novel technique for complex defects. Ann Plast Surg 2015 [Epub ahead of print].
[118] Berthet JP, Canaud L, D'Anoville T, Alric P, Marty-Ane CH. Titanium plates and dulamesh: a modern combination for reconstructing very large chest wall defects. Ann Thorac Surg 2011 Jun;91(6):1709–16.

[119] Girelli L, Luksch R, Podda MG, Meazza C, Puma N, Scanagatta P, Pecori E, Diletto B, Galeone C, Massimino M, Pasterino U. Surgical approach to primary tumors of the chest wall in children and adolescents: 30 years of mono-institutional expérience. Tumori 2015 Sep 10:0.
[120] Krüger M, Zinne N, Zhang R, Schneider JP, Heckmann A, Haverich A, Petersen C. Multidirectional thoracic wall stabilization: a new device on the scene. Ann Thorac Surg 2013;96:1846–1849.
[121] Krüger M, Zinne N, Zhang R, Schneider JP, Heckmann A, Haverich A, Petersen C. Multidirectional thoracic wall stabilization: a new device on the scene. Ann Thorac Surg 2013 Nov;96(5):1846–9.
[122] Lack V, Oetzmann von Sochaczewski C, Naidoo K, Loveland J. Pentalogy of Cantrell with thoracoabdominal ectopia cordis: attempted surgical correction and review of recent literature to aid prognostication prior to surgery. Ann Plast Surg 2015 [Epub ahead of print].
[123] Majdak-Paredes EJ, Shafighi M, Fatah F. Integrated algorithm for reconstruction of complex forms of Poland syndrome: 20-year outcomes. J Plast Reconstr Aesthet Surg 2015 [Epub ahead of print].
[124] Mayer OH. Chest wall hypoplasia--principles and treatment. Paediatr Respir Rev 2015;16: 30–34.

8 Miscellaneous infection

8.1 Introduction

Besides several main topics, thoracic surgery also covers a diversity of diseases and procedures, which cannot be summarized under one single heading. Among those, **Juan Tovar** from Madrid updates the variety of treatment options for pleural empyema. **Marija Stojkovic and Thomas Junghanss** from the Department of Clinical Tropical Medicine in Heidelberg comment on the topic of lung echinococcosis, which is contributed by **Akin Kuzucu** from Turkey. The age-related etiology of chylothorax requires different measures in terms of diagnosis and treatment. The German neonatologists **Anja Bialkowski and Christian F. Poets** discuss the congenital chylothorax, while the pediatric surgeons **Bethany J. Slater and Steven S. Rothenberg** focus on the aquired variant. Open as well as video-assisted procedures for thymus-related diseases are presented by **Lan Vu and Hanmin Lee** from San Francisco. **Jose Ribas Milanez de Campos and Hugo Veiga Sampaio da Fonseca** share their experiences in treating hyperhidrosis, while **Markus Krüger** adds comments to this particular chapter of the two Brazilian thoracic surgeons.

Juan A. Tovar

8.2 Empyema (including lung abcess)

Pleural surfaces are lubricated by a minimal amount of clear fluid that facilitates displacement with minimal friction during respiration. This fluid is filtered from the pleural capillary network and reabsorbed by the lymphatic vessels. Disturbances in the balance between secretion and reabsorption cause pleural effusion and this can happen in various clinical conditions. In the presence of infection, the effusion turns into "empyema" and the fluid becomes purulent with bacteria, fibrin and other debris.

In most cases pneumonia is at the origin of empyema that, for this reason is known as "parapneumonic". Purulent effusions can also have other origins like esophageal perforation, mediastinitis, subphrenic sepsis or postoperative infection. These are not considered in the present chapter.

In the past, pneumonia was a leading cause of morbidity and mortality both in adults and children and, although the advent of antibiotics dramatically changed the results of its treatment, it still remains a serious problem. A proportion of children with pneumonia develop pleural effusions that may evolve into empyema. For unknown reasons, the incidence of empyema is increasing in industrialized countries and the etiology of the infection shifted from *Streptococcus pneumoniae*, the more common germ isolated in the past, to *Staphylococcus aureus, Streptococcus pyogenes* or *Pseudomonas aeruginosa, Klebsiella* or other Gram negative and anerobic bacteria that became more prevalent due to the widespread use of antibiotics [1]. The nature of the pleural infection with abundant bacteriolysis and the frequent use of antibiotics prior to thoracentesis explain why the majority of samples recovered do not yield positive cultures. PCR studies, however, have shown that *Streptococcus pneumoniae* and *Staphylococcus aureus* remain the most prevalent germs in children [1].

Bacteria reach the pleural space from the infected lung (rarely from a ruptured lung abscess) and attract leukocytes that secrete pro-inflammatory cytokines, particularly Interleukin-8 (IL-8) and Tumor Necrosis Factor-α (TNF-α). These further permeabilize capillaries and pleural surfaces and cause imbalance of the sequence secretion/reabsorption.

In a first, **exudative** stage (stage I), pleural fluid is clear or thin, has a pH above 7.20, glucose above 60 mg/dL and a lactic dehydrogenase (LDH) less than three times the maximum normal serum level (<1000 U/L). Unless adequately treated, pleural effusion progresses into the **fibrinopurulent** stage (stage II). Bacteria coming from the infected lung are more abundant in the fluid and massive migration of leukocytes occurs. This stage is characterized by progressive secretion of inflammatory mediators with increased pro-coagulant activity and decreased fibrinolysis. The fluid becomes purulent and fibrin clots and peels line the surfaces creating isolated spaces with progressively thicker walls or septa. At this stage, the fluid has a pH below 7.20, glucose below 60 mg/dL and LDH higher than three times the maximum normal serum level (>1000 U/L) [2].

Finally, if still not successfully treated, empyema enters into stage III or the **organization** stage in which proliferation of fibroblasts in the fibrin depositions takes place and collagen synthesis generates thick scar tissue that perpetuates pleural septation while entrapping the lung and limiting its expansion and function [3].

Probably all patients with pneumonia have pleural effusions but in the vast majority of them these resolve under appropriate treatment without further complications. However, in some cases, fever does not go away under antibiotic therapy and pleuritic pain and/or respiratory difficulty may appear. Percussion and auscultation may indicate pleural involvement and plain X-rays of the thorax demonstrate the presence of fluid in the pleural space, particularly when they are taken in lateral decubitus (Fig. 8.2.1). In cases in which bronchopleural fistula has occurred as a consequence of lung necrosis and abscess, pyo-pneumothorax is apparent. Pleural thickening and scoliosis are also visible in the late phases of the process. Round hollow areas delimited by a thin shell (pneumatoceles) are visible in the parenchyma in some cases of *Staphylococcus* pneumonia.

The introduction of intercostal ultrasonography (US) facilitated early detection and assessment of the amount of clear pleural fluid during the exudative stage. US

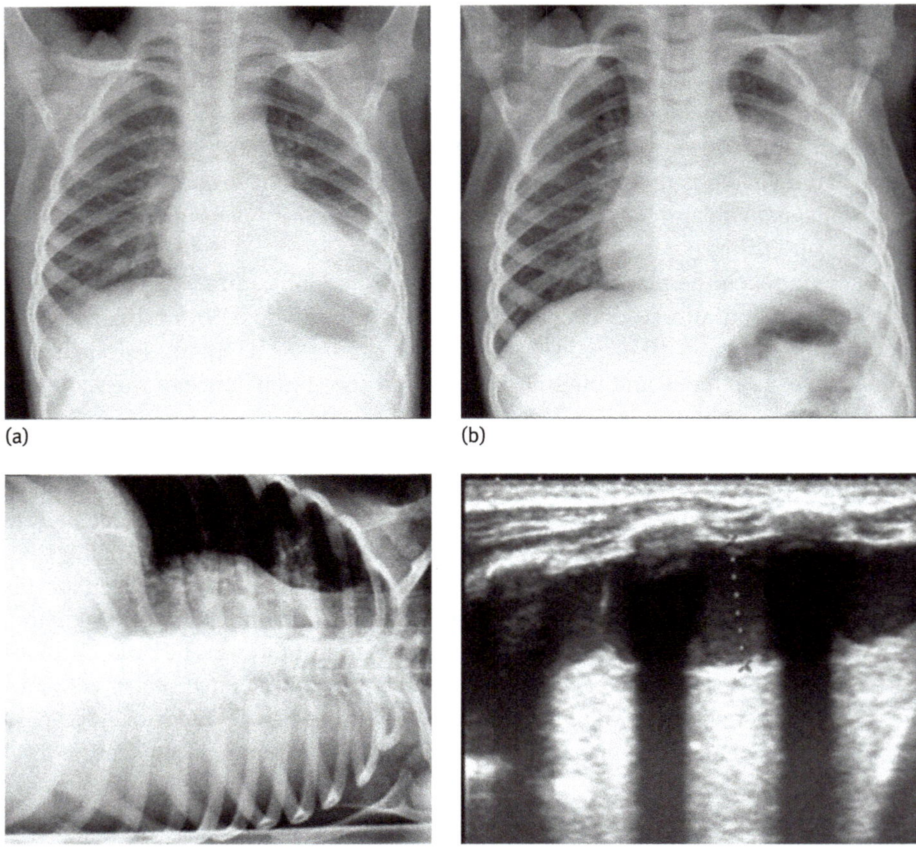

(a) (b) (c) (d)

Fig. 8.2.1: Plain X-ray of the thorax showing basal pneumonia with parapneumonic Stage I effusion on the left in a 3-year old boy. (a) at presentation, (b) 48 hours later. The amount of fluid increased greatly, as better shown by the film taken lying on the left side (c). Intercostal ultrasonography or US (d) shows a fluid rim of more than 10 mm.

imaging also demonstrates thick strands of fibrin and loculations during the fibrinopurulent stage (Fig. 8.2.2) and lung entrapment in the late, organization stage.

Other imaging procedures may occasionally be indicated, but certainly not in all patients and not in the early phases of the disease [4]. A CT-scan is useful for accurately locating closed spaces difficult to drain percutaneously, but it involves considerable irradiation (equivalent to 20–400 plain X-rays films) and tends to overrate the severity of the disease. It should hence be restricted to complicated cases and to those in which drainage is difficult because of multiple loculation [1, 5].

Knowledge of the natural course of pleural empyema should guide the therapeutic decisions. The exudative phase is reversible and can respond to appropriate

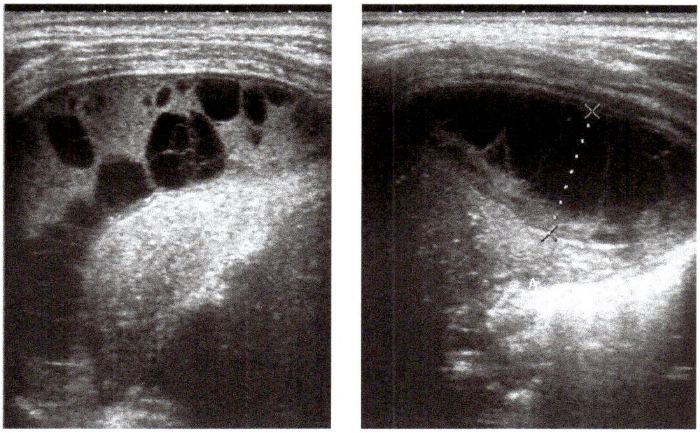

(a) (b)

Fig. 8.2.2: Intercostal US in a child with pleural fibrinopurulent, Stage II parapneumonic effusion. Large rim, thick peel and loculation are clearly shown.

antibiotic treatment alone. This should be directed empirically to the usual germs: i.v. Ampicillin 250–300 mg/kg/day in four doses or G-Sodium Penicillin, 300,000–400,000 IU/kg/day in six doses are preferred at the beginning, adjusting drugs to bacteriologic findings when available [6].

In most children with simple parapneumonic effusion, pyrexia and fever disappear and little attention is given to the pleural fluid. Only if the fever persists, pleuritic pain and/or respiratory difficulty develop, is assessment of the amount of fluid by plain X-rays or US indicated. When the rim between the thoracic wall and the lung exceeds 10 mm, thoracentesis at this stage may help to assess the nature of the effusion. Falling pH, glucose in the fluid and the presence of germs upon Gram staining are suggestive of progression towards fibrinopurulent stages and may indicate, together with clinical signs, dyspnea and persisting fever, drainage during this phase of "simple empyema". However, thoracentesis is indicated only in a proportion of patients and therefore, measurements of pH, glucose, LDH or Gram staining are of little help in many other cases.

When, in spite of adequate treatment, pyrexia and fluid persist, more than one thoracentesis would be necessary. In these cases, intercostal drainage is certainly preferable to multiple taps [1]. Pediatricians, pneumologists, intensive care specialists or invasive radiologists take charge more often in these first phases of the treatment of empyema, and pediatric surgeons are rarely involved at this stage. US-guided insertion of Fr10–12 soft drains using a guide wire introduced through a needle (Seldinger technique) is preferred. Unidirectional drainage with underwater seal is mandatory, and meticulous care of the tube is applied.

When the effusion reaches the fibrinopurulent stage, the empyema is considered "complicated" and requires more active treatment since, unless drained and cleansed, it might end up causing fibrosis and lung entrapment. Intravenous antibiotic therapy should then be based on Cefotaxime (200–300 mg/kg/day in four doses in addition to either Cloxacillin 150–200 mg/kg/day in four doses or Clyndamycin 30–40 mg/kg/day in four doses) [6]. Intercostal insertion of a 10–14 F drain is often sufficient for adequate drainage. It is generally placed in the mid-axillary line at the level of the fifth or sixth intercostal space in order not to interfere with the comfort of the child. US or CT-scan information may indicate other locations or more drains.

The ideal setting for insertion of the drain is the operating room and sedation or general anesthesia is mandatory. The tube should be connected to an underwater seal and aspiration of no more than –20 cm H_2O is considered to be beneficial. Milking and irrigation of the tube are necessary to clear out the debris that might otherwise obstruct it. The tube is removed when there is minimal drainage and the symptoms fade away. This happens in most fibrinopurulent empyemas although in some cases drainage and hospitalization have to be maintained for a relatively long period of time.

For this reason and because drainage alone may be insufficient due to loculation and drain obstruction, the treatment of stage II and stage III "complicated" empyema evolved into other modalities of treatment: video-assisted thoracoscopic surgical (VATS) drainage and cleansing of the pleural space or fluidification of the fibrin inflammatory debris by chemical treatment (fibrinolysis).

The introduction of VATS in the 90s had a huge impact in the treatment of empyema in adults and children. Direct view of the inflammatory lesions facilitated taking down the septa, extracting the peels, reducing the bacterial charge and appropriately irrigating and draining the thorax. A 5-mm port located at the mid-axillary line on the fifth or sixth intercostal space (unless imaging indicates a better location) is used for the 30° lens, and aspirator-irrigator and forceps are introduced by two or more 10-mm additional ports. The septa are taken down, the peel is separated (Fig. 8.2.3) and extracted, the pleural space is generously irrigated and the lung is freed, creating, if possible, a single cavity in which to optimally locate the drain or drains.

The advocators of VATS claimed that, since general anesthesia was most often used for simple intercostal drain insertion, accurate pleural cleansing and positioning of the tubes were better achieved under vision with a relatively minor invasion. In spite of VATS being a formal thoracic operation under general anesthesia with the consequent risks of hemorrhage, nerve or lung lesions and air leaks, this approach rapidly gained the favor of pediatric surgeons and pediatricians, who for the first time had the opportunity to view the nature and the extent of the pleural inflammatory environment. In addition, some randomized pediatric studies showed that VATS was superior to simple drainage in terms of length of drainage, hospital stay and need for additional fibrinolysis [7, 8].

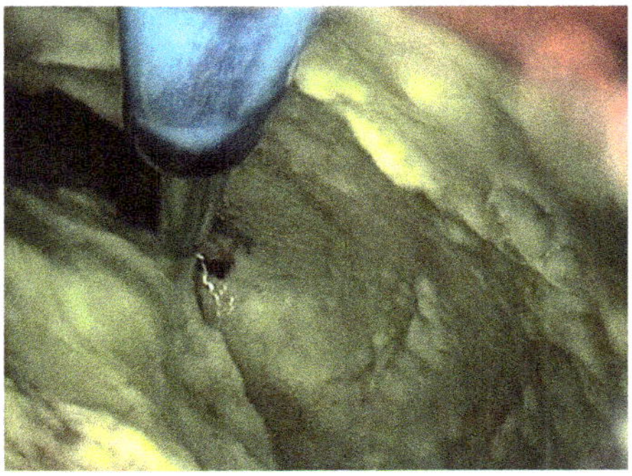

Fig. 8.2.3: Picture taken during thoracoscopy for Stage II fibrinopurulent pleural empyema in a child. The thick peels and inflammatory material are being irrigated, aspirated and prepared for extraction. The involvement of both parietal and visceral pleural surfaces is clearly displayed.

However, fluidification and cleansing of the exudates has been widely attempted in the past by irrigating the infected pleural space with diluted bleach and other antiseptics and the availability of new and more effective agents able to dissolve fibrin clots (fibrinolytics) rejuvenated this approach. After draining the fluid through the intercostal tube, a solution of streptokinase, urokinase or human tissue plasminogen activator (alteplase) is injected and left for some hours with the tube clamped. After a new period of drainage, the procedure is repeated several times in the ensuing days.

Streptokinase is an enzyme secreted by several species of *Streptococcus* that is able to activate human plasminogen and trigger plasmin proteolytic cascade that lyses fibrin clots. For the treatment of empyema it is injected at doses of 70–120 mL of a solution of 250,000 IU/100 mL, clamping the tube for the ensuing 4 hours, re-establishing the drainage under suction and repeating the procedure daily for 4 or 5 days.

Urokinase is another plasminogen activator originally isolated from human urine that is administered as a solution containing 1000 IU/mL in sterile saline in boluses of 40 mL (10 mL in patients below 10 kg). The tube is clamped for 4 hours and drainage resumed under negative pressure for the next hours. The treatment is repeated twice a day for 3 days. Unfortunately, urokinase is not available in all countries and particularly, not in the US.

A recombinant version of human tissue plasminogen activator (alteplase) is injected through the tube at a dose of 4 mg in 40 mL of sterile saline, followed by tube clamping for 1 hour and re-establishment of the drainage under suction until the next day. The procedure is repeated two more times.

Only a few randomized studies addressed the issue of the superiority of fibrinolysis over drainage and cleansing alone in children with pleural empyema. One of them did not show substantial advantage using streptokinase but the other one showed significantly better results with urokinase [9, 10].

It appears therefore that both fibrinolysis and VATS are more effective than drainage and irrigation alone as the first approach for complicated empyema in children. A retrospective analysis of the existing evidence showed that VATS could have some advantages but the degree of evidence met by randomized comparisons was not met by such analysis [11]. Level-A evidence-based studies were therefore mandatory to compare these approaches.

To our knowledge, only four controlled, prospective, randomized studies have been carried out in children to this day. The first one included 30 patients each in two VATS and urokinase fibrinolysis branches and concluded that there were no differences in the results but also that VATS was significantly more costly [12]. The second one studied 27 patients in each of the streptokinase or VATS branches and showed that VATS was significantly superior in terms of time until removal of the chest tube, hospital stay and duration of symptoms. In exchange, VATS was again significantly more costly [13]. The third study used either alteplase fibrinolysis or VATS in two groups of 18 patients each and could not demonstrate any difference between both groups except for the hospital costs, which were again higher in the VATS branch [14]. Finally, the fourth multicenter study was carried out on children below 15 years with septated empyema and included 53 treated by VATS and 50 with urokinase fibrinolysis. There were no differences between groups and the overall hospital stay was longer than in the other previously quoted studies probably because only stage III patients were included [15].

Therefore, in the present state of knowledge, both fibrinolysis and VATS are equally effective for the treatment of pleural empyema in children. However, taking into account that VATS is a major and more costly operation, drainage and fibrinolysis should be the preferred first approach for this condition [16]. VATS may still be indicated when drainage cannot be accomplished after appropriate fibrinolytic treatment.

Persistent broncho-pleural fistula or lung abscess should be treated whenever possible with antibiotics, appropriate drainage and fibrinolysis. Operative measures may be unsuccessful due to the necrotic-inflammatory environment met in such cases [5].

Major open operations for decortications are very rarely indicated in children except in cases in which multiple loculations with sepsis and severe lung encasing, a very unlikely event, compromise survival. In rare instances, persistent bronchopleural fistula might justify such treatments. Under such circumstances, thoracotomy, cleansing, closure of fistula and appropriate drainage achieved good results [17, 18]. With the current therapeutic protocols this is an extremely rare event.

The plasticity of the thorax and intra-thoracic organs in children accounts for the scarcity of functional sequelae in cases of empyema. A recent study on lung function in children treated for empyema showed only minimal FVC%, FEV1 and FEV1/FVC in comparison with controls. Empyema children did not show any difference in maximal exercise capacity [19]. In another study performed on 26 children after a mean of 8 years post-empyema treatment, there was no functional impairment, spirometry was normal in 80% and although X-rays were minimally abnormal in 36% and minimal MRI residuals were found in 82%, the functional significance was negligible [20].

Akin Kuzucu

8.3 Echinococcosis

8.3.1 Introduction

Parasitic diseases are important causes of morbidity and mortality in humans worldwide. Although most parasites that affect the lung are endemic to tropical and subtropical regions, immigration and travel practices have resulted in transfer of these diseases to other areas. Echinococcosis is one of the most geographically widespread zoonoses in the world. Human echinococcosis occurs as a result of infection by cestodes of the genus *Echinococcus*. Four *Echinococcus* species are known to be pathogenic for humans. The two most important of these are *E. granulosus* and *E. multilocularis,* which cause cystic echinococcosis (CE) and alveolar echinococcosis (AE), respectively. The other two species that affect humans are *E. vogeli* and *E. oligarthus*. These cause an infestation known as "polycystic echinococcosis" and are of minor importance.

8.3.2 Cystic echinococcosis

The most common tapeworm condition of the lung is cystic echinococcosis (CE), or "hydatid disease," caused by *E. granulosus*. This illness is concentrated in sheep-raising areas, such as the Mediterranean region, eastern Europe, Africa, South America, the Middle East, Australia, New Zealand and China (Fig. 8.3.1). Although,

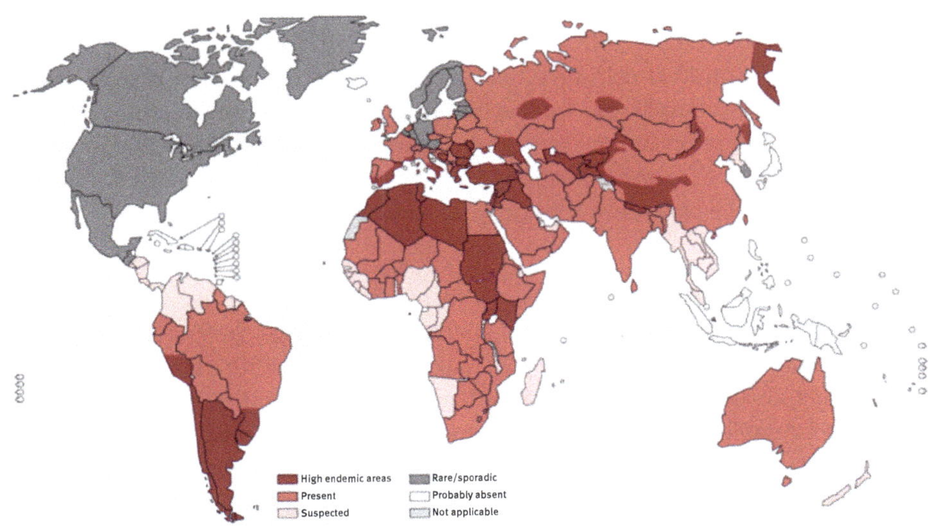

Fig. 8.3.1: Distribution of *Echinococcus granulosus* worldwide (Copyright© WHO).

the numbers of infections in animals and humans have decreased with time as a result of education and various control measures, CE continues to be an important public health problem in many countries.

8.3.2.1 Life cycle and morphology

Like all cestodes, *E. granulosus* requires two different host species to complete its life cycle. The definitive hosts are dogs and other canine carnivores, and the intermediate hosts are a variety of warm-blooded vertebrates (e.g. sheep, cattle, goats, pigs, camels and humans). The adult worms inhabit the small intestine of the definitive host and do not make the host ill. The adult worm releases eggs within the intestine, and these pass out with the definitive host's feces. Humans may become infected with *E. granulosus* accidentally through contact with this final host (usually a dog), particularly during playful close contact between children and dogs, or via ingestion of food or fluids that are contaminated with egg-containing feces. After an *Echinococcus* egg is ingested by the intermediate host, the embryo (known as the oncosphere, or first larval stage) is released into the host's gastrointestinal tract. Embryos then embed in the lining of the tract, and ultimately penetrate the mucosa and enter the mesenteric vascular system. They undergo blood-borne distribution in the portal circulation, and most embryos lodge in the intermediate host's liver. Each embryo then transforms to a cystic metacestode (second larval stage) filled with fluid. Each of these cysts is surrounded by the host's reactive tissue, known as a pericyst. Inside the pericyst, the cystic metacestode (endocyst) has an acellular outer wall or "laminated membrane" and an inner layer or "germinative membrane" that is a monolayer of viable pluripotent cells. While embedded in the viscera, brood capsules and protoscolices bud from the germinative membrane of some metacestodes (Fig. 8.3.2).

When a dog (or other definitive/final host) ingests a cyst in viscera of the intermediate host, the protoscolices are released from the cyst. These attach to the dog's intestinal wall, develop into mature adult tapeworms, and complete the life cycle. Since the life cycle relies on carnivores eating infected herbivores, humans are usually a "dead end" for the parasite and do not play a role in the biological cycle.

8.3.2.2 Pulmonary involvement

Most embriyos become trapped in the hepatic sinusoids, and therefore 70% of echinococcal cysts form in the liver. Embryos that bypass hepatic filtration enter the lung via the right circulation (hepatic vein, inferior vena cava, and pulmonary arteries). They either complete their cystic transformation in the lung or else pass through via the pulmonary vascular system and develop in another organ. Alternative pathways for this parasite to enter the lung are the lymphatic circulation or via a portocaval anastomosis in the portal system. As well, pulmonary or intrathoracic extrapulmonary

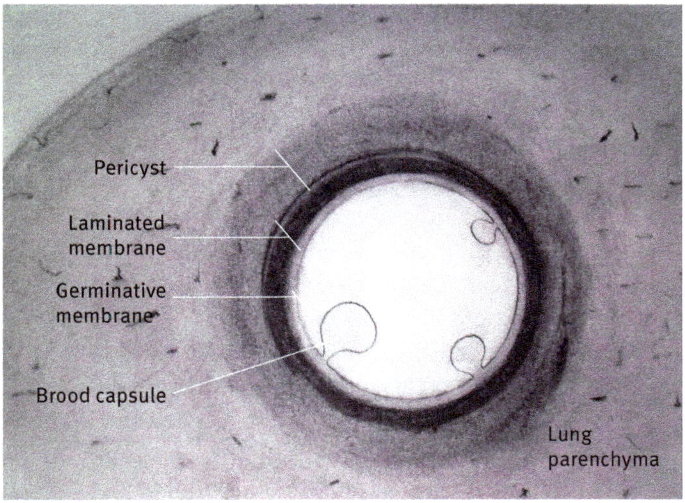

Fig. 8.3.2: Echinococcal cyst and its components.

involvement can occur secondary to intrathoracic rupture of cysts from the dome of the liver.

The lung is the second most common site of *E. granulosus* lodgment, with incidence varying between 15% and 30% [21, 22]. Much less frequent sites are the spleen, kidneys, orbit, heart, brain and bone, which account for approximately 10% to 15% of cases combined [22]. *E. granulosus* infestations may be acquired in childhood; however, because of the slow-growing nature of echinococcal cysts, most liver and lung cysts become symptomatic and are diagnosed in adulthood.

Most patients with CE have single-organ involvement and harbor a solitary cyst. In rare cases, primary echinococcosis develops in intrathoracic extrapulmonary structures, such as the pleural cavity, mediastinum, and chest wall. If a echinococcal cyst in the liver ruptures into the inferior vena cava, or a echinococcal cyst in the right ventricle ruptures, this can lead to secondary echinococcosis in the form of cyst/s, and potentially subsequent embolism and endovascular echinococcosis [21, 23, 24]. In rare cases, massive embolism of the pulmonary arteries occurs [21].

8.3.2.3 Clinical presentation

The clinical presentation of pulmonary CE depends on the size and location of the cyst/s, and whether these structures are intact or ruptured. Most small intact echinococcal cysts in pulmonary tissue remain asymptomatic. Large echinococcal cysts are more likely to cause chest pain, cough, or dyspnea by compressing the lung parenchyma and surrounding tissues. In young patients, the lesions can expand asymptomatically until they reach giant size (>10 cm in diameter) because the remaining healthy lung tissue is able to provide sufficient ventilation.

With complicated pulmonary CE (i.e. ruptured cysts), the clinical picture is variable and depends on the nature of the perforation. Echinococcal cysts in lung tissue can rupture into the pleural space or into a bronchus. Perforation into a bronchus can lead to expectoration of vomit-like cystic fluid and remnants of parasite-derived cyst wall. Rarely, complete expectoration of the cystic contents can result in spontaneous cure. However, in most cases, solid remnants of the collapsed endocyst are left in the cavity and become a source of recurrent bacterial infection. Purulent sputum and fever are strong indicators of bacterial infection of the cyst cavity, including pericystic lung tissue or abscess formation, situations that can result in sepsis. In some cases, ruptured CE causes severe complications, such as massive hemoptysis or anaphylactic shock.

In contrast to perforation into a bronchus, rupture of a echinococcal cyst into the pleural cavity usually causes pneumothorax, pleural effusion, or empyema. Cyst rupture into the pleural cavity can also result in tension pneumothorax, secondary larval spread, or allergic and anaphylactic reaction [25]. Pneumothorax almost always indicates the presence of a bronchopleural fistula.

8.3.2.4 Diagnosis

Cystic echinococcosis is usually diagnosed based on a combination of (1) identification of the cyst/s through various imaging techniques, (2) results of serological tests, (3) identification of protoscolices or hooks of *E. granulosus* by microscopic examination, (4) analysis of DNA markers in the cyst fluid or cyst wall (e.g. by polymerase chain reaction [PCR]), (5) macroscopic or histopathological detection of the pathognomonic structure of a cyst obtained through surgery or biopsy, and (6) history of possible exposure. Most cases of pulmonary CE are diagnosed from incidental radiographic findings on routine chest radiography.

8.3.2.5 Imaging-based approach

Most cases of CE are initially detected by finding cysts using different imaging techniques. Ultrasonography plays an important role in the diagnosis of abdominal CE. For this reason, ultrasonography-based classification systems have been developed to correlate CE cyst stages with natural history. According to the staging system of the WHO Informal Working Group (WHO-IWG), these cysts are classified as active (CE1 and CE2), transitional (CE3) or inactive (CE4 and CE5) [26]. Even though CE cyst staging systems have been developed for liver cysts, this classification also applies for echinococcal cysts in other organs. Today, the terms “complicated” (ruptured) and “uncomplicated” (unruptured) have been widely adopted for CE cysts of the lung. The WHO-IWG CE staging system may be used to replace these terms and help standardize clinical trials and treatment recommendations. Many radiologic findings of CE of the lung are similar to those of CE of the liver. However, in CE of the lung, chest radiography and chest computed tomography are preferred over ultrasonography for staging, and in contrast to hepatic cysts, pulmonary cysts usually do not calcify, and daughter cyst formation is rare.

On X-ray films, uncomplicated (CE1 stage) cysts appear as homogeneous, dense, round or oval lesions that have well-defined borders, are between 1 cm and 20 cm in diameter, and are surrounded by normal lung tissue (Fig. 8.3.3 A). Computed tomography (CT) reveals the fluid contents within an intact echinococcal cyst (CE1 stage) (Fig. 8.3.3 B). On CT images, the cyst wall, which represents the combined pericyst and endocystic wall, ranges in thickness from 2 mm to 1 cm. Cyst fluid usually appears close to the attenuation of water.

If the pericyst communicates with the tracheobronchial tree, air enters and dissects the pericyst and endocyst structures, producing radiographically visible air between the pericyst and the detached wall of the endocyst. This radiological appearance is known as a meniscus or air crescent sign (Fig. 8.3.4 A), an inverse crescent sign, or a signet ring sign. Each of these indicates detachment and is believed to be a harbinger of impending rupture of the endocyst (CE3a stage). If the cyst has ruptured, separation of the cystic membrane creates a wide spectrum of radiologic images. If the ruptured cyst communicates with the tracheobronchial tree, some of the fluid evacuates and air enters the space between the pericyst and the laminated membrane causing an air-fluid level. In some cases, the cyst wall appears to be crumpled and floating on top of the residual fluid, resulting in the well-recognized water lily or camalote sign (CE3a stage) (Fig. 8.3.4 B). The appearance of collapsed membranes inside the cyst with a serpentine configuration or with a twirled and twisted configuration

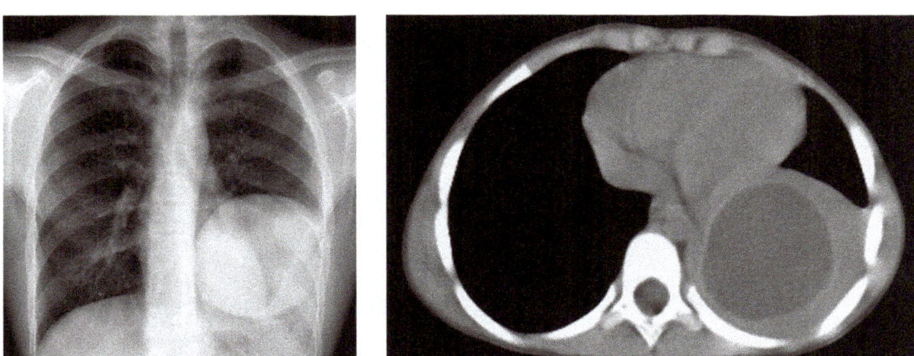

(a) (b)

Fig. 8.3.3: (a): Chest radiograph showing a well-defined, circular opacity surrounded by normal lung tissue in the left lower lung lobe (CE1 stage). (b): A computed tomography scan demonstrating a large solitary cyst and atelectasis in the pericystic lung tissue (CE1 stage).

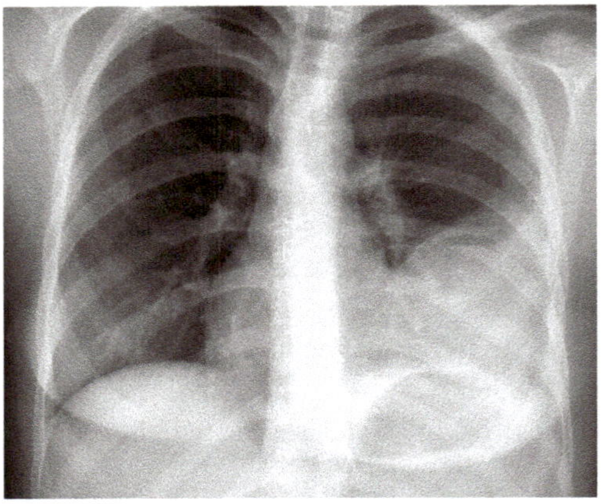

(a)

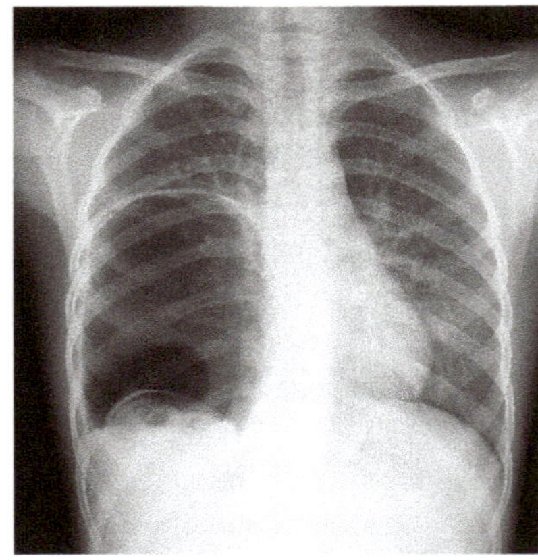

(b)

Fig. 8.3.4: Chest radiograph revealing the air crescent sign (CE3 stage) (a) and a ruptured echinococcal cyst with a water lily sign (CE3a stage) (b).

after partial expectoration of cyst fluid is called the serpent (or snake) sign or spin (or whirl) sign, respectively (CE3a stage) (Fig. 8.3.5). Several other radiological signs of CE on CT and magnetic resonance imaging (MRI) have also been described. These include the rim sign, air bubble sign, Cumbo's sign, cyst wall sign, ring enhancement sign, and halo sign.

A ruptured cyst may not have the characteristic imaging appearance of an echinococcal cyst. The inflammatory reaction in tissue adjacent to the lesion may mask

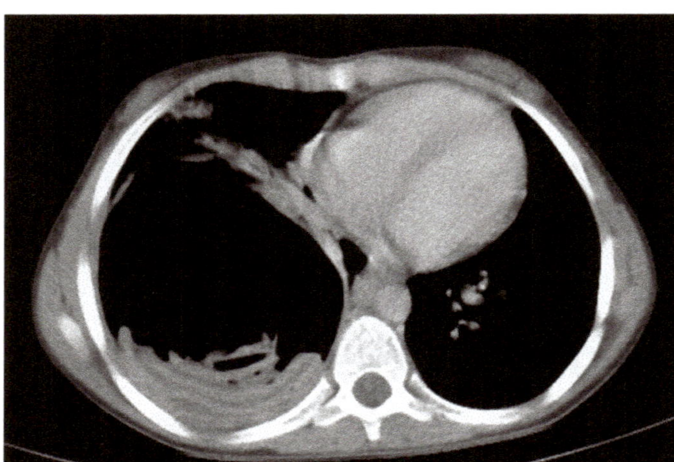

Fig. 8.3.5: A computed tomography scan showing a ruptured echinococcal cyst containing detached membranes inside the cystic cavity (the as whirl (or spin) sign (CE3a stage).

the ruptured cyst, and the overall radiologic appearance may not be indicative of the lesion. In some cases, the cyst membranes liquefy and the pericyst thickens (CE4 and CE5 stages). In this situation, the typical cystic nature may be lost and the radiological appearance on plain films may be similar to that of a bacterial lung abscess. CE4 stage cysts may give an appearance of a ball of wool sign, indicating the degenerative nature of the cyst (Fig. 8.3.6).

On MRI, T1-weighted images of echinococcal cysts show hypointense cystic content and an isointense wall relative to cyst content, whereas T2-weighted images show hyperintense cystic content and a hypointense wall [22]. However, currently, MRI is not frequently used for diagnosing pulmonary CE.

Bronchoscopy can be a useful diagnostic tool in challenging cases where a ruptured pulmonary echinococcal cyst does not have the characteristic clinical and radiologic appearance (CE4 and CE5 stages), [27]. If a ruptured cyst membrane causes occlusion in the bronchial system, it may be possible to visualize and eliminate the cyst remnants using bronchoscopy.

8.3.2.6 Laboratory tests

In the diagnosis of echinococcosis, laboratory tests are complementary to clinical findings and radiological studies. In most instances, eosinophilia can be normal or slightly increased and generally only occurs if the cyst is ruptured and there is leakage of antigenic material. As therapeutic puncture or diagnostic puncture are contraindicated in CE of the lung, direct diagnostic methods, such as examination of cyst

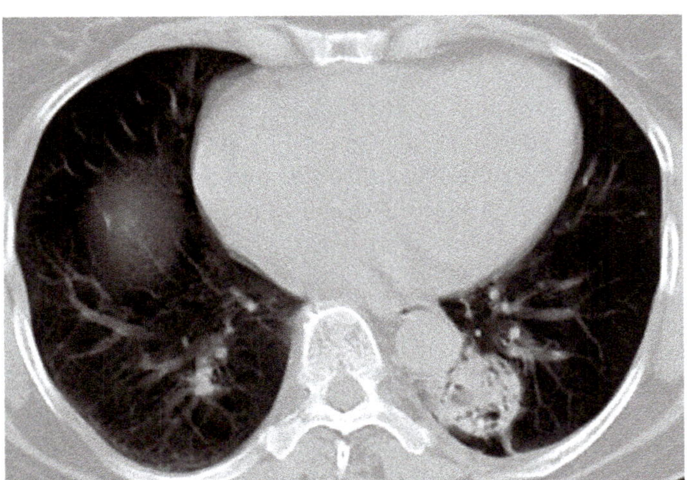

Fig. 8.3.6: A cyst with heterogeneous contents, in particular the so-called "ball of wool sign" (CE4 stage).

contents/fluid, are not performed frequently. Direct examination can only be done after surgical intervention or fine-needle biopsy in suspected cases of complicated cases that have not been definitively diagnosed.

In the past, intradermal testing (Casoni and Weinberg's respective complement fixation tests) was widely used to diagnose echinococcal disease, but these assays are rarely used currently because of low sensitivity and specificity. Today, several immunodiagnostic tests are available that can be used to confirm a clinical diagnosis; however, there are two main categories of problems with test methods that involve crude *E. granulosus* antigens: (1) false-positive results occur in the presence of other helminth infections, cancer, and immune disorders, and (2) false-negative results occur due to poor antigen presentations. Serology is less likely to be positive if the cysts are intact, calcified or nonviable, and children more frequently exhibit negative serology. False-negative results can also occur because of the location of a lesion. It is important to note that CE of the lung is more likely to be accompanied by false-negative serology than CE of the liver [28]. The most widely available tests confirm the diagnosis in 80% to 94% of hepatic CE cases, and in 65% of pulmonary CE cases [29].

Enzyme-linked immunosorbent assays for immunoglobulin G (IgG-ELISA), indirect hemagglutination antibody test (IHAT), latex agglutination test (LAT), and immunofluorescence antibody test (IFAT) are the immunological methods most commonly used in diagnosing echinococcosis. In all of these tests, cross-reactivity may be observed, particularly in cases of CE and alveolar echinococcosis (AE). The *Echinococcus* western blot IgG may be used to exclude cross-reactivity in positive sera. This assay correctly differentiates between CE and AE; however, cross-reactivity is not completely excluded [30].

It is accepted that immunodiagnostic tests do not replace clinical and radiological diagnosis; these tests are considered helpful diagnostic adjuncts and are useful, if necessary, for follow-up of operated or medically treated patients. Increased antibody titers may be detected even in patients with active cysts (CE1 and CE2 stages) who are negative prior to surgical intervention. Specific antibodies are known to increase as early as the first week after surgery and generally reaching a maximum toward the end of the first month [31]. In such cases, the titers decrease slowly over 12–18 months post-surgery [29].

8.3.2.7 Surgical treatment

Surgery is the main treatment for pulmonary CE, as the parasite must be eliminated to achieve a complete cure. In patients with pulmonary CE, the principle of surgery is to preserve as much lung tissue as possible. It is important to always use the most conservative surgical methods possible, and removal of all parasitic material and closure of bronchial openings is usually adequate treatment, even if a patient presents with giant cysts, multiple cysts, or lung abscess. Radical resection of the lung must be avoided unless the pulmonary parenchyma is seriously damaged or infected, or atelectatic areas are assessed as irrecoverable. In some cases, it can be difficult to determine the optimal surgical procedure when a giant echinococcal cyst has compressed a considerable amount of lung parenchyma for a long period. Such a decision may have to be made in the operating room. The parenchyma around an echinococcal cyst is often affected by the lesion and may exhibit chronic congestion, hemorrhage, bronchopneumonia, or interstitial pneumonia. These inflammatory changes in the lung tissue often resolve after surgical cyst removal. Patients with cystic lesions tend to show good recovery of lung tissue after surgery. Considering this, the size of cyst/s, number of lesions, and presence of infection should not be considered indications for radical resection, such as lobectomy. In particular, children and adolescents with CE usually have excellent pulmonary tissue capacity for lung expansion after surgery.

Lung-conserving approaches when treating pulmonary CE include pericystotomy and enucleation of the endocyst, aspiration-pericystotomy and removal of the endocyst with or without capitonnage, or pericystectomy. Regardless of the surgical procedure performed, spillage of cyst contents must be avoided to prevent intraoperative dissemination of protoscolices and eventual recurrence. During surgery, once a cyst is identified it is surrounded by pads soaked in 10% povidone-iodine or hypertonic saline solution to protect the operatory field from spillage and subsequent seeding of new cysts. Hypertonic saline solution is the preferred agent, as it is considered to have scolicidal properties. If enucleation is planned, the pericyst is opened, careful blunt dissection is performed between the pericyst and the endocyst, and the cyst is enucleated entirely. During the dissection, the airway pressure is lowered to prevent the cyst from protruding through the pericystic opening. This procedure carries high risk for cyst rupture and dissemination, and is generally preferred when treating small cysts only.

Another option once a cyst is identified is to aspirate the echinococcal fluid with a wide-bore needle. In this procedure, the pericyst is opened after aspiration, and then the entire cystic membrane is removed. In both of the two approaches, once the surgeon is certain that all cystic membrane has been removed, large bronchial openings are closed, the cavity is irrigated with normal saline solution, and the cavity is obliterated with separate purse-string sutures. These are placed from the deepest level to the surface of the cavity (i.e. capitonnage). Some authors suggest that capitonnage offers no benefit with respect to outcome [32], but this technique is the safest way to avoid prolonged air leakage and to protect the cavity from infection and abscess formation. In pericystectomy, endocysts are removed together with the host-derived capsule (pericyst). This procedure carries high risk of intra and postoperative complications such as bleeding or prolonged air leakage, and greater loss of parenchyma in which the cyst is situated.

Bilateral pulmonary CE can be managed with either a one- or two-stage surgery involving bilateral thoracotomy, or with median sternotomy. When bilateral thoracotomy is performed in patients with bilateral uncomplicated pulmonary CE (i.e. no ruptured cysts), it is best to first treat the side with the larger cyst/s or greater number of cysts. If there is a ruptured cyst on one side and an intact cyst on the other side, the intact cyst is treated first unless the ruptured lesion is causing urgent serious symptoms. In selected cases, lung and liver cysts may be treated during the same operation via thoraco-phrenotomy.

Recently, some reports have described video-assisted thoracic surgery in the treatment of pulmonary CE in selected patients [33, 34]. In these cases, the thoracoscopic approach is performed using the same principles as are followed with the open technique: protecting tissues from contamination, completely removing all parasitic contents, and closing any bronchial openings that are present. Patients who have small cysts or ruptured cysts that pose minimal risk of spillage may be favorable candidates for video-assisted thoracic surgery. The main advantage offered by thoracoscopy is less trauma and discomfort for the patient. However, information about long-term outcomes is needed before this procedure can become widely accepted.

8.3.2.8 Medical treatment

According to WHO Informal Working Group on Echinococcosis (WHO-IWGE) guidelines [35], chemotherapy is indicated for inoperable primary liver or lung CE, for patients with multiple cysts in two or more organs, for patients with peritoneal cysts, and to prevent secondary echinococcosis. Two benzimidazole compounds, mebendazole and albendazole, are the only effective drugs for treating uncomplicated echinococcal cysts, and as an alternative to surgery. Mebendazole is given at a dose of 40–50 mg/kg/day in three divided doses after meals (maximum daily dose 6 g). Albendazole is given at a dose of 10–15 mg/kg/day in two divided doses (maximum dose 800 mg daily). These two drugs are benzimidazole carbamates, and this treatment is most often administered in 3- to 6-month cycles [35]. Benzimidazole carbamates have inhibitory effects on glucose uptake, which leads to depletion of glycogen storage, degenerative alteration in the germinal layer, and cellular autolysis. Albendazole is usually preferred for chemotherapy owing to its higher bioavailability, the lower daily doses required, and its better efficacy overall. Praziquantel, an isoquinolone, has also been proposed as a treatment for CE at a dose of 40 mg/kg orally once weekly, and concomitant with benzimidazoles [35]. Praziquantel has been used alone and in combination with albendazole; however, the efficacy of praziquantel as primary chemotherapy for CE is not clearly defined [36].

In general, small isolated cysts surrounded by minimal adventitial reaction respond best to medical therapy, whereas complicated cysts that have multiple compartments or daughter cysts, or those that have thick or calcified surrounding adventitial reactions are relatively refractory to treatment. Drug penetration of echinococcal cysts is negatively correlated with the thickness of the pericystic fibrous capsule. For this reason, children respond to medical treatment better than adults do. Research has shown that 50% to 70% of patients with CE show some degree of response to medical management [30]; however, the reported cure rates in this patient group are only 10% to 30% [30]. It has been suggested that the larger the diameter of the cyst, the greater the possibility that medical treatment will fail and tend to be complicated. Relapses after chemotherapy have been observed in 14% to 25% of patients with pulmonary CE [30]. Some authors have noted that pulmonary CE and cysts in younger patients relapsed less frequently than hepatic cysts and cysts in older patients [37].

Overall, medical treatment is generally not considered a reliable way of eradicating *E. granulosus* and is a long and tedious process that carries considerable risk. Anthelmintic therapy causes degenerative changes in the endocyst wall, which could increase the likelihood of rupture. The incidence of degenerative changes in pulmonary CE treated with albendazole is approximately 80% [37, 38]. The fundamental issue is not the efficacy of anthelmintic therapy for pulmonary CE, but whether this form of treatment leads to complications. In some cases, if a cyst does rupture but the cyst membrane and contents are completely expectorated, then the patient may be cured. Even if the parasite dies due to the drug and there is no acute, serious complication, the cyst membrane will usually remain in the cavity. This cavity often leads to secondary bacterial infection and other complications, which are associated with more problematic surgeries and postoperative courses, and longer hospital stays than uncomplicated cases [25, 39].

The timing of pulmonary CE cyst rupture after initiation of anthelmintic treatment is reported to vary considerably, from 10 days to 2 months [39, 40]. Clearly, any patient who receives medical therapy for these cysts must be followed closely for at least 2 months with careful monitoring for serious complications that could require emergent intervention. The WHO-IWGE also suggests that medical and laboratory examinations should be conducted for adverse reactions such as neutropenia, alopecia, and liver dysfunction [35]. These problems can be severe and irreversible, and the WHO-IWGE recommends that these assessments be done every 2 weeks initially, and then monthly [35]. It is important to note that close follow-up is usually not possible in cases of CE because these patients tend to be from rural areas where medical care is distant and often inadequate. When considering how to proceed with a case, all the potential problems with medical treatment should be weighed carefully.

Several reports have suggested percutaneous treatment of pulmonary CE as an effective alternative to surgical treatment in selected patients with this disease. However, in general, percutaneous aspiration of pulmonary cysts has been considered too high-risk because of (1) the possibility of cyst rupture associated with any puncture, and (2) complications related to rupture. According to WHO-IWGE guidelines, percutaneous drainage of an echinococcal cyst (a procedure referred to as PAIR: puncture, aspiration, injection, re-aspiration) is considered to be contraindicated for pulmonary CE [35]. The safety and efficacy of percutaneous treatment are related to the anatomical site of the cyst. The PAIR method is mainly used in the treatment of hepatic and extrahepatic abdominal echinococcal cysts.

Each organ afflicted with CE has its own associated symptoms and therapeutic requirements. It is generally agreed that, regardless of whether symptoms are present, the first-line treatment for pulmonary CE is surgical, and medical therapy should only be used to prevent recurrence or in patients who cannot tolerate surgery. Close follow-up is recommended at 6-month intervals for at least 5 years [21].

8.3.3 Alveolar echinococcosis

There is less human exposure to *E. multilocularis* than to *E. granulosus*, but the precise extent of AE is unknown. For humans, *E. multilocularis* is the most pathogenic species of *Echinococcus*, and causes a potentially fatal, chronically progressive infestation. The life cycle is similar to that of *E. granulosus*, but the definitive and intermediate hosts involved are usually wild animals. The life cycle of *E. multilocularis* involves wild canines, usually foxes and wolves, as definitive hosts, and mainly rodents as intermediate hosts. Despite this parasite's predominantly sylvatic life cycle, domestic animals, such as dogs and cats, may also become infested and can transmit this agent to humans.

E. multilocularis, also known as *alveolar echinococcosis*, is more common in colder areas, such as the Arctic and some regions of Asia and west-central Europe. The primary anatomical location of this agent is the liver. Isolated extrahepatic locations (e.g. spleen, peritoneum, lung, vertebra, brain, kidney, heart, adrenal gland, and muscle) account for only 2% to 4% of all cases [41, 42]. Primary lung involvement is reported to be extremely rare [41–43]; however, *E. multilocularis* tends to spread to the lung and other organs in approximately one-third of affected patients via infiltration and metastatic formation [41].

A characteristic feature of AE is its exogenous, tumor-like proliferation that leads to infiltration of the affected organ/s, and to severe disease and even death in progressive cases. The prevalence of this disease is lower among children. Based on case data that the European Echinococcosis Registry (EurEchinoReg) surveillance network collected from 11 countries of western and central Europe and Turkey, the proportion of affected patients younger than 20 years is 2.1% (12/559) and the median age is 56 years (range, 5–86 years) [41].

Clinical symptoms of AE usually follow a long asymptomatic period (i.e. 5 to 15 years), and primarily include some clinical patterns that typically suggest digestive and hepatic disorders. Pulmonary symptoms, such as chronic cough, chest pain, hemoptysis, almost always occur after hepatic involvement.

Essentially the same radiological and serological procedures are used to diagnose CE and AE. Treugut et al. studied 20 cases of pulmonary involvement of *E. multilocularis* and described two radiological forms [44]: (1) a form with multiple ill-defined irregular lesions (up to 3-cm diameter) lying peripherally, some with stippled calcification; and (2) a form caused by liver disease penetrating the diaphragm and giving rise to various changes in the right lung base. Serological tests are more reliable for diagnosing AE than CE. The diagnosis can be confirmed by parasite identification in surgical or biopsy material.

When possible, the treatment for AE is total resection (i.e. removing the entire lesion from the liver and other affected organs by following the rules of radical tumor surgery). In cases where this is not feasible, long-term medical treatment with albendazole (in most cases lifelong) is the alternative. Even after complete excision, a minimum 2-year course of chemotherapy is recommended, and a minimum of 10 years of monitoring for possible recurrence is advised [35].

Marija Stojkovic, Thomas Junghanss

Comment

Echinococcosis is filed under the so-called Neglected Tropical Diseases (NTSs). Where the disease is prevalent, patients have limited access to care; where it is rare – in most rich countries – patients continue to encounter health care facilities with limited experience in the management of echinococcosis [45, 46].

Worth reiterating over decades because of its importance for patient management: *Echinococcus (E.) granulosus* and *E. alveolaris* are taxonomically close relatives, they cause, however, entirely different diseases: Cystic echinococcosis (CE) grows by pressure atrophy, alveolar echinococcosis (AE) by cancer-like infiltration and necrosis of surrounding tissues. Of importance for thoracic surgeons: AE of the lungs is extremely rare and almost entirely due to distant metastases or infiltrative expansion of hepatic AE [45].

Not much progress has been made over the years in CE/AE serological diagnostics. Lack of sensitivity of serological tests – very prominently in pulmonary CE – and cross-reactivity between CE and AE still causes mis- and over-interpretation of serological results. Differentiation between CE and AE may be possible with specific immunoblot patterns, but largely relies on imaging. If this fails, confirmation requires material of the lesion for microscopy, molecular methods, and histopathology which is a problem in pulmonary CE/AE. On imaging of the liver AE pseudocysts (large necrotic cavities) with transdiaphragmatic growth should not be confused with true CE cysts (which have a cyst wall with a smooth inner lining). Among the differential diagnoses of pulmonary air-filled space, occupying lesions TB caverns are worth mentioning. Asymptomatic pulmonary CE cysts are regularly discovered through CXR screening for active TB in immigrants.

Search for antigens suited for serological follow-up of CE-patients after interventions, e.g. surgery, has so far been unsuccessful. Follow-up to confirm cure or detect relapses remains in the realm of imaging.

In imaging substantial progress has been achieved, most importantly in staging CE cysts. The WHO cyst classification is increasingly valued as a tool for treatment decision and criteria have been developed to assign treatment modalities to cyst stages [45, 47]. Of major benefit to patients is accumulating evidence that WHO CE 4 and CE 5 cysts do not need any treatment at all if uncomplicated and yearly follow-up is guaranteed for 5–10 years (watch & wait) [45, 47].

WHO cyst classification is ultrasound-based and was primarily developed for hepatic CE cysts. By and large it can, however, be translated into CE cysts of any organ including the lungs. With the known limitations of ultrasound in the assessment of pulmonary

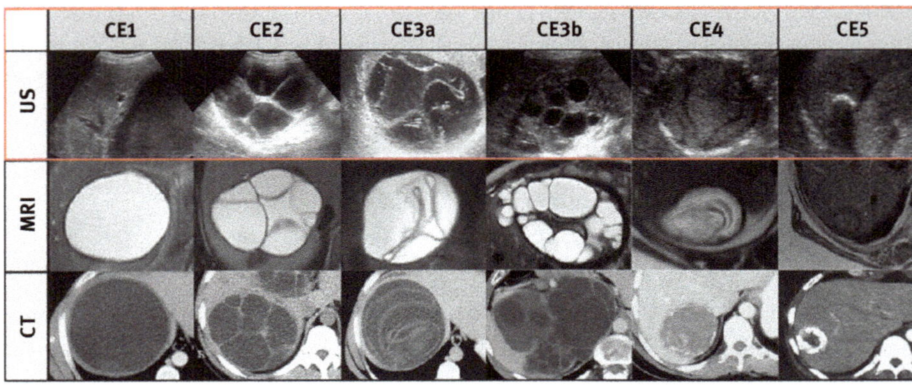

Fig. 8.3.7: "Best case" of CT/MR imaging. CE1: unilocular, simple cysts with liquid content and often with the CE1-specific "double line sign", CE2: multivesicular, multiseptated cysts, CE3a: cysts with liquid content and the CE3a-specific detached endocyst, CE3b: unilocular cysts with daughter cysts inside a mucinous or solid cyst matrix, CE4: heterogenous solid cysts with degenerative, CE4-specific canalicular structure of the cyst content, and CE5: cysts with degenerative content and heavily calcified wall. doi:10.1371/journal.pntd.0001880.g004 [48]

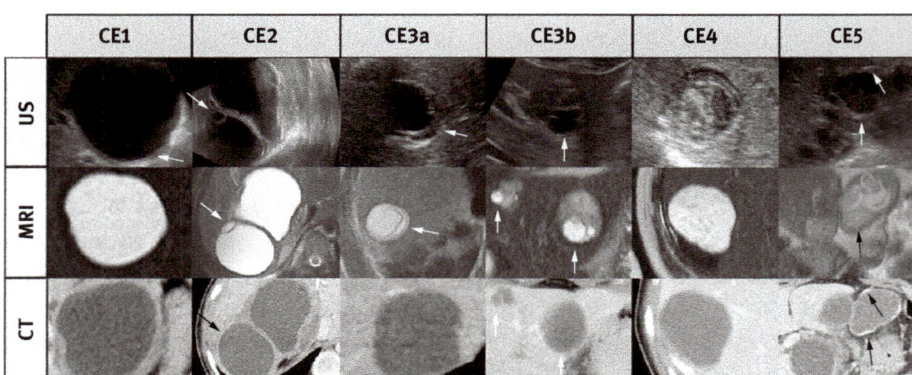

Fig. 8.3.8: "Worst case" of CT/MR imaging. The "double line sign", typical for CE1 is often seen in US (CE1/US, arrow), less reliably in MRI and CT. Daughter cysts and detached endocyst ("water-lily-sign") is often missed by CTs, but clearly visible in US and MRI (see CE2, CE3a, arrows). Daughter cysts inside a solid cyst matrix are often not recognized by CT (CE3b, arrows). The CE4-specific canalicular structure is often not visible on CT images. These cysts may be misinterpreted as type CE1 cysts, i.e. staged "active" instead of "inactive". The identification of calcifications is the domain of CT imaging. MRI does not differentiate well between thick hyaline walls and calcifications. US picks up calcifications only when a dorsal echo shadow is produced (see CE5, arrows). MRI: HASTE sequence, CT: post contrast enhanced images. doi:10.1371/journal.pntd.0001880.g005 [48]

pathology, computed tomography (CT) is the commonly used alternative. CT does not, however, reproduce the critical features of CE cysts, most importantly pathognomonic signs for diagnosis and staging and fistulas [48, 49]. The shortcomings of CT have been shown for hepatic CE cysts (see figures below; from [48]) and are equally applicable to CE cysts of the lungs. In assessing pulmonary CE MRI is clearly superior to CT.

On the basis of CE cyst staging, treatment decisions have become more adapted to individual patient needs. Current recommendations are summarized in the WHO IWGE of 2010 [47] and in a tabular form in [45].

We have long known that drug treatment with benzimidazoles, preferably albendazole, is far from satisfactory, both with regard to efficacy and side effects. A European consortium has looked into the cyst stage dependence of the efficacy of benzimidazoles in hepatic CE and found that it varies widely across stages [50]. On the basis of these results, the evidence base of indications of benzimidazole has improved. Monitoring of liver function tests and leucocytes is a must during benzimidazole therapy. Apart from peri-interventional prophylaxis the evidence base for benzimidazoles in pulmonary CE continues to be poor and they need to be applied cautiously if at all; rupture of the cyst being the main problem.

CE sugery needs to be creative. There are three important rules that need to be obeyed [45]:

> *The surgeon must be familiar with the architecture of CE cysts across stages – from unilocular highly active cysts filled with clear hydatid fluid which may be under very high pressure (WHO stage CE1) to completely consolidated inactive increasingly calcified cysts (WHO stage CE4 and CE5; which can mostly be left alone – watch & wait approach)*
>
> *The content of CE cysts (endocyst and hydatid fluid-containing protoscolices in millions) has to be removed* ***without*** *contact with any of the patient's tissues*
>
> and
>
> Intubation with a double-lumen endo-bronchial tube or an endobronchial blocker to avoid spillage of hydadid fluid and solid cyst material into the contra lateral lung should a wide cysto-bronchial fistul become patent during manipulation.

Anja Bialkowski, Christian F. Poets

8.4 Chylothorax in neonates

The diagnosis of chylothorax is usually made based on a pleural effusion characterized by a triglyceride level >1.1 mmol/L (with enteral fat intake) and a cell count >1000/µl with an estimated lymphocyte fraction >80%. CCT is the most common type of pleural effusion in neonates with an estimated (not population-based) incidence of 1:7.300 – 1:10.000. In our own population-based study, the incidence of CCT was only 1:24.000, which is similar to that reported by Haines et al. for a chylothorax survey in the UK. A male/female ratio of 2:1 is reported in some studies, the reason for this is unknown.

The etiology of CCT is often unclear. Associations with congenital heart disease, chromosomal disorders (e.g. Down, Turner, or Noonan syndrome), prenatal infection, birth trauma, thrombosis of the superior vena cava or other malformations (e.g. primary congenital pulmonary lymphangiectasis) have been reported. Recently, Bellini et al reported physiologic and pathophysiologic dynamics of pleural effusion and chylothorax highlighting three basic mechanisms leading to pleural effusion: increased transpleural filtration pressure, impaired lymphatic drainage, and increased permeability.

In previous case series, mortality was around 15%–20%, whereas mortality in our cohort was 11% and largely explained by existing co-morbidities. Decreased mortality may reflect more comprehensive pre- and postnatal management in recent years. Prenatal treatment consists of in utero pleural puncture or drainage to reduce the risk of lung hypoplasia, but the safety and efficacy of prenatal interventions yet needs to be elucidated. Postnatal treatment can be quite demanding for the medical team and often needs a very long time. As there are no generally accepted standardized guidelines published we here try to summarize the literature and our experience: if chylothorax is known antenatally the neonatal resuscitation team should expect to find all levels of respiratory distress after delivery and therefore should be well prepared. In some cases drainage or at least puncture of the pleural effusion, sometimes even on both sides, immediately after delivery, will promptly help to reduce respiratory support parameters. After stabilization of the neonate there are several other supportive measures to be considered. In case of high fluid loss via the drainage, arterial hypotension can occur. Volume loss should be monitored and substituted continuously until chylothorax resolves. Substitution can be done with isotonic solutions but also with albumin, immunoglobins or antithrombin depending on their blood levels to reduce secondary complications (lymphopenia and hypogammaglobulinemia with the risk of developing systemic infection, hypoalbuminemia and thrombosis). Reduction in chylous production can also be attempted either by withholding enteral nutrition and providing total parenteral nutrition, or by feeding a medium-chain triglyceride diet.

In our hospital we withhold enteral nutrition for one week and then re-evaluate chylous loss (if there is no drainage we monitor respiratory distress and ultrasound guided pleural effusion to decide the next step). If it is markedly reduced we would then start to feed the neonate with a medium-chain triglyceride diet. If there is still high chylous output via the drainage we either wait another week or start the neonate on octreotide.

In the past, beneficial effects of octreotide or somatostatine on chylous fluid production have been claimed in several case series. Published dosing regimens for octreotide and somatostatine are quite variable, reflecting insufficient knowledge on peptide hormone pharmacokinetics in infants with CCT. Our data suggest that patients treated with these drugs were more seriously ill, with significantly longer duration of pleural drainage and more infants with culture-positive sepsis or antithrombin administration. However, efficacy of this treatment needs to be evaluated in a prospective interventional trial.

If octreotide is used it can either be given iv continuously, most likely via a central catheter starting with 1 ug/kg/min and increasing up to maximum of 10 ug/kg/min every day, or it can be administered i.v. or s.c. three times a day at a dose of (50–) 100 µg/kg/d (max 240 µg/kg/d). Safety of peptide hormone treatment has also never been prospectively evaluated in newborns with CCT. So far, NEC, transient hypothyroidism, transient increases in liver enzymes and hyperglycemia have been reported in CCT infants treated with these peptide hormones. If the neonate is fully enterally fed with medium-chain triglyceride diet and chylothorax is resolved, there is the possibility to change back to breast milk or formula. The best time to exchange diets is not known but most centers aim for at least 4–6 weeks on medium-chain triglyceride diet before starting to exchange.

Several years prior to our study, we established a standardized treatment algorithm at our institution, quite similar to the one recently reported by Downie et al. for CCT or by Panthongviriyakul et al. for post-operative chylothorax. But to date, no standardized approach has been evaluated prospectively and there is yet no evidence that this standardized approach results in improved outcome.

In severe cases surgical treatment is sometimes necessary and needs to be discussed interdisciplinarily. Limits to define severe cases have not been established to a satisfying level so far. One option is to ligate the thoracic duct which can be done thorascopically. Pleurodesis is another possibility to stop chylous effusion and is either done mechanically or chemically (with talcum, doxycyclin, povidone iodid, OK-432 or fibrin glue). The last option is to insert a pleuroperitoneal shunt. All these methods have so far not been examined in randomized prospective studies and there is also no evidence that they result in improved outcome.

In summary, congenital chylothorax is a disease which can be demanding for all involved participants. A standardized management is needed to attain the best outcome for every patient.

Bethany J. Slater, Steven S. Rothenberg

8.5 Aquired chylothorax

Cylothorax is a fairly rare disorder with a high morbidity and mortality rate if left untreated [61]. The etiologies are variable consisting of both congenital and acquired causes (usually traumatic or post-operative). Postcardiac surgery accounts for 65%–80% of chylous effusions in children. In addition to direct injury of the duct, occlusion of the superior vena cava from thrombosis of external compression can lead to increased central venous pressure being transmitted back to the thoracic duct. The diagnosis is made with a chest X-ray demonstrating an effusion. Aspiration of the fluid reveals milky fluid in a patient who is being fed or clear fluid with a triglyceride level greater than 110 mg/dL and lymphocytes greater than 80% of the white blood cells in a fasting patient.

Initial management typically consists of placement of a chest tube to drain chyle from the pleural space and reduce compression of the lungs, keeping the patient NPO to decrease production of lymphatic flow, and possibly adding medication such as the somatostatin anologue, octreotide [62]. However, medical therapy is associated with a high failure rate and chyle loss can lead to serious metabolic, nutritional, volume, and immunologic abnormalities. T cell depletion leads to cell-mediated and humoral impairment increasing the risk of bacterial and viral infections [63].

Chylothorax is a complex problem to manage, and treatment can be a difficult. While conservative therapy with chest tube drainage may be successful, it may be prolonged and result in long-term hospitalization and associated morbidity. Continued drainage and complications from loss of chyle are the main indications for surgery in children with chylous effusions. It is usually recommend to pursue surgical treatment if a chyle leak has not responded to conservative therapy after approximately 2 weeks. However, the method and timing of surgery remains controversial.

Although there have been a variety of surgical procedures proposed for treatment, such as mechanical or chemical pleurodesis or placement of a pleuroperitoneal shunt, ligation of the thoracic duct has led to repeatedly successful results, and is those most frequently performed surgical procedure [64, 65]. Historically, ligation has been performed through an open thoracotomy, which leads to significant post-operative pain and potentially future chest wall deformity. Recently, authors have published case reports and series demonstrating the safety and efficacy of the thoracoscopic approach to thoracic duct ligation [66–68]. We reported our experience with 21 patients with chylothoracies refractory to conservative management [69]. All cases were completed successfully thoracoscopically. Operative time ranged from 20 to 55 minutes, and there were no intra-operative complications. One patient with congenital bilateral chylothoracies required a left partial pleurectomy. The chest tube duration post-operatively ranged from 4 to 14 days. Two patients failed the ligation and required a subsequent thoracoscopic pleurectomy and chemical pleurodesis respectively. A combination of direct sealing, local pleurodesis, and fibrin glue application resulted in successful sealing of the leak in all other cases. In a few of the cases, drainage did persist for up to a week, but then it diminished and sealed.

Surgical procedures are performed with the patient under general anesthesia and either left main-stem intubation or tracheal intubation and CO_2 insufflation. All procedures are performed in the right chest with three ports. The patient is placed in a modified prone position with the right side elevated 30%–45%. Depending on the size of the child this can be accomplished with padded roles or a beanbag. An axillary role should be used in all cases. The right arm should be placed up toward the head. The surgeon and assistant are positioned on the left side of the table toward the patient's front. The main monitor is placed on the right at the level of the lower thorax. The initial 4-mm port for the camera is placed in the 7th intercostal space in the posterior axillary line. A 3-mm port is placed in the mid axillary line approximately two–three interspaces below the camera port for a 3-mm Maryland. The final port (3 or 5 mm) is placed in the mid axillary line approximately at the level of the camera port. (Fig. 8.5.1) Ideally, these ports are placed so that the instrument tips will approximate a right angle (90 degrees).

The pleural cavity is insufflated with a low flow low pressure of CO_2. All intrathoracic adhesions and the inferior pulmonary ligament are divided to allow the lung to completely expand at the end of the procedure and allow adequate exposure. With the added magnification and direct view afforded by the thoracoscope, the site of the

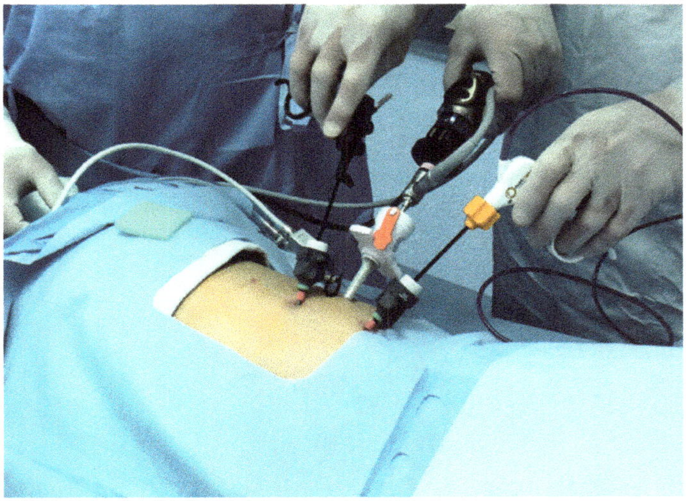

Fig. 8.5.1: Port placement for thoracoscopic thoracic duct ligation.

chyle leak can often be visualized. If this is the case, the site of the pleural rent can be repaired with a tissue sealer device, suture ligature, or clips. If the site of the leak is not readily apparent, a blind ligation of the thoracic duct is performed at the level of the esophageal hiatus where the thoracic duct passes posterior and lateral to the esophagus. (Fig. 8.5.2, Fig. 8.5.3) There should be a marked decrease in the amount of fluid accumulating in the pleural space. Once the ligation is complete, a mechanical pleurodesis is performed, fibrin glue is inserted, and a chest tube is left.

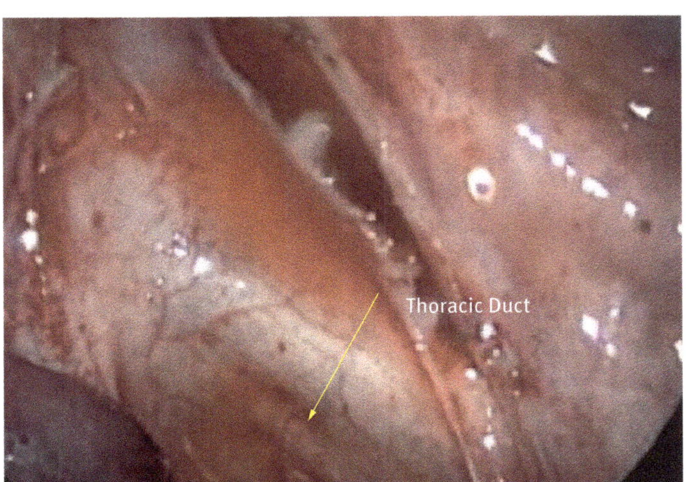

Fig. 8.5.2: Intraoperative picture of the thoracic duct visualized with the thoracoscope.

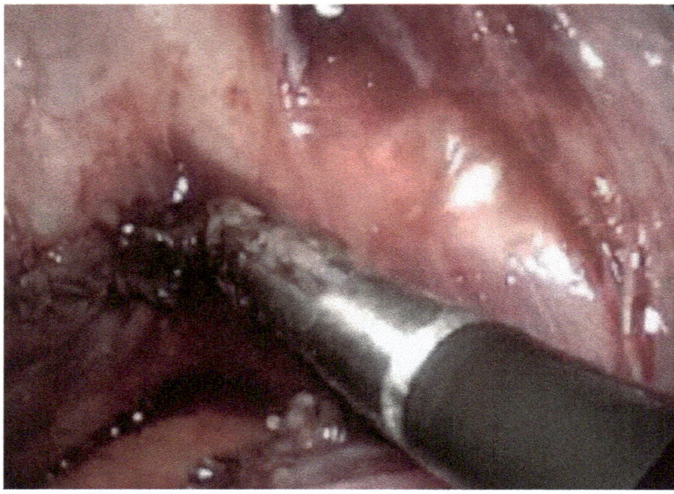

Fig. 8.5.3: Intraoperative picture of a 3-mm sealer being used to seal the thoracic duct at the level of the esophageal hiatus where the thoracic duct passes posterior and lateral to the esophagus.

There is little morbidity from this minimally invasive approach. In addition, this technique affords excellent visualization and magnification of the posterior thorax, decreased post-operative pain and less pulmonary dysfunction. The success of this technique may warrant earlier surgical intervention, particularly when performed quickly and efficiently to avoid a prolonged anesthetic. Even if unsuccessful, there is little to be lost by an initial thoracoscopic approach.

Acquired chylothorax is a complex problem to deal with and treatment can be a difficult. There is a significant hidden morbidity because of the large fluid and nutritional losses associated high volume leaks. While conservative therapy with chest tube drainage is often successful it may be lead to long-term hospitalization and associated morbidity. Thoracoscopic ligation of the thoracic duct offers a more invasive but perhaps less morbid way of treating this disease. It can be performed even in post-cardiac surgery patients. The site of the leak can be identified in the majority of cases and tissue sealing technology appears to be effective in sealing the duct. The minimally invasive nature of the procedure allows for early operation to avoid the often chronic and debilitating fluid and protein losses associated with a major chyle leak.

Lan Vu, Hanmin Lee

8.6 Thymus

Thymectomy was first recognized as a therapy for patients with myasthenia gravis (MG) in 1911, when Dr. Ferdinand Sauerbruch removed the thymus of a young woman with hyperthyroidsims and myasthenia gravis. Twenty-five years later, Dr. Albert Blalock performed the first successful thymectomy of thymic tumor and further suggested the role of thymectomy in patients with nonthymomatous myasthenia gravis. He postulated that the thymus had a role in the pathogenesis of myasthenia gravis. We now understand myasthenia gravis as an autoimmune neuromuscular disorder, mediated by autoantibodies to the acetylcholine receptor complex (AChR antibody positive). The antibodies are thought to originate in the hyperplastic germinal centers of the thymus. Myasthenia gravis is a heterogenous autioimmune disease and some patients who are AChR antibody negative have antibodies to another target on the surface of the muscle membrane, the muscle-specific receptor tyrosine kinase (MuSK). In addition, a small percentage of patients have seronegative myasthenia gravis (negative assays for both AChR and MuSK antibodies). The clinical manifestation of myasthenia gravis consists of fluctuating muscle weakness and fatigability in one or combination of different skeletal muscle groups (ocular, facial, limb, bulbar, and respiratory). The clinical features and electrophysiologic findings are similar between seronegative and seropositive patients.

The majority of patients with myasthenia gravis have thymic abnormalities. About 60%–70% of patients with AChR positive disease have thymic hyperplasia. In addition, the incidence of thymoma is estimated to be 21% and more likely to occur in male patients and those where the onset of myasthenia gravis occurred after 40 years of age. However, there have been at least two case reports of thymoma in pediatric patients with myasthenia gravis. Thymectomy is mandatory in patients with thymoma. This chapter will focus on the role of thymectomy in management of nonthymomatous myasthenia gravis.

Juvenile myasthenia gravis is defined as onset of disease before 18 years of age. Based on age of onset, juvenile myasthenia gravis is subdivided into prepubertal and postpubertal types. The postpubertal group shares the same clinical and laboratory features of the young adult patients. The prepubertal group, on the other hand, has a higher rate of seronegativity, higher proportion of ocular only disease, higher rate of spontaneous remission, and an equal sex ratio [70]. The pathophysiology of the myasthenia gravis is similar between children and adults and therefore the management of juvenile myasthenia gravis is extrapolated from evidence published in the adult population with some key caveats that will be discussed.

Medical management of myasthenia gravis follows these three main therapies: symptomatic treatment, chronic immunotherapy, and rapid immunotherapy. Initial therapy includes an oral actehylcholinesterase inhibitor, usually pyridostigmine, which prevents the degradation of acetylecholine at the neuromuscular junction, prolonging the effects of acetylcholine. Acetylcholinesterase inhibitors provide variable short-acting symptomatic relief and are most effective in improving limb and bulbar symptoms. Most patients with generalized myasthenia gravis will need additional therapy. Immunomodulating agents have been successful in achieving disease remission in some patients. However, the severe adverse effects of chronic immunomodulators including bone growth retardation and risk of adult osteoporosis with glucocorticosteroids and impaired fertility and late development of malignancy with azathioprine, mycophenolate mofetil, and cyclosporine, have limited their chronic use in pediatric patients. Rapid immunotherapies, plasmapheresis and intravenous immune globulin, are also immunomodulators, but have a quick onset and transient benefit and therefore are only used in certain situations, such as myasthenic crisis, preoperatively to prevent a postoperative crisis, bridge to slower acting immunotherapies, and sometimes to maintain remission in patients whose symptoms are not controlled on chronic immunomodulators.

Thymectomy has become widely accepted as long-term and sustainable therapy for myasthenia gravis. Remission is not immediate and has been shown to increase with longer duration of follow-up. The evidence for the benefits of thymectomy has been mostly based on class III observational case control or cohort studies. The published studies have been limited by differing baseline characteristics of surgical and nonsurgical groups, the lack of blinding, variation in the surgical technique, and variation in follow-up [71]. The first prospective randomized trial comparing thymectomy and no thymectomy in adult patients with nonthymomatous autoimmune generalized myasthenia gravis treated with steroids is currently underway, involving 70 centers in 22 countries [72]. Of note, this trial excludes patient less than 18 years of age and studies only the transsternal approach to thymectomy and therefore, it is unclear if the results of this study would necessarily apply to the pediatric group of patients.

Patient selection for thymectomy is important to consider. Most experts have recommended thymectomy within the first three years of diagnosis based on the observation that remission rates are greater when thymectomy is performed early after the onset of disease. However, in general, the percentage of patients who go into the remission is higher early in disease. Therefore it is unclear if thymectomy improves remission rates or remission occurs as the natural history of the disease. Given the fact that spontaneous remission occurs more frequently in prepubertal children with myasthenia gravis, thymectomy is only recommended for peripubertal and postpubertal children. The incidence of thymic pathology is more common in patients with AChR antibody positive disease and therefore, thymectomy is usually reserved for this group of patients. However, one retrospective study did find comparable remission rates in patients with AChR antibody positive disease and those with seronegative disease. The benefit of thymectomy was not seen in patients with MuSK antibody only positive disease. The majority of studies on thymectomy for nonthymomatous myasthenia gravis have included only patients with generalized disease. There is a reported decrease rate of conversion from ocular only to generalized myasthenia gravis after thymectomy. Generally, in the pediatric population, thymectomy is recommended for postpubertal patients with AChR antibody positive and generalized disease within three years of the onset of symptoms.

Minimally invasive approach for resection of benign anterior mediastinal diseases was first introduced in the early 1990s. The goal of thymectomy is the removal

Tab. 8.6.1: Thymectomy for nonthymomatous myasthenia gravis: pros and cons of three approaches.

Technique	Transsternal	Extended Transcervical	Minimally Invasive
First described	1911	19th century in infants and young children for concern of respiratory obstruction and sudden death; revived in mid-1960s for treatment of MG	1994–1995
	Extended sternotomy	Cervical incision with use of manubrial retractor or mediastinoscopy	Right or left side approach, three ports
Pros	Full exploration of anterior mediastinum into the neck	Shorter hospital stay compared to sternotomy	Small incisions, shorter hospital stay compared to sternotomy and transcervical approach
Cons	Longer hospital stay from pain control and postoperative respiratory complications	Limited experience in pediatric patients; concern for inadequate access to the inferior anterior mediastinum	Concern for inadequate access to the superior anterior mediastinum

of all thymic tissue and the surrounding extracapsular mediastinal and cervical fat which may contain ectopic thymic tissue. The transsternal, extended transcervical, and videoscopic approaches have been shown to successfully achieve this goal, resulting in similar rates of remission and symptom relief in long-term follow-up and low operative mortality. The advantages of video-assisted thoracocopic surgery (VATS) include shorter hospitalization, lower respiratory morbidity, and better cosmesis compared to open technique (transcervical and transsternal) in the pediatric patients [73–75].

At our institution, thymectomy is primarily performed using VATS technique. The anterior mediastinum is accessed through the left side with the patient in the supine position and a bump under the left chest. The key steps to the VATS approach include 1) identification and preservation of the left and right phrenic nerves, 2) identification and removal of the contralateral gland, 3) removal of cervical extension of the gland, and 4) ligation of arterial blood supply, which can be from the internal thoracic, inferior thyroid arteries or both, and 5) avoiding injury to the innominate vein, where the thymic vein drains.

Benign thymic pathology accounts for 3% of pediatric mediastinal masses. Giant thymic cysts can present with respiratory symptoms of upper airway compression. More often ectopic thymic cysts are incidentally discovered as neck masses. Thymic abscesses are rare in the pediatric patient, usually occurring from bacteremia or infected thymic cyst. Approach to the anterior mediastinum in these patients depends on the severity of each individual patient's presenting symptoms.

Advances in the minimally invasive approach to nonmalignant thymic diseases in pediatric population have followed closely in the footsteps of adult patients. By minimizing the perioperative risks of thymectomy, video-assisted thoracoscopic surgery has become a viable option for treatment of juvenile myasthenia gravis in select patients. However, conclusive comparative studies to evaluate the different techniques are still needed.

Video showing a thoracoscopic thymectomy.
https://www.degruyter.com/view/supplement/9783110419825_Thymectomy.mp4

Jose Ribas Milanez De Campos, Hugo Veiga Sampaio Da Fonseca

8.7 Hyperhydrosis

8.7.1 Introduction

Primary hyperhidrosis (PH) is a somatic disorder that results from hyperfunction of the sympathetic nervous system [76]. It usually starts during childhood [77], has a symmetric distribution and a similar prevalence in both sexes and affects 2.8% of the population. PH can lead to social, professional and emotional problems that are associated with low levels of quality of life (QOL) [78].

The palmar and plantar regions are the most commonly affected sites in this age group. The mother usually notices the symptoms of PH, and when parents seek medical help, they cannot find data from the literature to help them make an objective decision regarding the best time to use surgical treatment (Fig. 8.7.1).

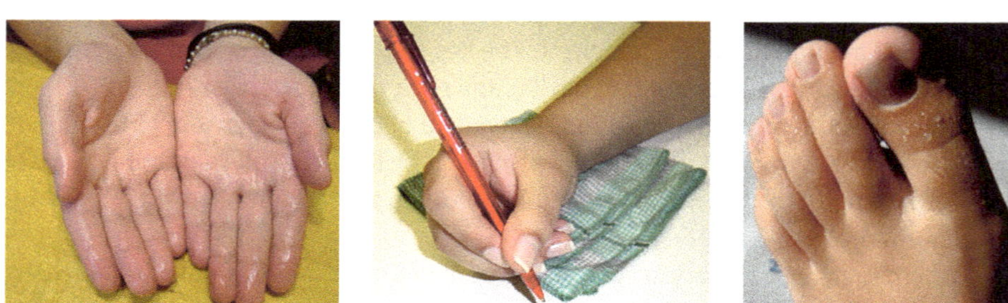

(a) (b) (c)

Fig. 8.7.1: Symptoms of primary hyperhidriosis.

8.7.2 Clinical management

Oxybutynin is a cholinergic antagonist that is used to treat pollakiuria and hyperreflectory urine bladder, and it is generally used at a dose of 10 to 15 mg per day. In children, oxybutynin has been routinely used to treat urologic conditions, particularly nocturnal enuresis. The first case reporting the collateral effects of oxybutynin in a man with urinary urgency was in 1988, which presented with a improvement of his symptoms of excessive sweating [79]. Many other reports were published [80–86], including with specific population such as children [87].

We did not use an objective measurement of sweating to evaluate the response to treatment because the methods available produce data at only a specific time [85]. There are no methods capable of evaluating the level of hyperhidrosis for an entire day. For this reason we suggest the child's perception of QOL as a surrogate for objective improvements in sweating [87]. Further-more, the goal of any treatment for primary hyperhidrosis is to improve the patient's QOL.

Considering that the main treatment for palmar and axillary hyperhidrosis is surgical and that the side effects of such therapy are significant, oxybutynin represents a possible alternative. In a prospective, controlled, randomized, blind trial in 50 patients with axillary and palmar symptoms between 18–50 years old, a comparison of the effects in quality of life of Oxybutynin against placebo was performed [89]. Hyperhidrosis improved in more than 70% of patients, and 46,8% of those presented great improvement. Plantar hyperhidrosis improved in more then 90%. Most patients (65%) showed improvements in their quality of life with minor side effects (dry mouth in 47%).

Short term results

In order to investigate the efficacy and impact in quality of life with the clinical use of Oxybutynin in children and adolescents, 45 persons between 7 and 14 years with palmar hyperhidrosis were evaluated before and 6 weeks after a clinical treatment using a progressive dose of Oxybutynin until 10 mg/day using a validated QOL protocol [87]. Before treatment, the totality of patients related a poor or very poor QOL (Tab. 8.7.1), justifying the need for intervention.

Tab. 8.7.1: Effect of hyperhidrosis on QOL before starting treatment (n = 45).

QOL before treat (score)	*n* (%)
Very poor	26 (57.8)
Poor (59–71)	19 (42.2)
Good (46–58)	0
Very good (33–45)	0
Excellent (17–32)	0

Tab. 8.7.2: Effect of treatment on clinical evaluation of palmar hyperhidriosis (n = 45).

Effect of treatment (score)	***n* (%)**
Worse (–)	0 (0.0)
No/slight improvement (0–4)	6 (13.3)
Moderate improvement (5–7)	17 (37.8)
Large improvement (8–10)	22 (48.9)

Tab. 8.7.3: Improvement in QOL after 6 weeks of treatment according to initial evaluatuion. *Fisher's exact test.

Level of improvement (score)	**Initial evaluation**		**p**
	Very poor (*n* = 26), *n* (%)	**Poor (*n* = 19), *n* (%)**	
Much better (17–32)	14 (53.8)	4 (34.8)	<0.001*
Slightly better (33–45)	7 (26.9)	11 (39.1)	
Same (46–58)	5 (19.3)	4 (26.1)	
A little worse (59–71)	0	0	
Much worse (72–85)	0	0	

The effect of treatment on the clinical evaluation of PH is presented in Tab. 8.7.2. More than 85% of children experienced improvement in hyperhidrosis, including 48.9% who experienced great improvement.

As shown in Tab. 8.7.3, the greatest improvements were observed in patients who initially classified their QOL as very poor. Approximately 80% of the patients who initially reported their QOL as poor or very poor had their condition much better or slightly better after treatment. None of the treated individuals reported deterioration in QOL after treatment.

As shown in Tab. 8.7.4, many of the patients reported clinical improvements at other sites of sweating after treatment. More than 50% of the patients reported a moderate or great reduction in sweating, regardless of the affected site.

The present results showed satisfactory outcomes of pharmacotherapy of hyperhidrosis in children. A clinical improvement in PH (slightly or much better) was observed in more than 85% of the children, which is superior to our previously reported results in adults [86, 90].

Oxybutynin yields good short-term results. It is a safe medication with limited tolerability because of antimuscarinic side effects, especially for doses exceeding

Tab. 8.7.4: Clinical Improvements in secondary sites of sweating. *Osmidrosis, abdomen and back, buttocks and legs, thorax.

Effect of treatment (score)	Plantar (*n* = 40), *n* (%)	Axillary (*n* = 7), *n* (%)	Osmidrosis (*n* = 5)	Other (*n* = 4)*
Worse (–)	0	0	0	0
No or slight improvement (0–4)	15 (37.5)	2 (28.6)	2 (40.0)	0
Moderate improvement (5–7)	12 (30.0)	3 (42.9)	2 (40.0)	2 (50.0)
Large improvement (8–10)	13 (32.5)	2 (28.6)	1 (20.0)	2 (50.0)

15 mg/day. The dose of 10 mg/day (for those weighting >40 kg) that we slowly and progressively reached in patients lowers the incidence of side effects (such as unbearable dry mouth), as patients progressively adapt to the antimuscarinic effects of the medication, and improves treatment adherence, as opposed to regimens in which full doses are initially started.

Long term results

These findings encouraged us to research long-term use outcomes in a large cohort (97 patients) who initiated pharmacologic treatment [91]. The patients' progress was monitored, and we focused on those who had a good initial response (6 weeks) and were treated for at least 6 months to investigate whether the improvement was maintained over the long term and whether tachyphylaxis occurred.

Comparing improvement between the 6-week assessment and the last evaluation (Tab. 8.7.5), 57.7% of patients remained in the same category of improvement, 18.9%

Tab. 8.7.5: Comparing self-assessment improvement of the main site of hyperhidriosis at 6 weeks of treatment and the last visit.

Improvement after 6 weeks	Improvement at last visit			Total
	Slight	Moderate	Great	
Slight	0 (0.0)	0 (0.0)	0 (0.0)	0 (0.0)
Moderate	3 (5.1)	13 (22.0)	14 (23.7)	30 (50.8)
Great	2 (3.4)	11 (18.6)	16 (27.1)	29 (49.2)
Total	5 (8.5)	30 (50.8)	30 (50.8)	59 (100.0)

worsened and 23.6% improved throughout the study. The change in subcategories was not statistically significant.

Oxybutynin had an improvement effect on other sites (i.e. not the main site) of hyperhidrosis as well. For example, for patients (n = 53) who complained of plantar hyperhidrosis, 48 (90.6%) improved moderately or greatly at the last consultation. There were two patients who complained of thoracoabdominal sweating, and at the last consult both graded their improvement in sweating as moderate. Only one patient reported craniofacial sweating, and at last consult he reported great improvement in sweating in this area. Regarding comparisons of complaints of dry mouth between the 6-week assessment and the last visit, 63.3% of patients remained in the same category (absent or light *versus* moderate or severe) throughout the study period, 20.7% improved, and 16% reported worsening.

At the final visit (median 19.6 months), 18.9% of patients experienced worsening in their improvement category (e.g. a patient who reported great improvement at 6 weeks but moderate improvement at the last visit). One possible reason for this is nonadherence. Because of the retrospective nature of this study, it is not possible to ascertain adherence using direct questioning or any other method. Another possible reason is tachyphylaxis, which, to the best of our knowledge, has not been reported.

Nevertheless, 23.6% of patients showed improvement in their response category, and more than 90% reported moderate or great improvement in hyperhidrosis over the long term. This apparent contradiction may be because worsening between categories does not necessarily lower overall patient satisfaction with medical care; that is, there may be some variation in the perceived amelioration of sweating, but it is not significant enough to cause patients to cease medication use. We believe that because of these overall encouraging results, patients who initially respond well to the medication may maintain treatment indefinitely.

Statistically significant difference was noted in outcomes of treatment between sites of hyperhidrosis (Tab. 8.7.6). Oxybutynin did not seem to have a better (or worse) effect if the most bothersome hyperhidrosis was on the hands or the axillae.

If patients have experienced good response after 6 weeks, it seems that they continue to benefit from therapy, as they maintain moderate or great improvement in palmar and plantar hyperhidrosis and in other sites of significant sweating.

Tab. 8.7.6: Improvement at last visit according to primary site of sweating.

Improvement	**Axilla**	**Palm (*n* = 50) (*n* = %)**	**Total (*n* = 59)**	**p-value**
Slight or moderate	3 (33.3)	25 (50.0)	28 (47.5)	0.48
Great	6 (66.7)	25 (50.0)	31 (52.5)	

Randomized double-blind, placebo-controlled studies must be undertaken to more rigorously assess the efficacy of pharmacologic treatment in children, although these data support our opinion that oxybutynin may be an appropriate and long-standing treatment option.

Nevertheless, the clinical outcomes of oxybutynin treatment are inferior to those of surgery. For example, video-assisted thoracic sympathectomy is associated with resolution or improvement in hyperhidrosis in 95% of patients, although 30% develop compensatory hyperhidrosis [78, 89], an irreversible increase in sudoresis affecting other sites. The main benefit of medical treatment is that compensatory hyperhidrosis does not occur, which reduces the likelihood of deterioration in QOL. Additionally, if pharmacotherapy is ineffective, the drug can be discontinued and surgery reconsidered.

8.7.3 Surgical treatment

In adults, video-assisted thoracic sympathectomy (VATS) is one of definitive treatment options; it is a safe procedure with good results, although it is associated with compensatory hyperhidrosis (CH), which occurs in virtually all patients with greater or lesser intensity, mainly on the trunk, with an unknown pathophysiology [92–94].

In children, VATS has been used in daily practice, apparently with the same safety and good results as adults, although there are few scientific studies, especially for its indication in children [93, 95–101]. It is also unknown whether surgery performed on children younger than 14 produces better results than clinical management after a longer period. The best way to evaluate this question is to measure the QOL in these groups after a long period of time.

We performed a prospective nonrandomized study which evaluated forty-five children with PH younger than 14 at the time of first consultation [93]. Thirty children underwent VATS, and 15 children were in the control group and not treated with anything.

Patients answered a questionnaire about their clinical improvement according to their subjective perception of improvement in hyperhidrosis on a scale from 0 to 2 (0 = no improvement, 1 = partial improvement, and 2 = no hyperhidrosis). The negative effect of hyperhidrosis on QOL before the treatment was classified into five different levels and calculated as the summed score from the protocol (range from 20 to 100): the higher the level, the greater the effect, and the poorer the QOL (>84, very poor; 68–83, poor; 52–67, good; 36–51, very good; and 20–35, excellent). Improvement in QOL after the treatment was classified using five levels (>84, much worse; 68–83, worse; 52–67, no change; 36–51, some improvement; 20–35, much better). Changes in PH after 4 years are presented in Tab. 8.7.7. Twenty-five patients (83.4%) in the VATS group experienced great improvement in PH, and five (16.6%) experienced partial improvement; 12 (80.0%) children in the control group had no improvement, and three (20.0%) had partial improvement.

Tab. 8.7.7: Improvement in palmar hyperhidriosis 4 years after surgery. *Fisher's exact test.

Treatment result	VATSG Freq. (%)	NOG Freq. (%)	p
No improvement	0 (0.0)	12 (80.0)	<0.001*
Parital improvement	5 (16.6)	3 (20.0)	
Absence of hyperhidriosis	25 (83.4)	0 (0.0)	
Total	30 (100)	15 (100)	

Tab. 8.7.8: Improvement in quality of life (QOL) after 4 years. *Fisher's exact test.

Level of improvement	VATSG Freq. (%)	NOG Freq. (%)	p
20–35 (much better)	23 (76.7)	2 (13.3)	<0.001*
36–51 (a little better)	7 (23.3)	4 (26.7)	
52–67 (the same)	0	4 (26.7)	
68–83 (a little worse)	0	5 (33.3)	
84–100 (much worse)	0	0 (00.0)	
Total	30 (100)	15 (100)	

CH was observed in 27 children who underwent VATS at the last assessment; 19 had slight CH and eight had severe CH. The most frequent locations were the abdomen [93] and back [100], then the thighs [82], buttocks [81], and lower legs [81].

Improvement in QOL is presented in Tab. 8.7.8. Two patients (13.3%) in the control group and 23 (76.7%) in the VATS group were much better than at the first evaluation.

The children who sought medical assistance were discontent with their PH. The degree of negative effect on their QOL was measured in our study using a specific QOL questionnaire on hyperhidrosis [102] that has been validated for adults and used in several published studies [103]. The degree to which hyperhidrosis worsens a patient's QOL depends on the severity of the condition and the patient's adaptation to each situation, even in childhood. Some children with milder hyperhidrosis have very poor QOL, but other children with very severe hyperhidrosis may report that their QOL is not so poor because they have adapted more successfully. All of the children in this study had poor or very poor QOL.

Almost all patients who are healthy can be treated with VATS except for small or obese patients, who might have a greater risk of CH after surgery and are a higher surgical risk [92].

We observed that children who reported CH presented such symptoms immediately after the surgery but only during periods of very hot weather, during exercise, and occasionally correlated with stress.

The results from the treatment of PH were more satisfactory in the VATS group. The children in the control group had QOL levels that were statistically lower. Palmar sudoresis was lower in more than 80% of the cases after surgery. The VATS group had an improvement of 76.7% with regard to QOL, but only a 20% improvement was noted in the control group.

The results of VATS are outstanding because more than 95% of patients become free of or show improvement in PH, although this improvement is often at the cost of CH (an irreversible increase in sudoresis in other parts of the body).

The factors that are currently associated with a worsening of QOL after thoracic sympathectomy for the treatment of hyperhidrosis are surgical failure and severe CH [104], which were not present in our series. In contrast, we observed improvement in only six patients, and nine patients were the same or worse in the QOL evaluation with conservative treatment (controls). We have shown that children younger than 14 with PH and low QOL have better results in improving their QOL after undergoing VATS.

Previous studies that have included children have not been objective and have all been retrospective. Cohen and colleagues [100] in 1998 evaluated 84 children and adolescents younger than 18 with PH who underwent sympathectomy between 1992 and 1995. The authors found that this surgery is safe and effective, with low morbidity and no mortality, and concluded that satisfaction with this procedure was high, despite compensatory sweating. Imhof and colleagues [105] followed 19 children between 1969 and 1997 who underwent thoracoscopic sympathectomy of ganglia T2 and T3 using a questionnaire that was sent by mail. Although QOL was not assessed, they concluded after long-term monitoring that sympathectomy in children is safe.

Lin [106] studied 350 children and adolescents aged 5 to 17 who underwent to videothoracoscopic sympathectomy of T2 ganglia for the treatment of PH between July 1994 and March 1998 and found minimal surgical complications and no surgical mortality. After a median follow-up of 25 months (range 5–44 months), anhidrosis was observed in 331 patients (94.6%), and 301 patients (86%) developed compensatory sweating on the trunk and lower limbs (armpit 12%, back 86%, abdomen 48%, legs 78%).

Steiner and colleagues [97] in 2008 compared the results of sympathectomy in a group of 116 children younger than 14 with those of another group of 209 adolescents and adults aged 15 and older more than 24 months after surgery using a questionnaire administered over the telephone. They found that sympathectomy solved the problem in most patients and generated a level of satisfaction in the postoperative long term of 84.5%.

Surgical technique

The patient is placed under general anesthesia and simple endotracheal tube with double-lung ventilation, in a supine position, slightly elevated at the shoulders with both arms abducted to 90 degrees. It is recommended a sequential approach, starting with the left side. Two 5-mm incisions are made; the first is a submammary incision made for the 30-degree camera, and the second incision is a midaxillary one for the surgical instruments. No carbon dioxide insufflation is necessary (Fig. 8.7.2).

The sympathetic chain is identified through the mediastinal pleura as a longitudinal cord, whitish, multinodular, making slight bulge in lateroposterior region of the thoracic vertebrae, over the heads of ribs.

The extent of intervention in the sympathetic chain depends on the clinical manifestations of the disease, as it follows: the second thoracic ganglion (G2) to patients with craniofacial symptoms, (G3) for patients with palms and soles HP; (G4) for palmar-axillary symptoms; and also solely (G4) for isolated palmar HP. In our opinion, clipping, cauterization or resection of the chain are feasible and with the same clinical results.

The lung is reexpanded under direct vision at the same time as the air is aspirated from the pleural space through a small catheter (16Fr). Hence, no thoracic drain is necessary. A chest radiograph was immediately requested postoperatively for complete

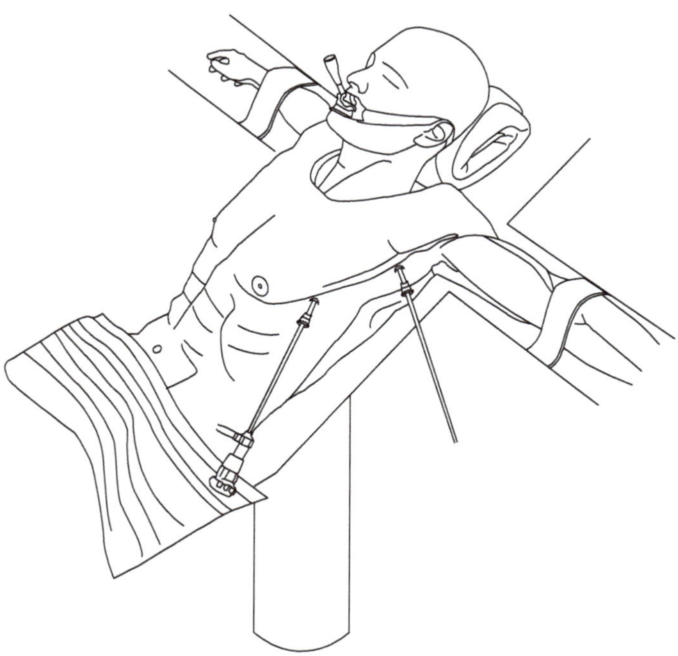

Fig. 8.7.2: Schema of the sequential approach to the sympathetic chain.

lung expansion. The follow-up includes a surgical revision after 7 days, a 30 days evaluation to verify early results, and then after 5 years for a later results evaluation.

8.7.4 Conclusions

Our study suggests that oxybutynin treatment is feasible, with significantly positive results for those who are able to maintain therapy for 6 weeks. After a median of 19.6 months, 90% of patients in this retrospective cohort had moderate or great improvement in excessive sweating.

For children with PH and poor QOL, oxybutynin appears to be a safe and effective initial treatment option to improve QOL and is a valid alternative to surgery. Further studies are required to determine the long-term outcomes of oxybutynin for treating PH.

For children with PH and poor QOL, VATS is better than conservative treatment because it produces better/definitive results with regard to sweating and greater improvement in QOL.

Marcus Krüger

Comment

The article by de Campos and da Fonseca provides an excellent overview of the treatment of hyperhidrosis in children. In the first section the article highlights the good results of medical treatment with Oxybutynin. The therapy with this cholinergic antagonist yields improvement of symptoms in more than 90% of patients with palmar hyperhidrosis. The side effects are mild with dry mouth as the main symptom. The authors indicate that in case of a good response after 6 weeks a long-lasting relief of the symptoms is likely. Randomized trials confirming these results are based on small patient groups (50 patients [88] and 62 patients [80] respectively). Therefore, the authors demand double-blind, placebo-controlled studies to provide better evidence for this therapy. One essential advantage of Oxybutnynin therapy is the absence of compensatory sweating. Compensatory sweating is the most frequent side effect of the surgical therapy. Compensatory sweating is difficult to treat and for some patients it can have a considerably negative impact on their daily life.

However, since the long-term results of video-assisted sympathectomy are superior, surgery is recommended for children who are unsatisfied with medical treatment and are older than 13 years. The authors present an interesting study comparing surgery and a control group in children younger than 14 years. Unfortunately, according to the actual article, the control group did not receive any treatment at all. Therefore, the superior results in the VATS group are not surprising. However, great improvement in 83.4% of the young patients 4 years after surgery represent encouraging results. For

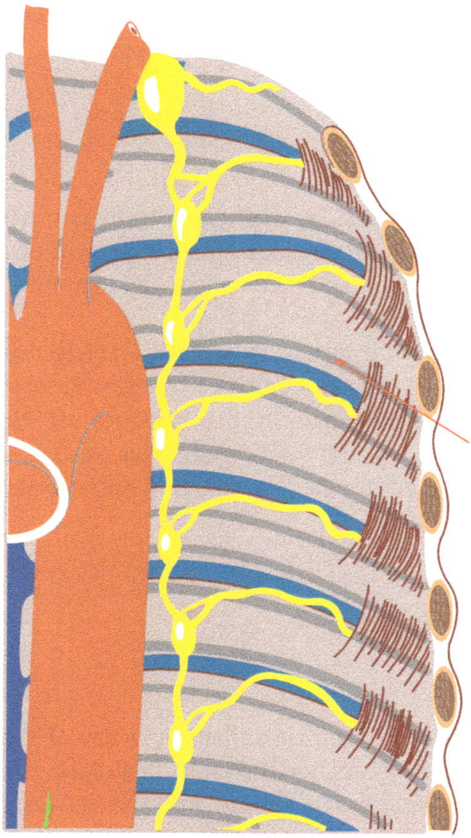

Fig. 8.7.3: Adapted standardized surgical technique, according the level of the thoracic ribs. G2 – between the levels R2 – R3, G3 – level of R3 – R4.

evaluation of these results more precise data concerning the age of the children at the time of surgery would be desirable.

The description of the operative technique is straightforward, focusing on the crucial points of the procedure. The authors describe a procedure with two 5-mm incisions and without carbon dioxide insufflation. The excellent results of the presented data support this operative technique. However, especially for surgeons who do not perform the procedure commonly, carbon dioxide insufflation may be helpful. For the description of the level of intervention in the sympathetic chain I would recommend the rib orientated nomenclature of the consensus committee of the International Society on Sympathetic Surgery (ISSS) and The Society of Thoracic Surgeons (STS) such as "clipped R5, top" or "cauterized, top R4, bottom R4" [107]. This would simplify the comparability of data of different working groups (Fig. 8.7.3).

Interestingly, the authors to not comment on advantages or disadvantages of the distinct technique of disruption of the sympathetic chain, such as clipping, cauterization, cutting or removing of a segment of the sympathetic chain. The clear advantage of clipping is the potential reversibility of adverse effects after removing of the clips. This is especially true regarding the compensatory sweating, which was also indicated by the authors as the most common adverse effect. Sugimura et al. [108] published their experience of 34 reversal procedures. In the case of clip removal within 6 months after the initial procedure, a marked relief of compensatory sweating was seen in 67%. The authors recommend to go without placing a thoracic drain and request an immediate chest radiograph with regard to full expansion of the lungs instead. Conceivably, a small thoracic drainage catheter for some hours postoperatively could supersede the chest radiograph for these young patients [109].

An interesting issue of surgery for hyperhidrosis is the possibility of intraoperative measurement of palmar blood flow and palmar temperature [110]. The preliminary results of an ongoing study at our institution using Laser Speckle Contrast Analysis (LASCA) Imaging are promising [unpublished data]. These measurements may influence the intraoperative decisions for selected patients.

In summary, this chapter on hyperhidrosis therapy for children illustrates the main issues very well and gives an insight into current developments in the field.

8.8 Further reading

[1] Balfour-Lynn IM, Abrahamson E, Cohen G, Hartley J, King S, Parikh D, Spencer D, Thomson AH, Urquhart D. Paediatric Pleural Diseases Subcommittee of the BTSSoCC. BTS guidelines for the management of pleural infection in children. Thorax 2005;60 Suppl 1:i1–21.
[2] Bryant RE, Salmon CJ. Pleural empyema. Clin Infect Dis 1996;22:747–62; quiz 63–4.
[3] McCauley L, Dean N. Pneumonia and empyema: causal, casual or unknown. J Thorac Dis 2015;7:992–8.
[4] Brims FJ, Lansley SM, Waterer GW, Lee YC. Empyema thoracis: new insights into an old disease. Eur Respir Rev 2010;19:220–8.
[5] Islam S, Calkins CM, Goldin AB, Chen C, Downard CD, Huang EY, Cassidy L, Saito J, Blakely ML, Rangel SJ, Arca MJ, Abdullah F, St Peter SD, Outcomes A, Clinical Trials C. The diagnosis and management of empyema in children: a comprehensive review from the APSA Outcomes and Clinical Trials Committee. J Pediatr Surg 2012;47:2101–10.
[6] Moreno-Perez D, Andres Martin A, Tagarro Garcia A, Escribano Montaner A, Figuerola Mulet J, Garcia Garcia JJ, Moreno-Galdo A, Rodrigo Gonzalo de Lliria C, Saavedra Lozano J. [Community acquired pneumonia in children: Treatment of complicated cases and risk patients. Consensus statement by the Spanish Society of Paediatric Infectious Diseases (SEIP) and the Spanish Society of Paediatric Chest Diseases (SENP).]. An Pediatr (Barc) 2015.
[7] Gates RL, Hogan M, Weinstein S, Arca MJ. Drainage, fibrinolytics, or surgery: a comparison of treatment options in pediatric empyema. J Pediatr Surg 2004;39:1638–42.
[8] Kurt BA, Winterhalter KM, Connors RH, Betz BW, Winters JW. Therapy of parapneumonic effusions in children: video-assisted thoracoscopic surgery versus conventional thoracostomy drainage. Pediatrics 2006;118:e547–53.
[9] Singh M, Mathew JL, Chandra S, Katariya S, Kumar L. Randomized controlled trial of intrapleural streptokinase in empyema thoracis in children. Acta Paediatr 2004;93:1443–5.

[10] Thomson AH, Hull J, Kumar MR, Wallis C, Balfour Lynn IM. Randomised trial of intrapleural urokinase in the treatment of childhood empyema. Thorax 2002;57:343–7.
[11] Scarci M, Zahid I, Bille A, Routledge T. Is video-assisted thoracoscopic surgery the best treatment for paediatric pleural empyema? Interact Cardiovasc Thorac Surg 2011;13:70–6.
[12] Sonnappa S, Cohen G, Owens CM, van Doorn C, Cairns J, Stanojevic S, Elliott MJ, Jaffe A. Comparison of urokinase and video-assisted thoracoscopic surgery for treatment of childhood empyema. Am J Respir Crit Care Med 2006;174:221–7.
[13] Cobanoglu U, Sayir F, Bilici S, Melek M. Comparison of the methods of fibrinolysis by tube thoracostomy and thoracoscopic decortication in children with stage II and III empyema: a prospective randomized study. Pediatr Rep 2011;3:e29.
[14] St Peter SD, Tsao K, Spilde TL, Keckler SJ, Harrison C, Jackson MA, Sharp SW, Andrews WS, Rivard DC, Morello FP, Holcomb GW, 3rd, Ostlie DJ. Thoracoscopic decortication vs tube thoracostomy with fibrinolysis for empyema in children: a prospective, randomized trial. J Pediatr Surg 2009;44:106–11; discussion 11.
[15] Marhuenda C, Barcelo C, Fuentes I, Guillen G, Cano I, Lopez M, Hernandez F, Perez-Yarza EG, Matute JA, Garcia-Casillas MA, Alvarez V, Moreno-Galdo A. Urokinase versus VATS for treatment of empyema: a randomized multicenter clinical trial. Pediatrics 2014;134:e1301–7.
[16] Gasior AC, Knott EM, Sharp SW, Ostlie DJ, Holcomb GW, 3rd, St Peter SD. Experience with an evidence-based protocol using fibrinolysis as first line treatment for empyema in children. J Pediatr Surg 2013;48:1312–5.
[17] Balci AE, Eren S, Ulku R, Eren MN. Management of multiloculated empyema thoracis in children: thoracotomy versus fibrinolytic treatment. Eur J Cardiothorac Surg 2002;22:595–8.
[18] Alexiou C, Goyal A, Firmin RK, Hickey MS. Is open thoracotomy still a good treatment option for the management of empyema in children? Ann Thorac Surg 2003;76:1854–8.
[19] Kontouli K, Hatziagorou E, Kyrvasilis F, Roilides E, Emporiadou M, Tsanakas J. Long-term outcome of parapneumonic effusions in children: Lung function and exercise tolerance. Pediatr Pulmonol 2015;50:615–20.
[20] Honkinen M, Lahti E, Svedstrom E, Jartti T, Virkki R, Peltola V, Ruuskanen O. Long-term recovery after parapneumonic empyema in children. Pediatr Pulmonol 2014;49:1020–7.
[21] Stojkovic M, Gottstein B, Junghanss T. Echinococcosis. In: Farre J, Hotez PJ, Junghanss T, Kang G, Lalloo D, White N. Eds. Manson's Tropical Diseases. 23rd. Ed. Elsevier Saunders Ltd. 2014;795–819.e3
[22] von Sinner W. Advanced medical imaging and treatment of human cystic echinococcosis. Semin Roentgenol. 1997;32:276–90.
[23] Gottstein B, Reichen J. Hydatid lung disease (echinococcosis/hydatidosis). Clin Chest Med 2002;23:397–408.
[24] Díaz-Menéndez M, Pérez-Molina JA, Norman FF, Pérez-Ayala A, Monge-Maillo B, Fuertes PZ, López-Vélez R. Management and outcome of cardiac and endovascular cystic echinococcosis. PLoS Negl Trop Dis. 2012;6:e1437.
[25] Kuzucu A, Soysal O, Ozgel M, Yologlu S. Complicated hydatid cysts of the lung: clinical and therapeutic issues. Ann Thorac Surg 2004;77:1200–1204.
[26] WHO Informal Working Group. International classification of ultrasound images in cystic echinococcosis for application in clinical and field epidemiological settings. Acta Trop. 2003;85:253–61.
[27] Komurcuoglu B, Ozkaya S, Cirak AK, Yalniz E, Polat G. Pulmonary hydatid cyst: The characteristics of patients and diagnostic efficacy of bronchoscopy. Exp Lung Res. 2012;38:277–80.
[28] Todorov T, Dakov L, Kosturkova M, Tenev S, Dimitrov A. Immunoreactivity of pulmonary echinococcosis 1. A comparative study of immunodiagnostic tests. Bull WHO 1979;57:735–40.
[29] Biava MF, Dao A, Fortier B. Laboratory diagnosis of cystic hydatid disease. World J Surg 2001;25:10–14.

[30] Pawlowski ZS, Eckert J, Vuitton DA, Ammann RW, Kern P, Craig PS, et al. Echinococcosis in humans:clinical aspects,diagnosis and treatment. In: Eckert J, Gemmell MA, Meslin FX, Pawłowski ZS, eds. WHO/OIE Manual on Echinococcosis in Humans and Animals:a Public Health Problem of Global Concern. Paris, France. 2001:20–72.
[31] Todorov T, Stojanov G. Circulating antibodies in human echinococcosis before and after surgical treatment. Bull World Health Organ. 1979;57:751–8.
[32] Turna A, Yılmaz MA, Haciibrahimoglu G, Kutlu CA, Bedirhan MA. Surgical treatment of pulmonary hydatid cysts: is capitonnage necessary? Ann Thorac Surg. 2002;74:191–5.
[33] Alpay L, Lacin T, Ocakcioglu I, Evman S, Dogruyol T, Vayvada M, Baysungur V, Yalcinkaya I. Is video-assisted thoracoscopic surgery adequate in treatment of pulmonary hydatidosis? Ann Thorac Surg 2015;100:258–62.
[34] Parelkar SV, Gupta RK, Shah H, Sanghvi B, Gupta A, Jadhav V, Garasia M, Agrawal A. Experience with video-assisted thoracoscopic removal of pulmonary hydatid cysts in children. J Pediatr Surg 2009;44:836–841.
[35] WHO. Guidelines for treatment of cyctic and alveolar echinococcosis. WHO Informal Working Group on Echinococcosis. Bull WHO 1996:74:231–242.
[36] Bygott JM, Chiodini PL. Praziquantel: Neglected drug? Ineffective treatment? Or therapeutic choice in cystic hydatid disease? Acta Trop. 2009;111:95–101.
[37] Franchi C, Di Vico B, Teggi A. Long term evaluation of patients with hydatidosis treated with benzimidazole carbamates. Clin Infect Dis 1999;29:304–309.
[38] Teggi A, Lastilla MG, De Rosa F. Therapy of human hydatid disease with mebendazole and albendazole. Antimicrob Agents Chemother 1993;37:1679–1684.
[39] Keramidas D, Mavridis G, Soutis M, Passalidis A. Medical treatment of pulmonary hydatidosis: complications and surgical management. Pediatr Surg Int 2004;19:774–776.
[40] Todorov T, Vutova K, Donev S, Ivanov A, Katzarov K, Takov D. The types and timing of the degenerative changes seen in the cysts during and after benzimidazole treatment of cystic echinococcosis. Ann Trop Med Parasitol. 2005;99:649–59.
[41] Kern P, Bardonnet K, Renner E, et al. European echinococcosis registry: human alveolar echinococcosis, Europe, 1982–2000. Emerg Infect Dis 2003;9:343–349.
[42] Piarroux M, Piarroux R, Giorgi R, Knapp J, Bardonnet K, Sudre B, Watelet J, Dumortier J, Gérard A, Beytout J, Abergel A, Mantion G, Vuitton DA, Bresson-Hadni S. Clinical features and evolution of alveolar echinococcosis in France from 1982 to 2007: results of a survey in 387 patients. J Hepatol. 2011;55:1025–33.
[43] Joliat GR, Melloul E, Petermann D, Demartines N, Gillet M, Uldry E, Halkic N. Outcomes After Liver Resection for Hepatic Alveolar Echinococcosis: A Single-Center Cohort Study. World J Surg. 2015;39:2529–34.
[44] Treugut H, Schulze K, Hübener KH, Andrasch R. Pulmonary involvement by Echinococcus alveolaris. Radiology. 1980;137(Oct):37–41.
[45] Stojkovic M, Gottstein B, and Junghanss T (2014) Echinococcosis. In: Manson's Tropical Diseases, 23rd Edition, Eds Farrar J, Hotez P, Junghanss T, Kang G, White NJ. Elsevier. Section 10, Chapter 56
[46] Brunetti E, Garcia HH, and Junghanss T (2011) Cystic Echinococcosis: Chronic, Complex, and Still Neglected. PLoS Negl Trop Dis 5(7): e1146. doi:10.1371/journal.pntd.0001146
[47] Brunetti E, Kern P, Vuitton DA, writing panel for the WHO-IWGE (2010). Expert consensus for the diagnosis and treatment of cystic and alveolar echinococcosis in humans. Acta Trop;114:1–16.
[48] Stojkovic M, Rosenberger K, Kauczor HU, Junghanss T, Hosch W (2012) Diagnosing and Staging of Cystic Echinococcosis: How Do CT and MRI Perform in Comparison to Ultrasound? PloS Negl Trop Dis 6(10): e1880
[49] Hosch W, Stojkovic M, Jaenisch T, Heye, T, Werner, J, Friess H, Kauffmann G W, Junghanss T (2008) MR imaging for diagnosing cysto-biliary fistulas in cystic echinococcosis. European Journal of Radiology. 66(2):262–7.

[50] Stojkovic M, Zwahlen M, Teggi A, Vutova K, Cretu CM, Virdone R, Nicolaidou P, Cobanoglu N, Junghanss T (2009) Treatment Response of Cystic Echinococcosis to Benzimidazoles: A Systematic Review. PLoS Negl Trop Dis 3(9):e524. doi:10.1371/journal.pntd.000052.
[51] Bialkowski A, Poets CF, Franz AR. Congenital Chylothorax: a prospective nationwide epidemiological study in Germany. Arch Dis Child Fetal Neonatal Ed 2015, Mar;100(2):F169–72.
[52] Straaten van HL, Gerards LJ, Krediet TG. Chylothorax in the neonatal period. Eur J Pediatr 1993;152(1):2–5.
[53] Büttiker V, Fanconi S, Birger R. Chylothorax in children: guidelines for diagnosis and management. Chest 1999;116(3):682–7.
[54] Rocha G, Fernandez P, Rocha P, Quintas C, Martins T, Proenca E. Pleural effusions in the neonate. Acta Paediatrica 2006;95:791–8.
[55] Roehr CC, Jung A, Proquitte H, Blankenstein O, Hammer H, Lakhoo K, Wauer RR. Somatostatin or octreotide as treatment options for chylothorax in young children: a systematic review. Intensive Care Med 2006;32:650–7.
[56] Das A, Shah PS. Octreotide for the treatment of chylothorax in neonates. Cochrane Database of Systematic Reviews 2007, Issue 1, Art No: CD006388.
[57] Helin RD, Angeles STV, Bhat R. Octreotide therapy for chylothorax in infants and children: A brief review. Pediatr Crit Care Med 2006;7(6):576–9.
[58] Panthongviriyakul C, Bines JE. Post-operative chylothorax in children: An evidence-based management algorithm. J Paediatr Child Health 2008;44(12):716–21.
[59] Ergaz Z, Bar-Oz B, Yatsiv I, Arad I. Congenital chylothorax: clinical course and prognostic significance. Pediatr Pulmonol 2009;44:806–11.
[60] Downie L, Sasi A, Malhotra A. Congenital chylothorax: Associations and neonatal outcomes. J Paediatr Child Health 2014;50(3):234–8.
[61] Peillon C, D'Hont C, Melki J, Fattouh F, Perrier G, Dujon A, et al. Usefulness of video thoracoscopy in the management of spontaneous and postoperation chylothorax. Surgical endoscopy 1999;13(11):1106–9.
[62] Rosti L, De Battisti F, Butera G, Cirri S, Chessa M, Delogu A, et al. Octreotide in the management of postoperative chylothorax. Pediatric cardiology 2005;26(4):440–3.
[63] Ferguson MK, Little AG, Skinner DB. Current concepts in the management of postoperative chylothorax. The Annals of thoracic surgery 1985;40(6):542–5.
[64] Lampson RS. Traumatic chylothorax; a review of the literature and report of a case treated by mediastinal ligation of the thoracic duct. The Journal of thoracic surgery 1948;17(6):778–91.
[65] Milsom JW, Kron IL, Rheuban KS, Rodgers BM. Chylothorax: an assessment of current surgical management. The Journal of thoracic and cardiovascular surgery 1985;89(2):221–7.
[66] Wurnig PN, Hollaus PH, Ohtsuka T, Flege JB, Wolf RK. Thoracoscopic direct clipping of the thoracic duct for chylopericardium and chylothorax. The Annals of thoracic surgery 2000;70(5):1662–5.
[67] Kumar S, Kumar A, Pawar DK. Thoracoscopic management of thoracic duct injury: Is there a place for conservatism? Journal of postgraduate medicine 2004;50(1):57–9.
[68] Kent RB, 3rd, Pinson TW. Thoracoscopic ligation of the thoracic duct. Surgical endoscopy 1993;7(1):52–3.
[69] Slater BJ, Rothenberg SS. Thoracoscopic Thoracic Duct Ligation for Congenital and Acquired Disease. Journal of laparoendoscopic & advanced surgical techniques Part A 2015;25(7):605–7.
[70] Ionita CM, Acsadi G. Management of juvenile myasthenia gravis. Pediatr Neurol 2013; 48(2):95–104.
[71] Gronseth GS, Barohn RJ. Practice parameter: thymectomy for autoimmune myasthenia gravis (an evidence-based review): report of the Quality Standards Subcommittee of the American Academy of Neurology. Neurology 2000;55(1):7–15.

[72] Newsom-Davis J, et al. Status of the thymectomy trial for nonthymomatous myasthenia gravis patients receiving prednisone. Ann N Y Acad Sci 2008;1132:344–7.
[73] Wagner AJ, et al. Long-term follow-up after thymectomy for myasthenia gravis: thoracoscopic vs open. J Pediatr Surg 2006;41(1):50–4; discussion 50–4.
[74] Bachmann K, et al. Long-term outcome and quality of life after open and thoracoscopic thymectomy for myasthenia gravis: analysis of 131 patients. Surg Endosc 2008;22(11):2470–7.
[75] Goldstein SD, et al. Thymectomy for myasthenia gravis in children: a comparison of open and thoracoscopic approaches. J Pediatr Surg 2015;50(1):92–7.
[76] Atkins JL, Butler PEM. Hyperhidrosis: a review of current management. Plast Reconstr Surg 2002 Jul;110(1):222–8.
[77] Bellet JS. Diagnosis and treatment of primary focal hyperhidrosis in children and adolescents. Semin Cutan Med Surg 2010 Jun;29(2):121–6.
[78] Lau WT, Lee JD, Dang CR, Lee L. Improvement in quality of life after bilateral transthoracic endoscopic sympathectomy for palmar hyperhydrosis. Hawaii Med J 2001 May;60(5):126–137.
[79] LeWitt P. Hyperhidrosis and hypothermia responsive to oxybutynin. Neurology 1988 Mar;38(3):506–7.
[80] Schollhammer M, Brenaut E, Menard-Andivot N, Pillette-Delarue M, Zagnoli A, Chassain-Le Lay M, et al. Oxybutynin as a treatment for generalized hyperhidrosis: a randomized, placebo-controlled trial. Br J Dermatol 2015 Jun 26.
[81] Lefrandt JD, Maurer JM. Oxybutynin for hyperhidrosis. Neth J Med 2007 Oct;65(9):356.
[82] Tupker RA, Harmsze AM, Deneer VHM. Oxybutynin therapy for generalized hyperhidrosis. Arch Dermatol 2006 Aug;142(8):1065–6.
[83] Maillard H, Fenot M, Bara C, Célérier P. [Therapeutic value of moderate-dose oxybutynin in extensive hyperhidrosis]. Ann Dermatol Venereol 2011 Oct;138(10):652–6.
[84] Wolosker N, Krutman M, Kauffman P, Paula RP de, Campos JRM de, Puech-Leão P. Effectiveness of oxybutynin for treatment of hyperhidrosis in overweight and obese patients. Rev Assoc Med Bras Jan;59(2):143–7.
[85] Wolosker N, de Campos JRM, Kauffman P, Yazbek G, Neves S, Puech-Leao P. Use of oxybutynin for treating plantar hyperhidrosis. Int J Dermatol 2013 May;52(5):620–3.
[86] Wolosker N, de Campos JR, Kauffman P, Neves S, Yazbek G, Jatene FB, et al. An alternative to treat palmar hyperhidrosis: use of oxybutynin. Clin Auton Res 2011 Dec;21(6):389–93.
[87] Wolosker N, Schvartsman C, Krutman M, Campbell TPDA, Kauffman P, De Campos JRM, et al. Efficacy and quality of life outcomes of oxybutynin for treating palmar hyperhidrosis in children younger than 14 years old. Pediatr Dermatol 2014;31(1):48–53.
[88] Ishy A, de Campos JRM, Wolosker N, Kauffman P, Tedde ML, Chiavoni CR, et al. Objective evaluation of patients with palmar hyperhidrosis submitted to two levels of sympathectomy: T3 and T4. Interact Cardiovasc Thorac Surg 2011 Apr;12(4):545–8.
[89] Wolosker N, de Campos JRM, Kauffman P, Puech-Leão P. A randomized placebo-controlled trial of oxybutynin for the initial treatment of palmar and axillary hyperhidrosis. J Vasc Surg 2012 Jun;55(6):1696–700.
[90] Wolosker N, de Campos JRM, Kauffman P, Neves S, Munia MA, BisceglIJatene F, et al. The use of oxybutynin for treating axillary hyperhidrosis. Ann Vasc Surg 2011 Nov;25(8):1057–62.
[91] Wolosker N, Teivelis MP, Krutman M, de Paula RP, Schvartsman C, Kauffman P, et al. Long-Term Efficacy of Oxybutynin for Palmar and Plantar Hyperhidrosis in Children Younger than 14 Years. Pediatr Dermatol 2015;32(5):663–7.
[92] de Campos JRM, Wolosker N, Takeda FR, Kauffman P, Kuzniec S, Jatene FB, et al. The body mass index and level of resection: predictive factors for compensatory sweating after sympathectomy. Clin Auton Res 2005 Apr;15(2):116–20.

[93] Neves S, Uchoa PC, Wolosker N, Munia MA, Kauffman P, de Campos JRM, et al. Long-Term Comparison of Video-Assisted Thoracic Sympathectomy and Clinical Observation for the Treatment of Palmar Hyperhidrosis in Children Younger Than 14. Pediatr Dermatol 2012;29(5):575–9.
[94] Yazbek G, Wolosker N, Kauffman P, Campos JRM de, Puech-Leão P, Jatene FB. Twenty months of evolution following sympathectomy on patients with palmar hyperhidrosis: sympathectomy at the T3 level is better than at the T2 level. Clinics (Sao Paulo) 2009 Jan;64(8):743–9.
[95] Lin TS, Huang LC, Wang NP, Chang CC. Endoscopic thoracic sympathetic block by clipping for palmar and axillary hyperhidrosis in children and adolescents. Pediatr Surg Int 2001 Sep;17(7):535–7.
[96] Cohen Z, Shinhar D, Kurzbart E, Finaly R, Mares AJ. Laparoscopic and thoracoscopic surgery in children and adolescents: a 3-year experience. Pediatr Surg Int 1997 Jul;12(5–6):356–9.
[97] Steiner Z, Cohen Z, Kleiner O, Matar I, Mogilner J. Do children tolerate thoracoscopic sympathectomy better than adults? Pediatr Surg Int 2008 Mar;24(3):343–7.
[98] Zacherl J, Huber ER, Imhof M, Plas EG, Herbst F, Függer R. Long-term results of 630 thoracoscopic sympathicotomies for primary hyperhidrosis: the Vienna experience. Eur J Surg Suppl 1998 Jan;(580):43–6.
[99] Noppen M, Dab I, D'Haese J, Meysman M, Vincken W. Thoracoscopic T2-T3 sympathicolysis for essential hyperhidrosis in childhood: effects on pulmonary function. Pediatr Pulmonol 1998 Oct;26(4):262–4.
[100] Cohen Z, Levi I, Pinsk I, Mares AJ. Thoracoscopic upper thoracic sympathectomy for primary palmar hyperhidrosis – the combined paediatric, adolescents and adult experience. Eur J Surg Suppl 1998 Jan;(580):5–8.
[101] Rashid HI, Osman HS, McIrvine AJ. Thoracoscopic (upper thoracic) sympathectomy for primary palmar hyperhidrosis in children. Int J Clin Pract Jan;52(8):537–8.
[102] Amir M, Arish A, Weinstein Y, Pfeffer M, Levy Y. Impairment in quality of life among patients seeking surgery for hyperhidrosis (excessive sweating): preliminary results. Isr J Psychiatry Relat Sci 2000 Jan;37(1):25–31.
[103] Milanez De Campos JR, Kauffman P, De Campos Werebe E, Andrade Filho LO, Kusniek S, Wolosker N, et al. Quality of life, before and after thoracic sympathectomy: Report on 378 operated patients. Ann Thorac Surg 2003;76(3):886–91.
[104] Schmidt J, Bechara FG, Altmeyer P, Zirngibl H. Endoscopic thoracic sympathectomy for severe hyperhidrosis: impact of restrictive denervation on compensatory sweating. Ann Thorac Surg 2006 Mar;81(3):1048–55.
[105] Imhof M, Zacherl J, Plas EG, Herbst F, Jakesz R, Függer R. Long-term results of 45 thoracoscopic sympathicotomies for primary hyperhidrosis in children. J Pediatr Surg 1999 Dec;34(12):1839–42.
[106] Lin TS. Transthoracic endoscopic sympathectomy for palmar hyperhidrosis in children and adolescents: analysis of 350 cases. J Laparoendosc Adv Surg Tech A 1999 Aug;9(4):331–4.
[107] Cerfolio RJ, De Campos JR, Bryant AS, Connery CP, Miller DL, DeCamp MM, McKenna RJ, Krasna MJ. The Society of Thoracic Surgeons expert consensus for the surgical treatment of hyperhidrosis. Ann Thorac Surg 2011 May;91(5):1642–8.
[108] Sugimura H, Spratt EH, Compeau CG, Kattail D, Shargall Y. Thoracoscopic sympathetic clipping for hyperhidrosis: long-term results and reversibility. J Thorac Cardiovasc Surg 2009 Jun;137(6):1370–6; discussion 1376–7.
[109] Leschber G, May CJ, Simbrey-Chryselius N. [Do thoracic surgery patients always need a postoperative chest X-ray?]. Zentralbl Chir 2014 Sep;139 Suppl 1:S43–9.
[110] Ng I, Yeo TT. Palmar hyperhidrosis: intraoperative monitoring with laser Doppler blood flow as a guide for success after endoscopic thoracic sympathectomy. Neurosurgery 2003 Jan;52(1): 127–30; discussion 130–1.

Index

www.ingramcontent.com/pod-product-compliance
Ingram Content Group UK Ltd.
Pitfield, Milton Keynes, MK11 3LW, UK
UKHW052008051026
15624UKWH00004B/628